MOTOR VEHICLE COLLISION INJURIES

MECHANISMS, DIAGNOSIS, AND MANAGEMENT

LAWRENCE S. NORDHOFF, JR., DC
DIRECTOR
AUTOMOTIVE INJURY RESEARCH INSTITUTE
PLEASANTON, CALIFORNIA

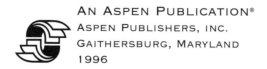

AN ASPEN PUBLICATION®
ASPEN PUBLISHERS, INC.
GAITHERSBURG, MARYLAND
1996

Library of Congress Cataloging-in-Publication Data

Nordhoff, Larry S.
Motor vehicle collision injuries: mechanisms, diagnosis, and management/
Lawrence S. Nordhoff, Jr.
p. cm.
Includes bibliographical references and index.
ISBN 0-8342-0727-3
1. Whiplash injuries—Chiropractic treatment.
2. Crash injuries. 3. Personal injuries.
4. Traffic accidents. 5. Chiropractic. I. Title.
RZ275.W48N67 1995
617.1'028—dc20
95-9527
CIP

The authors have made every effort to ensure the accuracy of the information herein, particularly with regard to technique and procedure. However, appropriate information sources should be consulted, especially for new or unfamiliar procedures. It is the responsibility of every practitioner to evaluate the appropriateness of a particular opinion in the context of actual clinical situations and with due consideration to new developments. Authors, editors, and the publisher cannot be held responsible for any typographical or other errors found in this book.

Orders: (800) 638-8437
Customer Service: (800) 234-1660

About Aspen Publishers • For more than 35 years, Aspen has been a leading professional publisher in a variety of disciplines. Aspen's vast information resources are available in both print and electronic formats. We are committed to providing the highest quality information available in the most appropriate format for our customers. Visit Aspen's Internet site for more information resources, directories, articles, and a searchable version of Aspen's full catalog, including the most recent publications: **http://www.aspenpub.com**
Aspen Publishers, Inc. • The hallmark of quality in publishing
Member of the worldwide Wolters Kluwer group.

Editorial Resources: Jane Colilla
Library of Congress Catalog Card Number: 95-9527
ISBN: 0-8342-0727-3

Printed in the United States of America

2 3 4 5

This book is dedicated to those
professionals seeking better
understanding, and to my family.

Table of Contents

Chapter 12—Medicolegal Reports **243**
Lawrence S. Nordhoff, Jr.

Chapter 13—Going to Court? **253**
Shawn Steel

Contributors

Richard I. Emori, Dr Engr
President
Emori Engineering Corporation
Mitaka, Tokyo
Japan

Andrew A. Fischer, MD, PhD
Chief
Rehabilitation Medicine Service
Veterans Affairs Medical Center
Bronx, New York
Associate Clinical Professor
Department of Rehabilitation Medicine
Mount Sinai School of Medicine
New York, New York

Jay A. Kaiser, MD
Medical Director
Marin Magnetic Imaging
Greenbrae, California

Gerald P. Keane, MD
Clinical Instructor
Stanford University School of Medicine
Stanford, California
Partner
Physiatry Medical Group
Menlo Park, California

Camille LaPointe
Illustrator
San Anselmo, California

Daniel Murphy, DC, DABCO
Instructor
Auburn, California

Richard Nolan, MD
Hayward, California

Lawrence S. Nordhoff, Jr., DC
Director
Automotive Injury Research Institute
Pleasanton, California

Damon Sacco, MD
Diagnostic Radiologist
Marin Magnetic Imaging
Greenbrae, California

Kulveen Sachdeva, MD
Diplomate
American Board of Neurology and
  Psychiatry
Associate Member
American Board of Electrodiagnostic
  Medicine
San Ramon, California

Timothy Sellers, DC, DACBR
Partner/Owner
Chiropractic Radiology Associates
Partner/Owner
Portland School of Radiography
Portland, Oregon

Malik Slosberg, DC, MS
Professor
Life Chiropractic College West
San Lorenzo, California

Shawn Steel, MA, JD
Assistant Professor
Cleveland Chiropractic College
Los Angeles, California

Michael L. Underhill, DC, CCSP
Private Practice
Beaverton, Oregon

Tyrone Wei, DC, DACBR
Private Radiology Practice
Associate Professor of Radiology
National College of Naturopathic Medicine
Former Chairman and Assistant Professor of
    Radiology
Western States Chiropractic College
Portland, Oregon

Arthur H. White, MD
Medical Director
SpineCare Medical Group
San Francisco Spine Institute
San Francisco, California

Foreword

A book written about car accident injuries may occur from several perspectives. First, it may focus on legal issues involving diagnosis and management and how to settle injury cases. Second, this book could give great attention from the insurance claims adjuster perspective. Third, it could explore the automotive engineering and crash reconstruction perspective. Lastly, this text could be written solely from a clinical viewpoint, discussing common issues confronting the doctor in practice.

However, from a more practical and useful perspective, because many types of professionals are involved in these injuries, an ideal book would attempt to look at all issues confronting car accidents. In addition, this book would evaluate the international automotive and clinical literature to further balance these issues.

This book thoroughly covers diagnosis, management strategies, prognosis, and mechanisms of injury. The multidisciplinary panel of authors and their extensive review of the literature lend to its credibility.

In summary, I suggest that you do yourself and your clients a service and read this book. This book will help attorneys, both for the plaintiff and the defense, better serve the injured victim. Whether the injury is annoying to completely disabling, these cases should be fully compensated in settlement or in court. This text will improve diagnosis and management strategies for doctors, therefore improving management outcome, and will also help claims adjusters better understand these injuries.

Melvin M. Belli, Esq

Preface

There are few modern medical problems having the complexity, frequency, loss of life and productivity, and economic costs as motor vehicle collision injuries (MVCIs). With increased worldwide industrialization and the need for an increasingly mobile society, automobiles have become the primary source of transportation for many societies. Although cars built today are safer in design, the rate of crashes increases steadily with increases in population, number of vehicles, and miles traveled.

Most of the past automotive collision research has focused on crashes resulting in critical to fatal injuries, which cause the greatest loss of life influence to our society. In comparison, little has been written about minor, nonfatal collision injuries, which occur in over 90% of all crashes and account for over one half of the associated economic costs.

The authors have attempted to bring forth as much information learned from current international automotive crash studies, medical literature, and clinical experience as possible. In addition, the multidisciplinary panel of authors further lends this book credibility. The book can be used practically by doctors,

therapists, claims adjusters who want to understand MVCIs, and attorneys preparing for arbitration hearings, trial, or settlement with insurance carriers. This book explores the international perspective on collision injury mechanisms, diagnosis, management, and prognosis and attempts to improve the methods of current treatment protocol, describe legal implications, and clarify insurance policies. There are too many current myths, misconceptions, and erroneous judgments being made about these types of injuries. For example: "Drunks don't get injured as much"; "The amount of damage to the car always equals the amount of damage to the occupant"; "Few people have residual spinal problems from MVCI"; and "Injury claims are mostly related to secondary gains."

There is an intense need in our society, at present, for a book that covers multidisciplinary clinical management of mild to moderate motor vehicle collision injuries. Additionally, injury facts, collision dynamics, and factors that influence injury outcome must be evaluated from an international perspective. Up-to-date guidelines for management also need to be brought into one source of literature as a reference manual. It is hoped that this book will give medical doctors, chiropractors, therapists, attorneys, educators, and insurance company representatives a reference source for injury mechanisms, management, and prognosis. The authors have attempted to address most practical issues relating to mild-to-moderate injuries.

Lawmakers, medical and chiropractic professionals and associations, and insurance companies currently have little motor vehicle collision injury data available by which to make policies that ultimately affect every consumer. At present, guidelines are being developed and changed by many insurance companies with respect to how doctors are paid and how insurance companies handle the insured occupant in a crash.

The chapters have been organized in a way that allows the reader to focus on a particular area of interest. Chapter 1 is a comprehensive, well-referenced guide to common post-collision injuries, functional disorders, and types of problems that the clinician must diagnose. Various disorders such as headaches, neck sprain, thoracic outlet syndrome, and herniated discs are discussed with regard to pathophysiology and mechanisms of injury. Chapter 2 covers history and examination strategy for personal injury cases. The various history forms illustrated allow the physician to gather all injury-related factors that may be needed for diagnosis, treatment, and litigation (if it occurs). The physical examination section is a brief synopsis of types of orthopedic and neurologic examinations that may be employed by the doctor.

Chapter 3 covers radiology for noncomplicated neck injuries. Radiologic guidelines are discussed, as well as types of problems seen in a practice. Chapter 4 covers magnetic resonance imaging and computed tomography of neck injuries in detail, with examples of common problems seen in a doctor's office. Chapter 5 expands the reader's knowledge of neurodiagnosis of upper-extremity neuropathies frequently seen after

neck injury. Chapter 6 is written in two parts, the first part evaluating soft tissue repair mechanisms and healing time and the second part covering methods to document injury. Chapter 7 discusses how to manage a wide variety of mild- to moderate-level crash injuries. Guidelines for treatment—how frequent, how long, and when to discharge a patient—are discussed. Guidelines for when to admit a patient to a hospital are covered. Treatment options such as cryotherapy, manipulation, traction, myotherapy, and electrical modalities are discussed with respect to validity and timing in the repair cycle.

Chapter 8, which examines rehabilitation of common postinjury disorders such as neck sprains, bulging discs, thoracic outlet syndrome, and headaches, offers the reader methods to maximize the repair outcome. Chapter 9 offers guidelines to the doctor in private practice who has a patient who is not responding to treatment and continues to have persistent pain and/or disability. Chapter 10 looks at disability frequency and regions of the body that give disability to the occupant. A multiple-region, functional capacity form has been developed for determining disability and documenting treatment outcome. This form has been adapted specifically for collision injuries and takes into consideration both neck and lower back disabilities. Chapter 11 provides the reader with information about prognosis gained from a recent international study of motor vehicle collision injury. Factors that influence poor prognosis are discussed in detail. Chapter 12 gives the doctor a sample of a narrative report whose style and content will adequately represent the needs of the patient.

Chapter 13 covers the legal aspects of a personal injury case. Chapter 14 covers a broad base of crash statistics, giving the reader a broader perspective of the economic costs associated with these injuries, their frequency, and other crash topics. Chapter 15 reviews frontal collisions, side collisions, and rear-end crashes; vehicle and occupant dynamics during the crash; sizes of vehicles; influence of seat belts and head restraints on injury outcome; and the correlation between damage to the vehicle and injury extent to the occupant.

Chapter 16 covers human tolerance to motor vehicle collision injuries by body region. Injury-potentiating factors, such as age and gender of the occupant, are discussed in detail. Chapter 17 looks at the various health care providers who treat these types of injuries, associated costs, and how managed health care will affect future directions in research and reimbursement.

I thank all of the contributing authors and the staff of Aspen Publishers, Inc. My wife, Cathy, and my children deserve praise for their tolerance for my time spent over the past 4 years. The following people deserve thanks for their help in reviewing material, technical support, and computer work: Torri Nagy; Darlene Livingood; Lorna May; Rex Manson, DC; Steve Nagy, DC; and Evette Wilkes. Personnel in the following libraries are thanked as well: University of California Berkeley Transportation Library, Life West Chiropractic College Library, University of California San Francisco Medical Library, and Stanford Lane Medical Library.

Chapter 1

Diagnosis of Common Crash Injuries

Lawrence S. Nordhoff, Jr., Daniel Murphy, and Michael L. Underhill

INTRODUCTION TO DIAGNOSIS

This chapter focuses on diagnosis of minor (no risk of fatality) injuries and the subsequent disorders that frequently occur after motor vehicle collisions. We discuss the more common postinjury disorders seen in private practice, including the acute to chronic problems. Emphasis is placed on neck and back strains and sprains, headaches, myofascial pain syndromes, disc injury, and concussions. Special focus is given in this chapter to upper-extremity examination. This chapter does not present a "cookbook" approach to diagnosis. Instead, our goal is to provide a solid foundation for the treating doctor to use in evaluating and understanding patient injuries. It is hoped that this will result in a more accurate foundation for achieving improved treatment outcomes. Secondary benefits include improved communication skills with patients, attorneys, and insurance adjusters.

There are numerous hurdles in evaluating and treating motor vehicle collision injuries (MVCIs). Are doctors suitably trained in making an adequate diagnosis? What are the mechanisms of injury? What is a cervicogenic headache? These are some of the questions that we will address in our investigation into injuries frequent in mobile societies.

DIAGNOSIS RATIONALE

Regardless of the clinician's philosophical constructs, appropriate, responsible steps must be taken on the patient's behalf to determine appropriate diagnosis. The purpose of the treating doctor in making a diagnosis or clinical impression is fivefold in personal injury cases: (1) Identify and prioritize the presenting condition(s) or complaint(s). (2) Determine the cause(s) or mechanism(s) involved. (3) Determine whether the doctor or facility has the resources available to provide proper treatment and whether a professional referral is required. (4) Provide to the patient an explanation of his or her condition, treatment options, and consequences. (5) Provide the basis for reimbursement of current and future medical bills and help determine the basis for settlement whether or not the patient is represented by an attorney.

Diagnostic impressions are established at the initial patient evaluation and may change as a function of time, repair, and response to treatment. For example, cephalgia may be a constant diagnosis throughout the course of treatment because of the persistence of this symptom, whereas a strain is a time-dependent diagnosis because it may turn into a myofascial pain syndrome in a chronic state as part of the repair process. The following variables should be considered when making a diagnosis:

- time since injury (stage of repair)
- severity of injury
- subjective complaints of patient
- severity of symptoms
- anatomic region involved
- pre-existing complicating conditions
- mechanism of injury
- objective findings by doctor
- underlying pathophysiology of problem
- confirmatory evidence (clinical, radiologic imaging, electrodiagnostic)

For the sake of diagnostic simplicity it is best if the clinician assumes that most MVCI patients will present with

- two or more injuries
- two or more complaints
- more than one cause for each complaint

Referred symptoms, such as headaches, upper-extremity paresthesias, and lower-extremity symptoms, such as sciatica, provide a unique diagnostic challenge. Depending on the stage of repair, the number of conditions (i.e., disc, myofascial, joint dysfunction) that could initiate these referred symptoms are numerous, more complex, and difficult to narrow down than the typical strain injury diagnosis. When dealing with referring symptoms there are several ways to find the most likely source. The clinician may try to reproduce, provoke, or lessen the symptoms with digital pressure at known anatomic regions typical for the complaint, and through a series of orthopedic or neurologic testing. The doctor

may try some form of management strategy and observe the results. For example, if the patient is having headaches and the headaches resolve with treatment, then diagnostic correctness is assumed.

The diagnostic challenge is met when the patient comes into the office with radiating symptoms and the doctor is unable to reproduce the typical pattern of referring symptoms. For example, it is much easier for the physician to treat a patient with a headache when digital pressure on the lateral aspect of the atlas transverse process worsens the patient's headache. The authors agree with Cailliet,[1] who feels that symptom reproduction is important in diagnosis, especially when pain is referred.

After a diagnosis has been determined, the patient should be informed about treatment options before initiating treatment. Once the course of treatment is initiated, the diagnostic process does not simply end, but becomes an ongoing process. The practitioner has continued responsibilities to recognize changes in the clinical situation of the patient and to update the diagnosis accordingly. If complaints persist beyond a reasonable time frame, a new treatment plan should be developed, including working with or referring to another health care provider.

THERE IS NO TYPICAL PATIENT

Two principles are operative when considering the mechanisms and diagnosis of injury to an occupant involved in a car crash: (1) there is no typical crash and (2) there is no typical patient.[2] This implies that no matter how much the doctor educates himself or herself there is still some degree of the unknown.

Why is there no typical patient? One author notes that "identical injury-site loads may cause a wide variety of injuries, depending upon which of a particular individual's structural elements is the weakest link."[2] The *Physician's Desk Reference* describes a wide variety of symptoms that may occur (including side effects) in the population from taking the same medication. In much the same way, people respond differently to the same chemical and may present with different clinical pictures from the same biomechanical trauma. Outside previous medical records, what does the doctor or insurance carrier know about the patient's pre-existing condition? Current magnetic resonance imaging (MRI) studies indicate that in the asymptomatic back pain population 53% had a disc bulge at at least one level and 27% had a disc protrusion shown.[3] In addition, a car accident reconstructionist may give good estimates on crash velocity, but at the same time may not know what the occupant velocities are for specific regions or specific tissues within the body for a specific type and size of vehicle.

BACKGROUND DATA ON MINOR INJURIES

A recent National Accident Sampling System (NASS) of police-reported collisions showed that a person in a car crash will sustain on average 2.5 injuries, with 4.7% having 5 injuries and 11.3% having 6 injuries.[4] This study also showed specific regions of the body and risk of minor injury (Figure 1–1). Overall, 86% of all MVCIs are minor in severity, and 94.9% of spine injuries are minor, according to the Abbreviated Injury Scale (AIS-1).

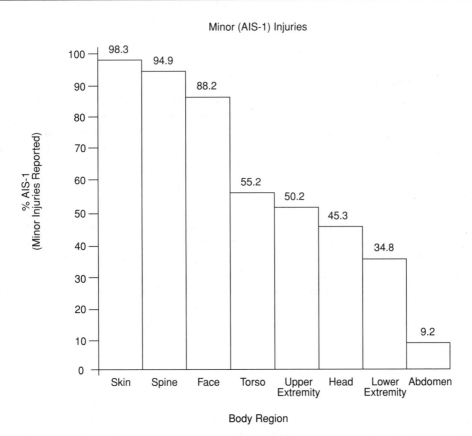

Figure 1–1 Frequency of police-reported mild (minor AIS-1) injuries in the United States. *Source:* Data from Luchter S., Multiple Injuries in Motor Vehicle Crashes, in 34th Proceedings, Association for the Advancement of Automotive Medicine, Scottsdale, Arizona, 1990.

INJURY AND SYMPTOM DISTRIBUTION

Several studies have correlated the type of injury with the vector of the crash. Figure 1–2 compares frontal, side, and rear-end crashes with injury frequency.[5] The consultation may be performed for the acute or chronic patient, and it is important to know the distribution of symptoms as it relates to regions so that the appropriate diagnosis can be made. Tables 11–1 and 11–2 show comparisons in acute and chronic patients. The most common complaints include neck pain, headaches, middle back pain, low back pain, and arm symptoms.

The Insurance Research Council (IRC)[6] analysis has shown in its analysis of insurance claims that when looking at reported claims by tort (BI) and no-fault (PIP) states that neck and back sprain/strains are the most common in the United States (Table 1–1). The IRC also has researched the most serious injuries reported by auto accident victims, with back and neck strains most commonly reported as being the most serious (Table 1–2).

HOW SOON DO SYMPTOMS APPEAR AFTER CAR CRASHES?

Many clinical, automotive, and epidemiologic studies report frequent delays in patients' having initial symptoms after sustaining an injury in an automobile collision,[7,8] accounting for many injuries not being reported to the police and thus not being entered into national crash data. Symptoms such as neck pain may be delayed for several days; other symptoms common to MVCI, such as headaches, back pain, and upper-extremity symptoms, may have their onset several months later.

Although there are many factors as to why these delays occur, one major factor is believed to be related to the spreading of posttraumatic edema.[9] Gravity and the spread of bleeding and inflammatory exudates along the myofascial planes cause secondary swelling and damage. One study of rear-end collision occupants using MRI to detect microscopic hemorrhage found active bleeding in the deep anterior and posterior cervical muscles 2 to 5 days after injury.[10]

The authors' experience has shown that about 95% of those occupants having been involved in a MVCI will have some degree of neck stiffness or pain within the first 2 weeks. Any abnormal delay in symptom onset requires further investigation and documentation by the doctor. The patient may report minor symptoms of initial aching or soreness that he or she assumes will improve over time. When symptoms do not improve or become worse over time, the patient finally enters the health care system. However, it is rare for the victim to have absolutely no neck pain or stiffness for 2 or 3 months and then suddenly develop it for no known reason. This pattern is different for other conditions.

Upper-extremity radicular symptoms from thoracic outlet syndromes, myofascial adhesions, trigger points, or disc syndromes are commonly experienced several weeks after the injury. Frequently upper-extremity pain and numbness begin later than the initial neck pain. Quintner's study[11] of 37 MVCI patients showed that 65% had onset of radicular symptoms within 3 months of the accident and 35% had onset beyond 3 months. These symptom delays primarily are due to biomechanical functional changes within spinal joints and myofascial structures as a result of alterations in ligamentous and disc stability. The mechanical changes in the zygapophyseal joints further irritate the nerve root and other pain-sensitive structures. Chemical irritation due to immobility, metabolite accumulation, and ischemia may further irritate the soft tissues.

In addition, as myofascial tissues begin to heal with scar tissue and to fibrose, causing alterations in tissue tone, they begin to irritate peripheral neural tissues. Over time, the neural tissue may become hypersensitive to stimuli. Perineural or thoracic outlet fibrosis in the exiting nerve roots may lead to long delays in radicular symptoms. In some in-

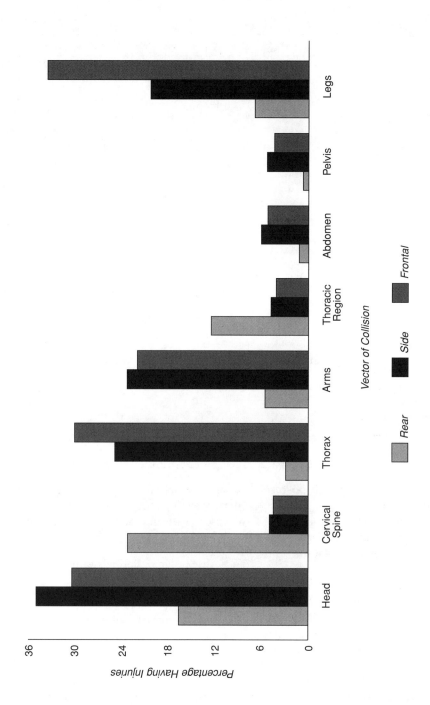

Figure 1–2 Vector of collision and injury frequency ranking. *Source:* Data from Foret-Bruno J.Y., et al., Risk of Cervical Lesions in Real-World and Simulated Collisions, in 34th Proceedings, Scottsdale, Arizona, Association for the Advancement of Automotive Medicine, 1990.

6   MOTOR VEHICLE COLLISION INJURIES

Table 1–1 Percentage of Claimants Reporting Various Types of Injuries in 1987 and 1992

	BI		PIP	
	1987	1992	1987	1992
Fatality	1%	1%	1%	1%
Permanent Brain Injury	*	*	*	*
Paralysis/Paresis	*	*	*	*
Loss of Body Part	*	*	*	*
Loss of Sense(s)	*	*	*	*
Internal Organ Injury	1	1	2	2
Fracture, Weight-Bearing Bone	4	3	4	4
Other Fracture	5	5	7	7
Scarring/Disfigurement	4	3	2	3
Concussion	6	4	7	5
Serious Laceration	3	2	4	3
Back Sprain/Strain	47	55	40	46
Neck Sprain/Strain	58	66	48	59
Other Sprain/Strain	11	13	12	14
TMJ† Dysfunction	1	1	1	1
Minor Lacerations	22	16	32	24
Psychological/Emotional	NA	2	NA	1
Other Injury	12	14	12	16
Unknown Injury	*	1	*	1
No Injury	1	1	1	1
No Response	*	*	*	*
Total Claimants	21,688	33,970	13,534	13,211

Note: Percentages total more than 100% because most claimants reported more than one type of injury.
*Percentage lower than 0.5%.

†TMJ, Temporomandibular joint.

Source: Reprinted from *Auto Injuries: Claiming Behavior and Its Impact on Insurance Costs* with permission of the Insurance Research Council, © 1994.

---

stances, patients may maladapt their posture to lessen neck or mid back pain.

Some symptoms may be delayed as a result of adhesion development and changes in the stability of the various ligamentous and myofascial attachments. It is not unusual for upper-extremity pain or paresthesias to become symptomatic or problematic 2 to 4 months after a MVCI.[1] Again, the clinical impression should be updated as changes in patient complaints and examination findings arise.

Neck pain and stiffness, headaches, and thoracic/lumbar spine pain account for the vast majority of symptoms that bring the patient into the doctor's office within the first 2 weeks after a MVCI. However, some condi-

tions may not show up for several weeks or may develop sometime later during the course of care and include the following:

- radicular symptoms
- disc bulge radiating symptoms
- myofascial pain syndromes
- thoracic outlet syndromes
- multiple crush syndromes
- postconcussion syndromes
- progression of degenerative joint disease

A frustrating aspect of MVCI is that the majority of these cases have no traditional orthopedic or neurologic objective findings (i.e., reflex abnormalities, upper motor signs) on examination.[9] For example, a study of 300 pa-

Table 1–2 Percentage of Claimants Reporting Most Serious Injury

Most Serious Injury	BI	UM	UIM	PIP	MP
Fatality	1%	1%	5%	1%	2%
Permanent Brain Injury	*	*	2	*	*
Paralysis/Paresis	*	*	1	*	*
Loss of Body Part	*	*	*	*	*
Loss of Sense(s)	*	*	*	*	*
Internal Organ Injury	1	1	2	1	1
Fracture, Weight-Bearing Bone	2	2	10	3	3
Other Fracture	3	3	9	5	5
Scarring/Disfigurement	2	1	4	1	1
Concussion	1	1	2	2	2
Serious Laceration	1	1	2	1	1
Back Strain/Sprain	25	27	17	24	24
Neck Strain/Sprain	40	40	15	31	32
Other Strain/Sprain	5	4	2	5	4
Miscellaneous Sprain/Strain†	1	2	1	1	1
TMJ‡ Dysfunction	1	1	3	*	*
Minor Laceration	7	6	1	13	13
Psychological/Emotional	1	1	2	*	*
Other Injury	9	9	23	10	9
Unknown Injury	1	1	*	1	1
Total	100%	100%	100%	100%	100%
Valid Responses	33,707	4,874	913	13,066	8,858

Note: When only one type of injury was reported, that injury is included as the most serious injury. Percentages are rounded to the nearest percentage point.

*Percentage lower than 0.5%.

†Miscellaneous sprain/strain claims involved instances where more than one type of sprain or strain (and no other type of injury) was checked, but the file reviewer did not indicate which one was the most serious injury.

‡TMJ, Temporomandibular joint.

Source: Reprinted from *Auto Injuries: Claiming Behavior and Its Impact on Insurance Costs* with permission of the Insurance Research Council, © 1994.

tients injured in rear-end collisions found only 2 patients who had diminished reflexes.[12] Still, a diagnosis must be made in order that appropriate treatment may be provided and reimbursed.

RANKING NECK AND BACK INJURY SEVERITY

Several international systems currently are used to rank car crash injuries. Some systems rank injuries by the risk of fatality, such as the AIS System. Other systems rank injuries by economic costs or associated disabilities. These ranking systems are used in federally funded studies and in many automotive research projects. These ranking systems are appropriate in the emergency department and the hospital, and for cost analysis and safety engineers. However, in private practice, where life-threatening injuries are seldom seen, these systems have little relevance or practical value to the doctor or insurance carrier. After doing an exhaustive search of the automotive literature, the authors felt that a more appropriate system for the physician in private practice treating the common neck and back injury should focus on issues such as pain severity, disability, types of tissues injured, and clinical standing. The following is a proposed minor, moderate, and serious ranking system that will easily expand most AIS-1 neck and back injuries:

Minor Injury (AIS-1)

- pain level 1 to 3 on Visual Analogue Scale (VAS)
- no time lost from work
- no palpable edema
- mild muscle spasm (relevant for 3 to 4 weeks after injury)
- pain in patient only at end of range of motion (ROM) testing
- local pain only (patient can touch painful area with finger)
- compression tests normal or only give mild joint pain
- no radiating symptoms
- excellent prognosis if early appropriate management

Moderate Injury (AIS-1)

- pain level 4 to 6 on VAS
- 1 to 4 days' time lost from work
- mild to moderate palpable edema
- moderate muscle spasm (relevant for 3 to 4 weeks after injury)
- mild pain in patient at middle of ROM testing and severe pain at end of ROM testing
- local pain only (uses hand or sweeps over larger area)
- compression tests give mild to moderate joint pain
- mild radiating symptoms that begin after 3 to 4 weeks
- prognosis good if early aggressive management but may be poor if delays in treatment occur or if victim is female in rear-end crash

Severe Injury (AIS-1)

- pain level 7 to 10 on VAS
- more than 4 days' time lost from work
- moderate to severe palpable edema
- absent supraclavicular notch in occu-pants involved in rear-end crashes associated with sternocleidomastoid muscle swelling (bogginess due to edema) and spasm
- measurable neck swelling (by tape measure or on radiographs) in occupants involved in moderate- to high-speed rear-end crashes
- severe muscle spasm (splinting)
- head grasp sign: patient grabs mouth, hair, or head with hand to help move from supine to sitting position
- moderate to severe pain in patient at middle of ROM testing; may be unable to move to normal limits of motion
- more diffuse, extremely severe pain the first day or the next morning and radiating arm or leg symptoms (onset less than 1 week)
- cervical compression tests create non-clinical radiating symptoms or reproduce typical arm symptoms
- difficulty sleeping (restlessness)
- radiographic instability on stress views
- includes all patients having clinically significant nonsurgical disc bulges
- typically patient in small car hit by heavier car; patient's head rotated at time of impact; patient elderly; female; higher-speed crash; patient has significant pre-existing complicating condition
- prognosis usually poor even with early aggressive management

Patients with complicated spinal fractures, severe disc injuries, or significant head injuries; patients having any pathologic signs or symptoms, evidence of severe spinal ligamentous instability on radiographs, grade III upper- or lower-extremity ligament tear, or extremity fracture or dislocation; and patients having persistent pain levels holding at 7 to 10 on VAS for more than 30 days with little help from analgesics, anti-inflammatories, or muscle relaxants should be categorized as having more serious injury (AIS ≥ 2). These cases are best managed by a multidisciplinary panel of providers. In these cases it is advantageous for the chiropractor to discuss the comanagement strategies, because the patient might be confused or alarmed as to why the referral is being recommended.

Abbreviated Injury Scale

Considering that the vast majority of car crashes result in mild to moderate injuries, it is worthwhile for the health professional to be aware of the most commonly used international system for categorizing and ranking MVCIs.[13] Although this system is not practical to the clinician, it provides the statistical basis for many reports and therefore should be noted. The AIS system was first published in 1971 as a result of efforts of the American Medical Association (AMA), the Association for the Advancement of Automotive Medicine (AAAM), and the Society of Automotive Engineers (SAE). The AIS has been adopted as the official injury collection data tool by all federally funded crash investigation teams in the United States.[14]

The AIS rating is based on anatomic injury and ranks single maximum injury severity[13] and its threat to the occupant's life.[15] It scores injuries and not their consequences.[16] It does not have a linear progression; does not address injury outcome, disability, or impairment; and does not indicate prognosis or associated costs. It does not include pain, swelling, or tenderness.[13] The main significance of the AIS rating is that higher values indicate higher risk to life loss.[17] For all types of injuries the average value is 1.22.[4] Table 1–3 shows the six AIS categories with the risk for death.[13,15]

MILD HEAD INJURY

The physician may see mild head injuries in the acute to chronic stage in the office setting, usually subsequent to a car crash or a fall. It is

Table 1–3 AIS Categories with the Risk for Death

AIS Rank	Degree of Injury	Risk for Death (%)
Mild–Minor Injury	AIS-1	0
Moderate Injury	AIS-2	0.1–0.4
Serious Injury	AIS-3	0.8–2.3
Severe Injury	AIS-4	10
Critical Injury	AIS-5	50
Virtually Unsurvivable	AIS-6	≤ 100

apparent that head injury patients see a variety of care providers in the United States, including medical doctors, chiropractors, and physical therapists for either primary or secondary complaints. Mild head injury (MHI) has been referred to in the literature as mild brain injury (MBI), diffuse axonal injury (DAI), cerebral concussion, and also in nonspecific terms such as closed head injury (CHI) and traumatic brain injury (TBI). In this section we focus on the common minor brain injury or concussion as it relates to motor vehicle collisions. We will concentrate on diagnosing the acute MHI and the chronic postconcussion syndrome (PCS), which may follow as a healed sequela to the MHI.

Analysis of several large studies concluded that approximately 7 million nonmajor head injuries occur annually in the United States.[18] In 1980, costs for treatment of acute head injury in the United States were estimated at $4 billion.[19] Rimel et al.[20] evaluated 538 minor head injuries and found that 46% were from MVCIs, 23% from falls, 18% from sports activities, 10% from assaults, and the rest from miscellaneous causes. Other studies have confirmed that most minor head injuries are due to motor vehicle collisions or falls.[21] The male to female ratio is around 2.5:1,[22,23] with alcohol intoxication noted in 28%[23] to 44%[24] of cases. Concussions usually are seen in motor vehicle collisions in which the head hits a broad, soft surface in contrast to most subdural hematomas, which occur from smaller, hard-surface impacts as commonly seen in falls and assaults.

Mechanisms of Head Injury

There are several factors that affect the incidence and severity of head injuries.

Human Factors

Precollision occupant body bracing in low-speed crashes (less than 8 mph), having an air bag inflated in a frontal crash, and using a seat belt can lessen the head impact velocity and reduce injury severity. However, alcohol intoxication, the presence of rigid surfaces, and pre-existing psychological problems can worsen injury outcome. See Chapter 16 on human factors.

Vehicle, Speed, and Collision Factors

Forces to the head during collisions can be influenced by the size, rigidity, and shape of the other vehicle or object hit as well as the collision speed, vehicle crashworthiness, and type of crash. Head impact speed is relative to the distance from the occupant's head to the interior of the car.[25] Malliaris et al. concluded after reviewing NASS data that at a crash velocity (delta V) of 10 mph an AIS-1 head injury would occur with every additional 5 mph additional speed and would increase the injury ranking one higher level.[26] Figure 1–3 illustrates the increase in head injury severity with velocity. A mean delta V of 27 mph was found to result in serious head injury.[25] It has been suggested that *twice* the rotational head velocity is required to cause a concussion with no head impact as is required from forces with head contact.[27] Seat belts will lessen the likelihood of head impact significantly at lower velocities, but once the delta V exceeds 30 mph, seat belts will lessen the risk of hitting the head only slightly.

Classification of Head Injury Severity

There are several methods of classifying head injury severity. Some emergency departments utilize the time of coma and/or the Glasgow Coma Scale, whereas all federally funded groups use the AIS system. Strub and Black[28] recommend a concussion severity scale that correlates posttraumatic amnesia time to prognosis, suggesting that 0 to 15 minutes of amnesia equals a slight concussion and 15 to 60 minutes equals a mild concussion. Rimel et al.[20] define MHI as that which produces unconsciousness for 20 minutes or less or a Glasgow Coma Scale score of 13 to 15 and hospitalization not exceeding 48 hours. The Glasgow Coma Scale, although used in most emergency departments, is not very useful for the doctor in private practice in ranking MHI.

As discussed earlier in this chapter, the most commonly recognized international system for ranking automotive collision injuries is the AIS. The AIS scores injuries and not the consequences of injuries such as pain or disability. The risk of fatality directly relates to the ranking in the AIS system. AIS-1 injuries, or minor head injuries, have no risk of death. One study shows that 88% of all brain injuries are concussions with 44% being AIS-1 (minor) and 47% being AIS-2 (moderate) injuries.[22]

Minor Head Injury (AIS-1)

Patients with minor head injury include occupants who are unconscious for less than 1 minute, have no skull fracture, and have up to 30 minutes of anterograde amnesia. Anterograde amnesia refers to no memory of events immediately following the incident.

Outside the AIS system these mild head injuries typically involve the occupant's head hitting a large padded surface or result from inertial loading at higher-speed collisions. These injuries involve low- to high-speed crashes and affect patients not having soft neurologic findings or skull fracture. Common symptoms include headache, dizziness, tinnitus, and visual symptoms.

Moderate Head Injury (AIS-2)

Patients with AIS-2 injuries are unconsciousness for 1 to 15 minutes and have over 30 minutes of anterograde amnesia. Simple, noncomplicated skull fractures are frequently associated with this level of injury. Outside the AIS system the moderate head injury is

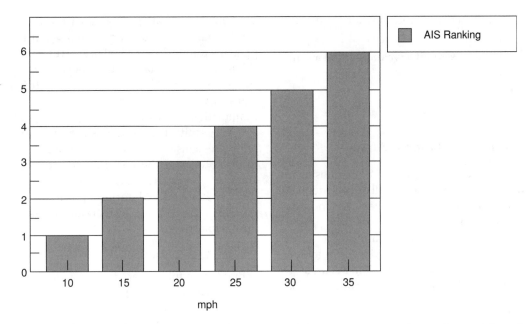

Figure 1–3 Head injury severity increases with increased changes in impact velocity. *Source:* Adapted with permission from Malliaris A.C., Hitchcock R., Hedlund J., A Search for Priorities in Crash Protection, Society of Automotive Engineers, Inc., paper 820242, 1982.

typically seen in higher-speed crashes, among older occupants, and among intoxicated occupants. Neurologic examination may reveal soft findings in some of these cases.

Symptoms Common to Acute Mild Head Injury

It has been estimated that as many as 10% of motor vehicle collision occupants will have MHI.[29] Rutherford et al.[30] found that women have a higher symptom rate than men at both 6 weeks and 1 year after the accident.

Symptoms common to MHI include the following:

- Headaches. Headaches[24,31–33] are seen in 12% to 80% of patients after MHI. Typical headaches are described as continuous, nonthrobbing, generalized, and constant pain that is caplike or headbandlike in distribution. There is recent evidence that there is an *inverse relationship* between head impact severity and head-ache frequency and severity.[34] Patients with minor head injuries appear to have more severe headaches than patients with severe head injuries.
- Scalp dysthesias[31]
- Dizziness/vertigo[18,24]
- Fatigue[31,32]
- Intellectual or cognitive impairment,[31,32,35] including impaired short-term memory, loss of concentration and attention, and diminished problem-solving skills
- Amnesia[36]
- Irritability[37]
- Disorientation

Less common MHI symptoms include the following:

- Blurry vision and diplopia[31]
- Sexual dysfunction[35]
- Sensitivity to noise[32]
- Tinnitus[31]

- Disturbances in coordination
- Disturbances in balance
- Upper-extremity weakness and numbness
- Hand tremor[38]
- Cluster headaches[39]

Examination of Mild Head Injuries

In the office, the first stage of diagnosing an MHI is to have the patient fill out an adequate head injury form (see Chapter 2 for form description). In addition, the front-desk personnel should be instructed to inform the doctor of any unusual patient behavior that may contribute to the evaluation. General areas to evaluate in MHI cases[18,37,40–42] are described below.

Mental Status

In the interview with the MHI patient, look for mental process changes from the preinjury state. During the interview and examination, the patient should be evaluated closely as to appropriateness of mannerisms, behavior, and responses to verbal questions and examination procedures. Investigate mental function including short- and long-term memory and alertness of the patient to time and place. Higher levels of cognition may be evaluated by having the patient count backward in threes starting from 100. Each counting response should be accurate and rapid in a normal patient. Observe carefully any early signs of a declining level of consciousness. These signs may include agitation, restlessness, loss of orientation, and lethargy and may be the first indicators of a developing hematoma.

Pupillary Responses

After excluding an eye prosthesis, a surgical procedure, or a traumatic event that may result in asymmetric pupils, the examiner proceeds with an eye examination. In a room that is dimly lit, look for pupillary responses with a penlight. It is important to bring the light in briskly from the side to see how the pupils re-

act. Close observation is necessary to detect subtle changes in pupillary responses. If the patient's pupils (P) are equal in size (E), round (R), and have normal reactive constrictive responses to light (L) and accommodation (A) bilaterally, the doctor can chart PERLA in the examination findings.

If the examiner finds sluggish or absent pupillary responses, the abnormal findings need to be noted and the patient referred to an emergency department, preferably at a trauma hospital. Abnormal pupillary responses may indicate intracranial pressure from hemorrhage.

Cranial Nerve Examination

Brain stem injuries are common after head injuries. Doing a complete cranial nerve examination is important. The most frequent problems found in a private practice are trigeminal nerve paresthesias and nystagmus.

Equilibrium Testing

Having the patient do a tandem walk may reveal a wide-based (cerebellar) gait.

Finger-to-Nose Testing

The doctor looks for speed and accuracy of the patient with the patient's eyes open and closed. Note any awkwardness or past-pointing.

Red Flags on MHI Differential Diagnosis

The most important signs that indicate referral include increasing sleepiness, progressively worsening headache, and occasionally intractable nausea. High blood pressure (more than 160/100 mm Hg) with low pulse rate is representative of head injury. Other symptoms indicating referral include limb weakness and cerebrospinal fluid drainage from nose or ears.

Skull X-Ray and CT Studies

Following head trauma, the treating doctor must make clinical decisions on what diagnostic tests—including X-rays and CT—are indicated, keeping in mind the best interests of the patient. Even so, about 3.7 million skull radiographs were taken in 1980 in the United States and less than 9% showed skull fracture.[43] Another study determined that even if a linear skull fracture is present in a patient with minor head injury, few or no intracranial sequelae are likely.[44]

A recent multidisciplinary panel and validation study of 7,035 patients in 31 hospitals developed a management strategy to reduce unnecessary radiography.[43] The panel divided the patients into three groups according to their rated risk levels. Low-risk patients included those with headaches, dizziness, scalp lacerations, hematomas, contusions, and abrasions with no neurologic abnormalities. The moderate-risk group, of whom 4% had intracranial complications, included those with a history of progressive headache, alcohol or drug intoxication, posttraumatic seizures, vomiting, posttraumatic amnesia, suspected fracture, multiple trauma, serious facial trauma, and concussion. One study found that approximately 8% of cerebral concussions are accompanied by skull fracture.[45] The high-risk category consisted of those patients having significant scalp lacerations, exposed skull bone, penetrating head injuries, and suspected depressed skull fractures. This review also revealed that children younger than 2 years of age are at high risk, having an 8.6% to 27% incidence of skull fracture.[43]

This panel also found that the low-risk group of patients had no intracranial injuries and therefore did not require X-ray examination. In this low-risk group, it was concluded that fractures in three to six patients per 10,000 could potentially be missed. Patients in the moderate-risk and high-risk categories should have CTs or skull X-rays. CTs should be ordered if skull X-rays show any fracture or the patient has persistent tachypnea (possibly indicating increased intracranial pressure). Other indications for CT included suspected cerebrospinal fluid drainage from the ears or nose, bruising under both eyes (raccoon eyes), or bruising over the mastoid process (Battle's sign).

Pathophysiology of Concussion

A concussion is an immediate mechanical event caused by direct or indirect trauma resulting in a loss of consciousness or a lessening of mental processes.[15] Concussion injuries have a mechanical pathogenesis[46] due to a distortion of the brain caused by internal shearing forces that lead to widespread axonal tract stretching within the white matter. "The available evidence indicates that diffuse axonal injury (DAI) in human beings occurs at the time of head injury and is not due to complicating factors such as hypoxia, brain swelling or raised intracranial pressure."[46] Cawing et al[47] define diffuse axonal injury as being due to focal tears and lesions of the brain stem and corpus callosum and to diffuse microscopic injury scattered throughout the cerebral hemispheres and the brain stem. Several studies have demonstrated that when the axon is injured, it expels a ball of axoplasm, which may manifest itself later as microscopically diffuse axonal retraction balls at injury sites.[40,48]

Gennarelli[49] feels that in the concussion, "much of the effect of strain on the axon is to its function and not to its gross structure." Gennarelli suggests that the pathophysiology of concussion is from brain motion within the skull, deformation and strains within the brain, and axon disruption. Strains are distributed centripetally, with maximal strains near the brain surface. It is estimated that there are approximately 100 billion neurons in a human brain, with a greater number of axonal interconnecting pathways.[50] Jennett and Teasdale[37] conclude that even in mild concussions there is some resultant structural damage to the brain.

Mild head injuries are not associated with any significant mortality; therefore, postmortem studies are not available. Consequently, it is common to use animals, such as monkeys, in studies using mathematical computations; the resulting data are then extrapolated to humans. This allows for predictions of injury types and tolerance levels. Additionally, human cadavers are used to evaluate impacts.

Repeated Head Injuries

It is well accepted in current medical literature that concussion injuries appear cumulative in MVCIs, as well as in some sports injuries.[28,51]

Chronic Postconcussion Syndrome

Chronic postconcussion syndrome (PCS) is never an immediate diagnosis following head injury. It is merely a diagnostic term that describes a constellation of findings typical of a patient who has developed a chronic dysfunctional condition or is having healed residuals following a concussion (head injury). The diagnosis of PCS entails a time factor and is typically made at about 3 months postinjury.

One hospital study of 1,115 adults concluded that as many as 50% of patients with minor head injury were at risk for developing PCS.[52] A significant number of these patients had headaches, dizziness, and memory problems during the first year after injury.[24] Recent evidence strongly supports the theory that there is an organic basis for PCS. An animal craniocervical injury study concluded that the etiology of postconcussion syndrome following whiplash injuries is organic and that the neck injury is the primary element in the cause of this syndrome.[53] (See Chapter 11 on head injury prognosis.)

Chronic PCS Symptoms

Common PCS symptoms may include those affecting higher levels of cognition and personality. The following chronic symptoms are common:[21,32,37]

- headache
- blurry vision
- loss of balance
- loss of coordination
- poor memory
- reduced drive/motivation
- language difficulty
- difficulty handling multiple tasks
- reduced attention span
- difficulty with problem solving
- performance inconsistencies
- absence of ability to anticipate
- slower reaction times
- sleep disorders
- more assertive than normal with others
- angry outbursts
- depression
- inflexibility
- less diplomatic than normal
- personality change and lack of social inhibition
- hand tremors
- tinnitus
- physical fatigue and reduced mental stamina
- more shallow relationships with people
- indifference to other people
- sexual dysfunction

Diagnosing PCS

As the patient's mild head injury heals and develops into its chronic form, the PCS, the challenge of making a diagnosis becomes more complex. The difficulty in accurate diagnosis is determining functional changes in the brain's processing ability secondary to a head injury. Brain function is more difficult to test than peripheral nerve function, mainly due to inaccessibility, more complex function, and less acceptance and understanding of the long-term disability that may occur as a result of MHI. There are two primary tools for the doctor to utilize in evaluating possible PCS patients: a complete history and referral for neuropsychologic testing.

In obtaining a history, the patient is best interviewed with ample time to address any mental processing problems that have occurred since the injury. Sometimes having a spouse, family member, or close friend along to give an outside opinion can be valuable in assessing the patient. In the history review, look primarily for new symptoms that are classic for this type of injury while ruling out other factors such as marriage or work difficulties. Obtaining an accurate history assists the health practitioner in determining whether a referral to a neuropsychologist is needed for further testing and possible therapy.

Neuropsychologic tests that may be performed on patients with PCS include memory and learning tests, motor skills tests, visuospatial and constructional performance testing, amnesia tests, and tests for language performance. Other tests also include reasoning and problem solving, as well as evaluating attention and concentration. Because of the multifaceted, complex nature of head injuries, these multiple neuropsychologic tests need to be done to demonstrate dysfunction. A 6- to 12-hour neuropsychologic evaluation usually is needed to document postconcussion problems properly.[54] Shorter evaluations will not address the complex nature of these injuries.

One study of 53 patients, 90% with MVCIs, 1 to 22 months after mild brain injury found that the head injury patients performed significantly more poorly than the uninjured group in organization tasks and attention to detail.[55] No difference was seen in patients who had lost consciousness and those who were only dazed. Litigation or its absence had no effect on outcome as well. A study by Ewing et al.[56] of ten patients 1 to 3 years after mild head injury, at a simulated altitude of 3,800 m to create mild hypoxia, found that vigilance and memory task performance were significantly below those of the control group.

There are a number of difficulties in evaluating a patient with postconcussion syndrome. One obvious reason is that the patient's functional capacity before the head injury is usually not known. Strub and Black[28]

believe that once a concussion has been diagnosed, the establishment of parameters to determine the severity and prognosis of the postconcussion syndrome can be difficult because of the considerable dispute reflected in the literature. The difficulty with many of the neuropsychologic tests is that the patient may not be stressed in the specific area of deficiency, or not stressed enough, and therefore deficits may not be observed. Levine[21] suggests that when testing, a time limit should be used to add further stress and enhance deficits.

POSTTRAUMATIC DIZZINESS, BLURRY VISION, AND TINNITUS

Several authors have described posttraumatic auditory and visual symptoms following MVCI.[57,58] A recent animal study that simulated 12-mph rear-end collisions concludes that these symptoms can be explained by the transient cerebrospinal fluid pressure injury effects on the lower cervical spinal ganglia.[59] Some patients may have delayed onset of symptoms for several days or weeks. Baker's study[60] of 100 MVCI cases found that 10% to 15% of the cases had paresthesias, tinnitus, and blurry vision, with most having trigger points typical of overloading in the splenius capitis muscle. These trigger points were treated and the symptoms resolved. A number of authors have attributed these symptoms to (1) irritation of the sympathetic nerves that penetrate the precervical fascia ending in the stellate ganglia; (2) contractured deep cervical fascia; (3) irritation of the cervical sympathetics; (4) disruption of cervical sensory spinal afferents; (5) vertebrobasilar artery compromise; and (6) abnormal afferent fiber impulses from the cervical joints and neck muscle receptors that end in the vestibular nuclei in the brain stem.[1,61]

Cervicogenic Dizziness

Several authors have researched cervicogenic disequilibrium, finding whiplash injuries common.[62,63] One study established that minor head or neck injury may be associated with postinjury dizziness.[64] For a person to maintain a normal equilibrium, the brain must have input from visual centers, the vestibular system, and the proprioceptive system from mechanoreceptors in the neck joints, muscles, and ligaments.[65] Head and neck motion should precipitate dizziness if it has cervicogenic origins.[63] Revel et al.[66] performed experiments with 30 patients having chronic neck pain and 30 control subjects. They found significantly poorer balance scores for the neck-pain group, indicating alterations in the cervical proprioceptive system. This meant that these neck-pain patients had difficulty in coming back to their reference position after active movement with a tendency to overshoot. Cervicogenic dizziness can be secondary to sympathetic nerve overstimulation, altered neck and lumbar proprioception, neck or lumbar muscle spasm, or vertebral artery problems.[62] It also has been reported that after neck injury, dizziness was found to be due to vestibular disturbances.[58]

Cervicogenic Blurry Vision

Oculomotor symptoms[67] such as blurry vision after whiplash have been reported, concluding that chronic symptoms are probably due to brain stem lesions, dysfunction of the cervical proprioceptive system, or sympathetic nerve irritation.

Cervicogenic Tinnitus

Approximately 8.5% of the general population has tinnitus.[68] House et al.[68] feel that causes for tinnitus include whiplash, neck myofascial spasm, temporomandibular joint (TMJ) dysfunction, concussions, and cranial or cervical fractures. Tamura[57] claims that "tinnitus may be produced by sympathetic stimulation of the caroticotympanic nerve which derives from the internal carotid plexus."

Barré-Lieou Syndrome (Cervicocranial Syndrome)

This syndrome is seen much less commonly than singular auditory or visual symptoms. Cervicocranial syndrome consists of three or more of the following: headache, tinnitus, vertigo, and ocular problems.[57] In this syndrome, symptoms are most commonly secondary to C-3 to C-4 root sleeve irritation. About 75% of patients tested will have C-4 segmental hypoesthesia; about 68% will have disturbances of touch, pain, and temperature sensations, many having bilateral symptoms. Root sleeve defects at C-3 to C-4 that irritate the sympathetics cause a combination of headaches, dizziness, tinnitus, and ocular symptoms, primarily seen with rear-end collisions.[57]

DIAGNOSIS OF POSTTRAUMATIC AUDITORY AND VISUAL SYMPTOMS

The patient history and interview are important parts of diagnosis, as is symptom reproduction examination. Attempting to reproduce these symptoms can be done in the office and involves a number of methods, including using deep digital pressure in the cervical muscles and sternocleidomastoid muscles, and having the patient rotate the head upward and back, looking for symptom recurrence or aggravation. Much like a rheostat, as the patient rotates the head the symptoms start mildly and then become more intense with increasing motion. One author suggests that in order to verify cervical proprioceptive input causing vertigo, have the patient sit in a swivel chair and hold his or her head while rotating the chair. If the twisting of the lower body as the head is held increases vertigo, inner ear problems can be ruled out.[69]

There are a number of conditions that should be ruled out in patients with auditory and visual symptoms. Over-the-counter and prescription medication use must be considered as a possible cause of these symptoms.

Primary disorders of the inner ear may be involved and must be ruled out. In older patients the possibility of transient ischemic attacks (TIA) should be weighed. Be alert to a history of cerebrovascular accidents (CVA) and myocardial infarction (MI). Consider referral of the patient to an eye, ear, nose, and throat specialist for further testing and evaluation if there is any diagnostic question.

POSTTRAUMATIC HEADACHE/ MIGRAINES

Headaches and/or migraines are the second most common complaint following automobile collisions. Headache may occur after a minor rear-end crash or higher-speed crashes. These headaches include muscle tension headache, muscle contraction headache, cervicogenic headache, and migraines. Sources for these posttraumatic headaches include sensory input from the postural and stabilizing myofascial structures of the neck, shoulder, and upper back. Most chronic headaches occurring after MVCIs share many of the same characteristics of muscle contraction or tension headache and some have symptoms similar to those of migraine headaches. It is the authors' experience that many post–head injury headaches originate from soft tissues and joints of the cervical spine.

Typical Headache Description and Common Associated Symptoms

Most headaches that originate from cervical soft tissue stimuli are described as being constant, slightly varying in intensity, nagging or aching, and may be made worse with certain body positioning or movements.

It is important for the doctor to realize that in most collisions in which the head hits the interior structures of the vehicle the occupant will have a concussion as well as a cervicothoracic injury. This is dependent on the area of skull impact and the orientation of the cervical spine and torso at the time of impact. Fioravanti et al.[70] found that about 67% of patients having headache as the chief complaint after trauma had associated and consistent symptoms of dizziness, vertigo, weakness, and tinnitus.

Types of Headaches Seen following Neck and Head Injury

Cervicogenic headaches, myofascial trigger-point headaches,[71] muscle contraction headaches, tension headaches, site-of-impact headaches, and migraines[72] are the most common types of headaches seen in practice, after headaches caused by neck and head injuries. Tension headaches and migraines have been found to correlate with cervical spine musculoskeletal dysfunction[73,74] and occipital neuralgia from muscle spasms of the suboccipital muscles,[31] both of which may occur after MVCI. Weiss et al.[75] did a study of 35 patients, 22 with MVCIs, mostly women, who developed chronic common or classic migraines after having a mild neck injury. Migraines now are generally considered a *primary neurologic disturbance* that affects vascular structures.[75]

Anatomic Sources for Headaches

The brain is not sensitive to pain, but other structures within the outer dural covering of the brain, scalp sensory nerves, mandible, cervical and attaching muscles, and cervical joint pain-sensitive tissues may all contribute to headaches. Overall, Saper[76] believes that there are more than 316 causes of headache. Headaches may arise from irritation of myofascial trigger points in the temporalis, masseter, sternocleidomastoid, splenius capitis, and trapezius muscles.[7] Whiplash injury causes excessive stretching of the upper cervical joint capsule, resulting in irritation of the dorsal root of the greater occipital nerve as it passes through the capsule.[7] Anatomically, the dorsal ramus of the C-2 spinal nerve and its extension the greater occipital nerve may be irritated by trauma, resulting in occipital neuralgia.[77]

Acute to chronic headaches, arising from or made worse following a neck or head injury may result from any of the following conditions:

- localized soft tissue inflammation
- upper cervical spine joint fixation
- muscle contraction, ischemia
- cervicogenic-uncovertebral-apophyseal joint headache
- occipital neuralgia, C-2 to C-3 radiculopathy
- cervicothoracic myofascial trigger points
- temporomandibular joint dysfunction
- thoracic outlet syndrome
- site-of-head impact headache

Cervicogenic Headaches

Several authors describe the anatomic basis for cervicogenic headaches.[78-80] A special area of gray matter in the brain stem that descends into the cervical cord receives nociceptive afferents from both the trigeminal nerve (fifth cranial nerve) and the sensory roots of C-1, C-2, and C-3. This gray matter has been termed the spinal fifth tract of the medulla[80] and the trigeminocervical nucleus.[79]

Bogduk notes that incoming nociceptive afferent information from the cervical nerve roots C-1 to C-3 communicates with second-order nociceptive neurons in the trigeminocervical nucleus. These second-order nociceptive neurons also receive noxious input from trigeminal afferents coming from the face. When they in turn send information to the thalamus there is confusion as to the actual source of the information, and frequently it is interpreted as arising from the trigeminal fields (ophthalmologic, maxillary, and mandibular distributions).[79] See Figure 1–4 for an illustration of the anatomic basis for cervicogenic headaches.

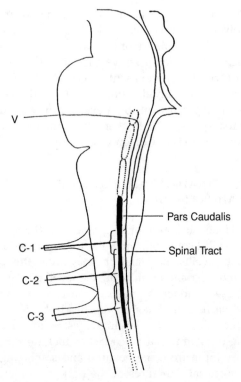

Figure 1–4 Sketch of the brain stem showing the location of the pars caudalis of the spinal nucleus of the trigeminal nerve, its continuity with the dorsal gray matter of the spinal cord, and the overlapping distribution of terminals of the spinal tract of the trigeminal nerve and those of the C-1, C-2, and C-3 spinal nerves in the trigeminocervical nucleus (*black bar*). *Source:* Reprinted from Bogduk N., The Anatomical Basis for Cervicogenic Headache, *Journal of Manipulative and Physiological Therapeutics,* Vol. 15, No. 1, with permission of Williams & Wilkins, © 1992, National College of Chiropractic.

The majority of frontal and scalp headaches get referred stimuli from the greater and lesser occipital nerves, which are derived from the C-2 to C-4 roots and the trigeminal nerves.[1] Wilson[81] shows evidence that nociceptive input from C-1 to C-3 roots may produce pain by irritating the trigeminal nerve system, which could refer pain into the head, neck, and face.

Cervical hyperextension with lateral-rotation neck injuries is known to cause specific

C-2 ganglion dorsal ganglia compression.[82] Bogduk and Marsland[83] found that C-2 to C-3 zygopophyseal joints may be a source of headaches as well. Seletz notes that the most commonly involved nerve root in cervicogenic headache is the C-2 root. In contrast with other cervical nerve roots, it is not well protected with pedicles and facets; furthermore, the nerve exits between C-1 and C-2, which is the point of greatest cervical rotation. He also notes that the C-2 root is the most likely to be interpreted as coming from the ophthalmologic field of the trigeminal nerve.[80] This gives the patient the feeling of hemicrania with pain radiating behind the eyeball. The neck-tongue syndrome may develop if the C-2 ventral ramus is injured, resulting in neck pain, numbness in the occipital region, and tongue paresthesia. These symptoms may occur or intensify when turning the head.[77]

Cervicogenic headaches typically are described as unilateral, located in the frontal-temporal area and precipitated by neck motion, with onset related to injury, neck pain, and stiffness.[84]

Site-of-Head-Impact Headache

Ebelin et al[85] did a 10-year study of 61 MVCI patients and concluded that head injury doubles the risk for long-term cervicocephalic syndromes, compared with the group that had whiplash injury but no head injury. Mandel[33] concluded that muscle tension headaches will occur in 70% of all patients with postconcussion syndrome. Occipital neuralgia occurs in up to 14% of patients with postconcussion syndrome.

The most common sites of head-impact headaches are located around the immediate area where the head was hit. The head contact usually involves hitting the steering wheel, dashboard, or windows. The headache frequently begins at the impact site and occasionally is referred to other areas. The healed injury site on the person's scalp is fibrotic and tender to touch, and deep digital pressure will reproduce or intensify the customary headache pattern if involved. Dizziness may also be associated with these headaches. Site-of-head-impact headaches are usually caused by direct damage to neural structures covering the skull or by scarring, entrapment, and irritation to sensory nerve fibers at the site.

Locating Sources of Posttraumatic Headaches

There are several ways to locate the causes of headaches that follow MVCI. Pain description in the patient's history is the most common basis for diagnosis. Other methods of diagnosis include attempting to reproduce headache pain by applying digital pressure to pain-sensitive structures that have a predilection for causing headaches. These can include the neck, face, upper back, and scalp regions. A headache reproduced by having the patient move the head in various motions also confirms a cervicogenic basis.

Reproduction of the patient's typical headache by joint stressing and digital pressure is probably the most accurate conservative method of pinpointing cervicogenic or soft tissue causes and determining the complexity of the diagnosis. A range-of-motion evaluation in the upper neck region, feeling for palpable texture of the soft tissues of the neck, and looking for trigger points will assist in confirming the diagnosis. The doctor uses deep finger pressure to locate tender and/or fibrotic areas and, while holding the pressure for 10 to 15 seconds, asks the patient to describe the effect of the pressure. If the patient has a headache prior to the deep pressure, look for intensification or lessening. If the patient does not have a headache, ask whether the pressure causes the headache to come on, and if so whether the headache is typical in location and quality of the headache normally felt.

Other causes of headaches must be excluded or ruled out, such as use of dietary stimulants, nutritional disorders, use of drugs that induce headache, anemia, endocrine disorders, emotional stress, and other illnesses. The history of the patient, including patterns of headaches, location of headaches, precipitators, aggravators, and family history, is helpful in providing a clinical picture. Poor posture and emotional stress can initiate or perpetuate headaches as well. The doctor must also rule out TMJ involvement, especially if the patient was in a rear-end collision. The TMJ is discussed later in this chapter. Briefly stated, if there is facial pain along with headache, suspect TMJ involvement. An MRI study in 100 patients with TMJ symptoms found that 88% had pathologic joint effusion and 94% had meniscus deformity.[86]

Drug-Induced Headache

The clinician must be aware that certain patients who chronically use analgesics for their headaches or other pain may develop a pattern wherein the body's normal adaptive response to the medication (when the vasoconstrictive chemical effect wears off) is rebounding vascular dilation, which results in a self-induced headache cycle. For example, frequent use of aspirin and acetaminophen products by chronic headache sufferers often perpetuates and worsens headache frequency and intensity.[87] The last thing that any physician wants to do is to turn a patient with episodic headaches into a chronic, daily headache sufferer. The drug-induced headache is often described as a dull, diffuse, bilateral, nonthrobbing headache that typically begins when the person awakes and then persists all day, with pain frequently noticed in the neck.[87,88]

STRAIN/SPRAIN DEFINITIONS RELATED TO THE NECK AND BACK

When relating neck and back strain/sprain injury severities, the traditional system of grades I, II, III for ranking extremity injuries does not apply. This is primarily due to the multilevels of paraspinal muscles, tendons, and ligaments in the neck and back and the inability of the examiner to isolate and stress any specific spinal ligament or muscle. Figure 1–5 illustrates the complex nature of the neck at the C-6 level.[89] The Insurance Research Council reports that according to a study comparing figures from 1987 with those from 1992, the number of claimants reporting strains and sprains is increasing (Table 1–4).[6]

Strain: A neck or back strain is a partial or complete tear of a muscle or tendon, implying that muscle/tendon fibers have elongated beyond the normal anatomic motion barrier and/or exceeded the muscle's tolerance level to velocity change. A strain can occur in the neck or back if moderate- to end-levels of motion are attained or if the load tolerance is exceeded. Neck or back strains typically are seen in lower-speed frontal and side crashes in which the occupant is braced.

Sprain: A neck or back sprain is a partial or complete tear of ligamentous structures, usually occurring after the outer muscles have stretched and torn. In the neck, middle back, and low back, the diagnosis of a paraspinal soft tissue sprain must include muscles and/

Table 1–4 Percentage of Claimants Reporting Sprain/Strain Injuries Only, Non–Sprain/Strain Injuries Only, and Those Having Combination Injuries

	% of All Claimants	
	1987	1992
BI Claimants		
Sprain/Strain Only	55%	60%
Sprain/Strain plus Non–Sprain/Strain	20	23
Non–Sprain/Strain Only	25	17
PIP Claimants		
Sprain/Strain Only	44	48
Sprain/Strain plus Non–Sprain/Strain	20	23
Non–Sprain/Strain Only	36	29

Note: Excludes "no injury" and "unknown injury" claimants.

Source: Reprinted from *Auto Injuries: Claiming Behavior and Its Impact on Insurance Costs* with permission of the Insurance Research Council, © 1994.

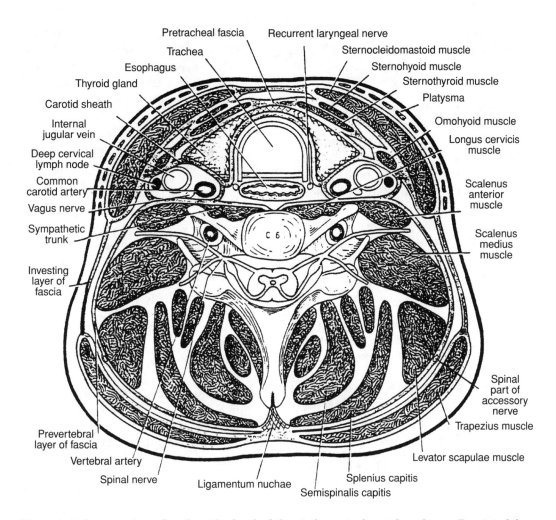

Pretracheal fascia

Trachea

Esophagus

Thyroid gland

Carotid sheath

Internal jugular vein

Deep cervical lymph node

Common carotid artery

Vagus nerve

Sympathetic trunk

Investing layer of fascia

Prevertebral layer of fascia

Vertebral artery

Spinal nerve

Recurrent laryngeal nerve

Sternocleidomastoid muscle

Sternohyoid muscle

Sternothyroid muscle

Platysma

Omohyoid muscle

Longus cervicis muscle

Scalenus anterior muscle

Scalenus medius muscle

Spinal part of accessory nerve

Trapezius muscle

Levator scapulae muscle

Ligamentum nuchae

Splenius capitis

Semispinalis capitis

C 6

Figure 1–5 Cross-section of neck at the level of the sixth cervical vertebra. *Source:* Reprinted from *Clinical Anatomy for Medical Students*, 3rd ed., by R.S. Snell, p. 712, with permission of Little, Brown & Co., © 1986.

---

or tendons and fascia, as these outer soft tissues are always involved in varying degrees. Neck and back sprains always include muscle and tendon injuries with the ligament trauma. If neck motion causes the ligaments to be overstretched, then both strain to the muscles and overstretching of ligaments occur simultaneously.

When the physician ranks the severity of a neck or back injury, he or she has to look primarily at the indirect effects of the injury, that is, the pain, disability, palpable edema, sleep loss, and other side effects of the injury. An adequate system for ranking injury severity for most auto injuries is given in a previous section, "Ranking Neck and Back Injury Severity."

Although the term *whiplash* is commonly used, it should be avoided as a clinical diagnosis because it is considered nondescriptive, merely implying a type of rapid head and neck motion involved in a rear-end crash.

Forces or loads that spinal joints and their attaching soft tissues can be subjected to in motor vehicle collisions include any of the following:

- bending loads seen in flexion, extension, and lateral flexion
- shear loads in translational or horizontal movement
- vertical tension loads in distraction movements, i.e., low-speed rear-end collisions
- axial loads in compression movements
- torsion loads with rotational movements

Influence of Seat Belt Use on Rate of Spinal Injury

The automotive and clinical literature consistently shows that normal use of seat belts changes the pattern of injury. Seat belts save lives and at the same time, while operating in the way they are designed to be used, increase the risk of sprain/strains. One recent study compares the rate of spinal strains by use of seat belts.[90] This hospital study of 863 cases reports 48% cervical strains, 0.03% thoracic strains, and 13% lumbar strains in occupants using seat belts. Occupants without seat belts report 28% cervical strains, 0.02% thoracic strains, and 7% lumbar strains.

Differentiating Spinal Sprains and Strains

Common methods of differentiating sprain/ strains include the following:

- Obtain a history, primarily to determine the mechanism of injury with emphasis on how far the head moved, i.e., head-restraint position. For example, if the occupant's head restraint was positioned properly to limit rearward neck motion, the anterior neck ligaments will not be overstretched. This does not include the rapid lengthening and shortening accordion effect in the neck, causing micro-

scopic joint injury within the joint. The clinician can correlate pain severity and crash speeds in broad terms, meaning that at higher crash velocities more injuries occur and thus the risk is higher for ligament injuries.

- Palpate the paraspinal soft tissues. Feel for muscle bogginess and edema, joint play end-feel, and pain response of the patient to palpation. Boggy end-feel when laterally bending the patient to the end range is common for ligament injuries. See Figure 1–6 for a breakdown of MVCI patients that evaluated joint protector muscles in the body by the vector of crash.
- Have the patient perform an isometric muscle contraction in neutral neck position without moving the neck and note any increase in pain. This may isolate muscle soreness from ligament involvement.
- Evaluate active and passive range of motion, which can be helpful in determining the type of injury that has occurred. A muscle strain will begin to cause pain in the midpoint to end of active resistive motion, whereas a sprain will generate pain primarily at the end of neck passive motion.

NECK INJURY

Otremski et al.[91] studied 1,197 crash victims and found that the typical patient with a neck injury was a middle-aged woman who had been wearing a seat belt when involved in a low-speed rear-end collision. A Japanese study found that in 167,721 automobile crashes, the most frequent injury site was the neck, occurring in 29% of the crashes.[92] Another recent study of 3,927 occupants showed that 18% sustain neck sprains with 80% having the neck injury as the primary complaint.[93] One study of an English emergency department showed 65% of crash victims had neck injuries.[94]

JOINT PROTECTOR MUSCLES

KEY:

HEAD & NECK:
1. Sternocleidomastoid
2. Scalenes anticus
3. Masticatory
4. Semispinalis capitis
5. Splenius capitis

SHOULDER:
6. Upper trapezius
7. Levator scapula
8. Intraspinatus
9. Teres minor
11. Teres major
12. Latissimus dorsi

13. Subscapularis
14. Deltoids
16. Serratus anterior

ELBOW & WRIST:
17. Brachialis
18. Triceps
19. Extensor digitorum
20. Flexor carpi ulnaris

HAND & THUMB:
21. Adductor pollicis

LUMBO-SACRO-ILIAC
22. Quadratus lumborum
23. Iliocostalis

HIP:
24. Gluteus medius
25. Gluteus maximus
26. Piriformis
27. Adductor longus
28. Pectineus
29. Tensor fascia lata

KNEE:
30. Vastus medialis
31. Semimembranosus

ANKLE:
32. Peroneus longus
33. Medial gastronemius

FOOT & FIRST TOE:
34. Flexor hallucis longus

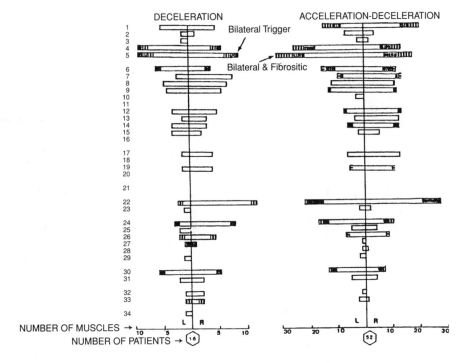

continues

Figure 1–6 Frequency and location of joint protector muscles following various vectors of collision. *Source:* Reprinted from Baker B.A., The Muscle Trigger: Evidence of Overload Injury, *Journal of Neurological and Orthopaedic Medicine & Surgery*, Vol. 7, No. 1, pp. 35–43, with permission of the American Academy of Neurological and Orthopaedic Surgeons, © 1986.

Figure 1–6 continued

JOINT PROTECTOR MUSCLES

KEY:
HEAD & NECK:
1. Sternocleidomastoid
2. Scalenes anticus
3. Masticatory
4. Semispinalis capitis
5. Splenius capitis

SHOULDER:
6. Upper trapezius
7. Levator scapula
8. Intraspinatus
9. Teres minor
11. Teres major
12. Latissimus dorsi

13. Subscapularis
14. Deltoids
16. Serratus anterior

ELBOW & WRIST:
17. Brachialis
18. Triceps
19. Extensor digitorum
20. Flexor carpi ulnaris

HAND & THUMB:
21. Adductor pollicis

LUMBO-SACRO-ILIAC
22. Quadratus lumborum
23. Iliocostalis

HIP:
24. Gluteus medius
25. Gluteus maximus
26. Piriformis
27. Adductor longus
28. Pectineus
29. Tensor fascia lata

KNEE:
30. Vastus medialis
31. Semimembranosus

ANKLE:
32. Peroneus longus
33. Medial gastronemius

FOOT & FIRST TOE:
34. Flexor hallucis longus

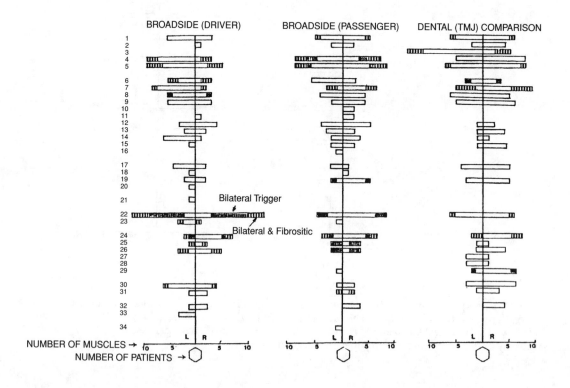

Mechanisms of Neck Injury

In developing an accurate diagnosis of neck injuries an understanding of the mechanisms involved is essential. There are three primary mechanisms of neck injury: (1) inertial loading of the head and neck, resulting in the neck soft tissues moving beyond stretch rate tolerance levels or distance overstretching of tissues beyond tolerance levels; (2) accordion lengthening joint effect in rear-end collisions; and (3) indirect, compressive loading into the neck from a head impact, such as on the windshield.

Malliaris et al.[26] report that the neck is the most injured body region in noncontact crash injuries. Rapid, high forces frequently result in muscle, tendon, fascial, ligament, and capsular stretching and tearing. Neck injuries are caused by tensile, shear, and compression stresses resulting from a mixture of overbending, axial compression, and rotational loading.[94]

Type of Crash and Neck Injury

The vector of collision can be related to the degree and type of injury sustained in a crash. The physician must realize that the seating position of the occupant at the time of the crash plays a significant role in causing injury. Lövsund et al.[95] found that the incidence of neck injury for occupants sitting in the rear seats was about 50% lower than that for front seat occupants. Each type of accident has components that are unique. Rear-end crashes with rapid acceleration result in rapid hyperextension injury, whereas frontal collisions or decelerations cause hyperflexion injury. Side crashes will cause lateral flexion and rotational musculoskeletal injuries. The consensus of medical and automotive literature is that the rear-end crash has the highest reported number of minor to moderate neck injuries. A study of 300 crash cases was reviewed[96] showing that the incidence of neck pain varies by vector of collision. In rear-end collisions 30.8% of the occupants had neck pain, 22.5% of the occupants in frontal collisions had neck pain, 16.9% of the occupants in right-side collisions had neck pain, and 10.7% of occupants in left-side collisions had neck pain. Another report concludes that in frontal collisions 7.6% of occupants and in rear-end collisions 18% of occupants had AIS-1 (minor) neck injuries.[97]

Most neck injuries are reported as either minor or serious.[98] In MVCI the chance of having a serious neck spinal injury has been estimated as 14 times greater than in the thoracolumbar region.[99] As Mackay states, "The neck, perhaps more than any other body region, exhibits age and disease effects which must profoundly influence the nature and level of tolerable applied force."[100] Adolescents, the elderly, and persons with spinal degeneration are subject to neck trauma at lower collision forces than are others.[101] The neck normally can flex and extend through a 120-degree range without injury, but small amounts of cervical rotation at either end of the range may cause serious injury.[102] Spinal ligaments appear to be compliant initially, but as the overall amount of motion increases the spinal ligaments become progressively stiffer.[103]

Hyperextension Cervical Spine Injuries

The occupant's head and neck may hyperextend 140 degrees in a rear-end collision.[58] If the rebound flexion is added to the 140 degrees of hyperextension, the entire motion range may near 200 degrees, well beyond the normal tolerance.

Experimental and clinical evidence suggests that it is the hyperextension neck injury (rear-end crash) that has been found to be more damaging to the soft tissues of the neck, resulting in higher occurrences of neck pain than either the frontal or side collisions.[94,103,104] A National Highway Traffic Safety Administration Agency (NHTSA) study shows that 26% of rear-end collision victims went to doctors offices afterwards, whereas of those in other types of crashes, only 10% went to see a doctor.[104]

Dunn and Blazar[105] found that the most injurious motion occurring in a collision is neck hyperextension and that even low-velocity rear-end collisions may produce significant forces that can cause musculoligamentous tears, hemorrhage, disc fiber damage, and vertebral body fracture. Trimble[106] estimates that approximately 20% of all rear-end collision occupants will have significant injury. Indeed, hyperextension neck injuries are typically seen in low-speed crashes.[9]

Most hyperextension injuries are primarily soft tissue strains or sprains. In more serious injuries they may also include cervical fracture and disc-vertebral body separation.[99] Head impact will increase the risk of cervical fracture threefold.[5] Upper cervical injuries occur with extension-compression injuries,[107] from either rear-end collisions involving low or absent headrests or frontal collisions in which the neck is hyperextended when the head hits the windshield. If the head is rotated at the time of the crash, the symptoms will usually be worse on the side to which the head was rotated.[108] Neck rotation narrows the intervertebral foramen and will create unequal preimpact ligament and muscle tension. This means that if a driver and passenger are looking at each other at the time of collision, the driver may have more pain on the right side and the passenger more intense pain on the left side.

A recent study by Deng and Goldsmith[109] on instrumented human head–neck–upper-torso replicas concludes that in rear-end crashes the longus colli sustains the greatest deformation, about 57%, which can cause injury. The scalenus anterior muscle was deformed in about 21% of cases, a higher percentage than for the longus capitis, sternocleidomastoid, and scalene posterior muscles.[109] Cailliet[7] and Jeffreys and McSweeney[9] explain that in hyperextension injuries the sternocleidomastoid, trapezius, splenius capitis, semispinalis capitis, scaleni, longissimus capitis, rhomboid, rectus capitis, superior and inferior oblique capitis, longus

colli, and longus capitis muscles are damaged. MacNab[108] concludes that if the neck is rotated 45 degrees at the time of collision, the amount of cervical extension is reduced about 50%. MacNab's cervical extension experiments in animals show tears of the longus colli muscle with occasional injury to the cervical sympathetic plexus.[108] Anterior longitudinal ligament (ALL) tears also have been associated with separation of cervical discs from vertebrae.[94]

Hyperflexion Cervical Spine Injuries

Hyperflexion neck injuries occur primarily in frontal crashes but frequently occur in rear-end collisions in which the head rebounds. (It would benefit the reader to review Chapter 15 if unclear about the specific crash dynamics involved.) In most frontal collisions the head and neck of an occupant will move forward rapidly in an arc, with the chest being restrained back by the shoulder harness. In addition to compressive forces of the neck on the torso, the head may hit the window or other object, further adding to the injury.

Hyperflexion neck injuries primarily produce ligamentous-disc trauma.[99] One animal study showed that hyperflexion injuries produce the most damage to vertebrae, discs, nerve roots, the posterior longitudinal ligament, the interspinous ligament, and zygapophyseal joints.[110] A postmortem study of 22 MVCI cases found that the majority of the posterior muscle ruptures occurred near the facet joints.[111] Twice as many vertebral fractures and dislocations occur in hyperflexion than in hyperextension neck injuries.[110] Cailliet[7] believes that in hyperflexion injuries the posterior longitudinal and interspinous ligaments will be damaged, as well as the zygapophyseal joints and erector spinae muscles.

A recent experimental human replica study concluded that in frontal crashes the splenius cervicis and splenius capitis muscles had the greatest muscle deformation, about 50%.[109] If the neck is flexed at the time of compression the T-1 to T-4 area will receive the greatest concentration of stress.[112] Lower cervical injuries occur with flexion-compression,[107] which might occur in frontal collisions in which the head hits the windshield, dashboard, or steering wheel.

Roaf reports that "normally speaking, pure flexion has the same effect on the vertebral bodies and intervertebral discs as pure compression, because the interspinous ligaments are strong and act as a hinge so that the force transmitted to the vertebrae is a pure compression force. However, if the flexion force is accompanied either by distraction, horizontal displacement or rotation, then the interspinous ligaments and ligamenta flava may rupture."[113]

Rotational Cervical Spine Injuries

Rotational neck injuries occur in any collision that involves vehicle rotation or when the occupant has the head turned at the time of the crash, causing torque. Rotational cervical injuries also may occur in oblique or offset frontal collisions in which the car rotates after the collision. Rotational spinal soft tissue injuries primarily affect the ligaments and facet joint complex.[99] Joint coupling results in complex cervical joint motion. Figure 1–7 compares cervical and upper dorsal injuries to the vector of collision.[114] Side and frontal collisions have different injury distributions.

Lateral Flexion Neck Injuries

The side collision is the most common type of collision resulting in lateral flexion injuries. See Figure 1–7 for the types of spine and cervicothoracic spine and soft tissue injuries in frontal and side crashes. Side crashes have a tendency to affect the middle to upper neck regions more than do frontal crashes. Frontal crashes have dramatic effects at the T-4 level. A recent study by Deng and Goldsmith[109] with human replica models showed that in lateral

flexion crashes, the longus capitis muscle had the greatest incidence of deformation, 57%, compared with the rest of the muscles. The coupling motion of neck rotation with lateral flexion has a significant role in determining the type of injury that will occur.

Posttraumatic Cervicalgia

Cervicalgia or neck pain is the most common complaint reported by MVCI patients. The doctor diagnoses the direct effects of injuries or healed residual musculoskeletal problems responsible for this complaint. This pain may be referred to the neck region from a disorder existing elsewhere or may represent the injury itself.[1]

The incidence of neck pain in the uninjured or preinjured general population has been estimated to be about 7%.[103] Bland[115] also reports that approximately 12% of women and 9% of men in the US population have neck pain at any given time. In the United States almost 20 million motor vehicle collisions occur annually[116] involving passenger cars, trucks, motorcycles, and trains, providing a continual source of neck pain cases.

How To Quantify and Qualify Neck Pain Extent and Character

There are several methods currently available to determine the extent and character of neck pain, including use of the following:

- history forms that include subjective pain descriptions (i.e., ache, hurt, burning, deep, stabbing, dull, etc.)
- pain drawings for location and description
- pain intensity scales
- pain frequency scales
- patient interview to clarify descriptive terms
- palpation to determine whether the patient's response is consistent with the verbal or written description

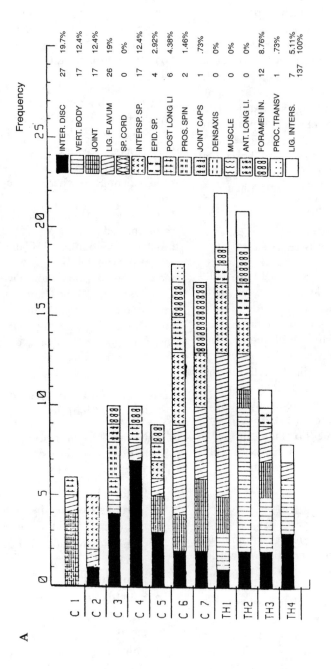

continues

Figure 1–7 Location of vertebral column injuries according to type of collision; A, frontal collision, B, side collision. *Source:* Reprinted with permission from Kallieris D., Mattern R., Miltner E., et al., Considerations for a Neck Injury Criterion, Society of Automotive Engineers, Inc., paper 912916, 1991.

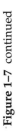

Figure 1–7 continued

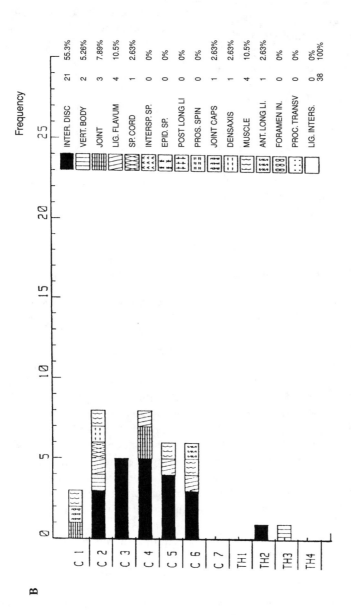

- pressure algometry (see Chapter 6, Part 2)

The importance of properly assessing a patient's neck pain cannot be overemphasized. Descriptive terms used by the patient often can help indicate the source of pain. The person who uses many terms to describe the discomfort may have psychologic problems as well. Pain location or referral descriptions can also suggest psychologic influence, especially when the patterns do not follow known anatomic pathways. Pain levels can also be used to monitor progress and determine the effectiveness of treatment. As intensity levels decrease, the patient's activity level and treatment (including frequency) may be modified.

Neck pain can be assessed clinically by using either pain drawings or various pain questionnaires. One of the simplest and yet highly accurate methods is use of the Visual Analogue Pain Scale, which rates the pain on a scale of 0 to 10.

Anatomic/Biochemical Basis of Neck and Back Pain

Most generated pain originates in the muscles.[1] Pain from musculoskeletal injury is initiated by noxious byproducts of posttraumatic repair and muscle spasm that affect sensory nerve endings.[1] Posttraumatic chemicals released include kinins, prostaglandins, and histamines, as well as potassium, which acts on the nerve fibers. If the ligament, tendon, or periosteal trauma results in localized muscle spasm, the spasm may continue to generate pain even though the other areas have healed. Sustained muscle contraction causes ischemia, resulting in nociceptive stimuli from the retained muscle metabolites eventually leading to pain.[1] Janda[117] reports that increased muscle tone can result from responses to pain or impaired coordination of muscle contraction, and the whole reflex arc can be activated. Cailliet[1] feels that "the neurologic pathway for muscular pain is probably via the sensory fibers that represent 30% of the motor root fibers."

Cervical zygapophyseal pain is one of the most common sequelae of patients' having auto injuries.[118,119] During the car crash the cervical spine motion may result in the meniscoids being impacted by the articular processes, pinching the meniscoids. In addition the joint capsules may be torn. Joint pain of the neck may result from thickening of the joint capsular ligaments. Tendons have intrinsic unmyelinated nerves that transmit pain sensations, as well.[1] Dwyer et al.[120] have outlined common sensory distributions for cervical zygapophyseal joints (see Figure 1–8).

Neck tissues capable of transmitting pain (nociception) include the following:[1]

- anterior and posterior longitudinal ligaments
- outer annular disc layers
- fasciae
- nerve root dura
- muscles
- ligaments
- zygapophyseal joints[119]

Non–pain-sensitive tissues include the nerve root as it leaves the intervertebral foramen, the central intervertebral disc, ligamentum flavum, and the vertebral body.

Lantz et al.[121] did experimental testing of cervical spines and concluded that in flexion-extension loading both facet joint capsules and capsular ligaments are subjected to high degrees of strain and deformation. These tissues, being densely innervated with free nerve endings, create increased neural activity, which may produce pain directly or cause contraction of the spinalis and semispinalis muscles of the neck, eventually causing spasm and pain.

Zimmerman[122] recently described several mechanisms that may cause lower back pain, all of which also cause neck pain:

1. Mechanical excitation of nociceptors in joint capsule, muscle, bone, and perivascular locations

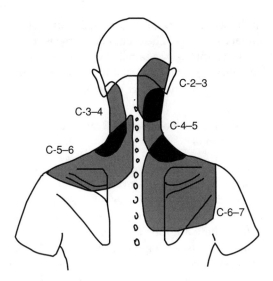

Figure 1–8 A composite map of the results in all volunteers depicting the putative characteristic distribution of pain from zygapophyseal joints at segments C-2–3 to C-6–7. *Source:* Reprinted from Dwyer A., Aprill C., and Bogduk N., Cervical Zygapophyseal Joint Pain Patterns I: A Study in Normal Volunteers, *Spine*, Vol. 15, No. 6, p. 456, with permission of J.B. Lippincott Company, © 1990.

2. Mechanical excitation of nociceptors in ligaments, particularly at insertion, secondary to muscle hypertonus or joint instability

3. Chemical activation of synovial, periarticular and muscle nociceptors due to inflammatory responses, ischemia, or biochemical deficits of the contractile apparatus

4. Chemical activation of synovial and periarticular nociceptors due to neurogenic inflammation mediated by neuropeptides released from afferent nerve fibers

5. Nerve or root entrapment due to disc herniation, narrow canal, swelling of articular or periarticular structures, bone proliferation, or microfractures

6. Reflex hypertonus of muscle induced and maintained by proprioceptive and nociceptive afferent inputs or by descending excitatory influences associated with emotional stress

7. Reactive neurogenic immobilization of the vertebral joints to induce guarding posture, resulting in inappropriate strain on the vertebrae

8. Psychosomatic enhancement of pain, mediated, for example, by muscular hypertonus or inappropriate posture[122]

Any of the following conditions may directly or indirectly cause neck pain after motor vehicle injuries. Several may occur simultaneously.

- direct pain from overstretched/torn sensory nerves
- localized soft tissue inflammation from neck sprain/strain
- biomechanical joint instability with resultant neural irritation or hypersensitivity
- uncovertebral joint ischemia
- cervical zygapophyseal joint capsule and meniscoids[119]
- nerve irritation
- cervical myofascial adhesions
- myofascial trigger points
- nerve rootlet compression
- disc injury or disc bulging against pain-sensitive tissue
- neural ischemia
- chemical byproduct accumulation and irritation
- stenosis

Neck Injury following Head Impact

There is considerable evidence in epidemiologic, postmortem, automotive crash, clinical, and engineering literature that neck injuries may occur secondary to direct impact to the skull.[123–127] Biomechanical and pathologic studies indicate that the neck and head are considered one functional unit.[128] Head impacts from blunt blows frequently seen in MVCIs impart much of their kinetic energy into the cervical spine. If the impact to the crown of the head does not cause a skull fracture, most of the load will be transmitted to the neck.[129] One postmortem MVCI study found that skull fractures were found to reduce the energy transformation into the cervical spine, thus more severe cervical spine injuries were seen if the skull had no fracture.[111] A review of literature by Steudel et al.[128] showed an incidence of cervical spine fracture with head injury ranging from 6% to 63%. Figure 1–9 illustrates the cervical spine loading differences seen when the neck is flexed or extended at the time of head impact, common for the frontal crash. It is imperative that the physician take lateral swimmer X-ray views in cases in which the neck is flexed, as fractures can be missed down to the T-4 level.

The head injury patient may not have the neck evaluated by the initial physician. Because of the potential seriousness of head injuries and focused attention by the doctor, it is common for the patient to miss having a neck examination. It is imperative that physicians who evaluate head injuries rule out neck injury. Nonfracture soft tissue and joint injuries in the cervical spine happen in most MVCI head injuries, varying with the degree and amount of force applied. Crash speeds are usually higher in instances when the head hits some interior part of the vehicle. Recently Yoganandan et al.[130] reported that the neck compressive forces from head–face impacts show as short-duration, high-amplitude waveforms for the head and large-duration, short-amplitude waveforms for the cervical spine, suggesting a decoupling action between the head and neck. The longer-duration peaks were probably due to failure and yielding[130] of various cervical spine tissues.

Cervical compressive injuries are part of all axial head injuries. When the head hits the windshield, roof, or other part of the car interior, frequently the flexion-extension-rotational-compression components all exist si-multaneously or occur sequentially during the impact sequence. The occupant's torso is compressing the neck against the head that has just impacted some object and is now stationary or moving in another direction.

Neck Injury in Low-Speed Rear-End Collisions

One common neck injury seen in clinical practice involves the 8-mph or less low-speed rear-end crash. Only in recent literature has the mechanism of this injury been analyzed in detail. There are four mechanisms of cervical spine injury (see Chapter 15 for details). Neck soft tissue injuries occur primarily from (1) the neck's moving beyond anatomic limits; (2) the neck's moving at a rate exceeding tolerance; (3) rapid lengthening and shortening movement; and (4) excessive cerebrospinal fluid pressures, which injure the spinal ganglia.

Hyde[2] concludes that rear-end crashes having less car damage repairs are more liable to cause "significant neck injuries (because they put the neck into hyperextension)" than those having more car damage repairs "(which are more liable to put the neck in tension)." The crash study by Emori and Horigruchi using human volunteers found that the human neck will extend nearly to the limit of anatomic tolerance in 2-mph rear-end collisions.[131] In another study, McConnell et al.[132] recently analyzed human test subject kinematics and responses to low-velocity rear-end collisions in which head restraints and seat belts were used. The clinical threshold for mild cervical strain injury was at 5 mph for male subjects.

Several probable mechanisms of neck, upper back, and low back injury can occur, including straightening of the cervical, dorsal, and lumbar spinal curvatures against the forward-moving seat back surface. Upward movement of the test subject's head and neck immediately "followed by a sudden and surprisingly vigorous descent of the trunk, may result in a rubberband effect of the kinematically straightened and stretched trunk/spinal

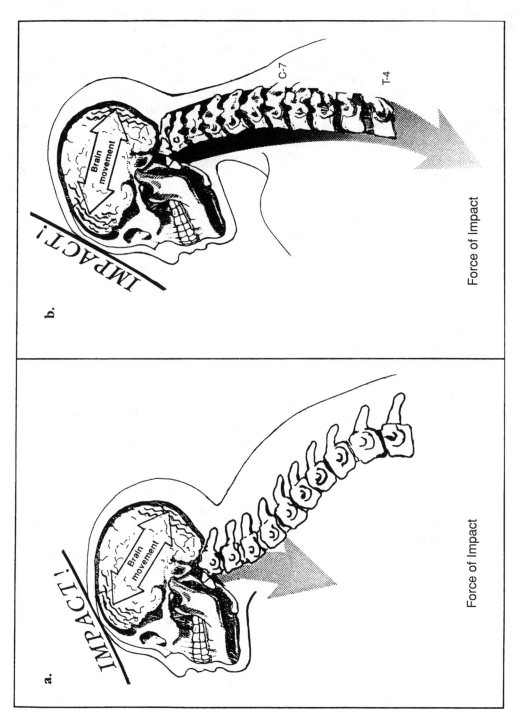

Figure 1–9 Neck injury following head impact. Neck extension (a) and flexion (b) angulations focus energy in different regions of the spine.

structures as the upwardly moving pelvis becomes restricted by the lap belt."[132] It appears in the study by McConnell et al.[132] and the study by Scott et al.[133] that the principal mechanical stress on the cervical spine related to rear-end collisions in the low- to very-low-velocity range is a rapid compression-tension cycle directed axially through the cervical spine and neck musculature as the neck sequentially compresses, extends, and accelerates the head in tension and then flexes, all occurring within the normal physiologic range-of-motion limits of the neck. The authors suggest that cervical/upper thoracic/lumbar muscle strains are caused by "rapid, short excursion, forced muscular compliance to unanticipated tension, occurring at an onset rate beyond the physiologic tolerance of the affected muscles' intracellular microstructures."[132] Tests show that even when tolerable (nonfracturing/nondislocating) load levels are applied to the cervical spine, the mechanical behavior of the neck is altered. This is believed to be due to the disc's ability to uptake and/or release fluids. The disc is able to handle only a set rate of loading.[134] This may explain the high frequency of neck pain sufferers in low-speed rear-end collisions.

CERVICAL AND LUMBAR DISC INJURY

Posttraumatic cervical[135,136] and lumbar disc[137] herniations are occasionally seen in clinical practice in MVCI cases. The primary areas involved include the C-5 to C-6 and L-4 to S-1 levels, with most MRI imaging showing old pre-existing disc degeneration.[137] Hyde[2] feels that "disc degeneration must be present for disc herniation to occur but not all degenerative disc disease results in disc herniation." Most studies that evaluate the incidence of disc degeneration and/or disc herniation involve retrospective surgical studies that compare the general population rate to the population having a history of being involved in a car accident. A recent study by Hammer et al.[138] found that MVCI patients who underwent anterior cervical discectomy and fusion had twice the rate of surgery as that of the general population. They also found that the annual incidence of MVCI patients requiring cervical disc surgery was 3.5 per million population, and the mean age at operation of those patients having previous MVCI was significantly higher than the mean age of patients not having been involved in a MVCI. Another surgical study of 253 disc herniation patients found that the majority had a history of flexion-extension injury or of having been in a car crash.[139] The surgical cases mentioned above for MVCI herniated discs represent a small fraction of the total number of cases that were managed nonsurgically.

The study by Hammer et al.[138] provides evidence that MVCI causes structural changes that predispose the cervical disc to premature degenerative disc disease. Cervical disc injuries may occur in motor vehicle collisions in which rapid rotational accelerating forces cause tearing of annular fibers or in cases in which a seat belt acts as a focal point for bending the body.

The majority of patients who have herniated cervical discs are female.[136] Patients who exhibit early (within the first week), predominant, radiating symptoms down either upper or lower extremities should be suspect for a disc bulge in the cervical or lumbar region. This is particularly true for occupants exhibiting neck, abdominal, or hip seat belt bruising.

A recent postmortem study of 22 MVCI cases found common isolated avulsions of the annular fibers from the rim of cervical vertebral bodies, with annular ruptures extending into the central disc in adults.[111] This study also showed that in adolescents cartilaginous end-plate avulsions were typical. Sances et al.[137] believe that herniated discs may be produced by trauma, usually at the C-5 to C-6 level, produced by mild flexion and rotational forces. Primary sites of lesions have been reported to be at the C-5 to C-7 region.[136] One report ranks cervical disc protrusions by frequency of nerve root involvement, with C-7 most frequent and C-6, C-5, and C-8 occurring in descending order.[140] Axial compressive neck injuries, during which the occupant's head sustains a blunt blow, may cause a symmetric disc protrusion with bilateral symptoms.[141]

Factors Related to Disc Injury

The intervertebral disc fibers spiral in opposite directions, having lower injury tolerance to shearing, translation, or displacement forces.[142] Laboratory experiments show varying results, depending on the model used, age of cadavers, and testing procedures. One review of the influence of posterior articulations on the stress to the intervertebral discs concluded that the integrity and degeneration of the facet joint provide less stability of the disc, resulting in smaller amounts of rotational forces needed to cause tearing of the disc in these cases.[113] A study of 40 MVCI patients concludes that the most common level of injury is at C-5 and C-6, with the primary mechanism being flexion.[143] The occupant who is using a three-point seat belt also will have a higher likelihood of incurring inertial loading disc injury than the unrestrained occupant because the belt restrains the pelvis, lower back, and chest, thus focusing kinetic energy onto the neck region. See Chapter 16 for further discussion on seat belts.

Symptoms of Cervical Disc Injury

A surgical study of 253 patients with lateral cervical disc protrusions found that about 80% had neck pain, 77% had radicular pain, 35% had shoulder pain, 8% had interscapular pain, and 13% had headaches.[139] Approximately 53% had numbness in one arm, and only about 5% had bilateral numbness. Approximately 36% had weakness in one arm and about 1% in both arms. A study of 61 cervical disc patients found that 92% had upper extremity pain.[144] Frequently in patients with disc protrusions there is constant minor to moderate neck pain with occasional periods of severe pain, usually aggravated by particular movements of the head. Rockett[145] concludes that the patient with acute cervical disc protrusion will usually lean the head toward the side of the root being compressed. Neck and interscapular pain may be exacerbated by rotating and extending the head toward the painful side.[145]

Occasionally after disc injury there is delayed onset of pain. Panjabi et al.[146] report that disc injuries can affect spinal mechanics of the same joint as well as other levels, altering the loading characteristics between the apophyseal joints and discs. This may later lead to cartilage degeneration, facet atrophy, and narrowing of the intervertebral foramen, as well as generating pain. In occupants older than age 50, the likelihood of herniation of a cervical disc decreases. This is substantiated by the anatomic study by Bland[115] of 153 cervical spines. His analysis revealed that by age 45 there is little if any nucleus pulposus left to herniate.

All MRI reports must be correlated clinically. For example, a 4-mm L-5 to S-1 disc bulge having no nerve root compression shown on a supine MRI can be very significant for a patient who describes severe leg pain primarily when sitting, when the disc is loaded under a lot more pressure than when supine.

UPPER-EXTREMITY REFERRING SYMPTOMS FOLLOWING MVCI

Upper-extremity symptoms, such as shoulder, arm, or hand pain or paresthesias, commonly occur after MVCIs. These symptoms may occur as a direct result of trauma, such as compressive forces from the driver's holding onto a steering wheel, or they may be observed in patients having radiating symptoms from cervical spine disorders. The literature shows (see Tables 11–2 and 11–3) that the incidence of posttraumatic symptoms sometime during acute to chronic stages will be in the range of 22% to 40%. The primary factors contributing to upper-extremity symptoms include dynamic or static traumatic forces that compress or stretch neural tissues, resulting in inflammation, ischemia, or fibrous adhesions that develop as part of the normal reparative process. Other factors may be injury to sclerodermal tissues and vascular involvement. Rehabilitation may be difficult if the doctor does not properly diagnose the cause of the upper-extremity symptom.

The most common initiator of upper-extremity symptoms is sclerodermal tissue irritation/inflammation. Sclerodermal sources of pain or paresthesias include any connective tissue lesions that do not originate directly from muscle (myotomal) or skin (dermatomal). Sclerodermal tissue involvement includes pain originating from capsular ligaments, spinal ligaments, discs, and fasciae. The authors have found that many times the sensory complaints in MVCI cases do not follow typical dermatomal mapped patterns; instead they overlap into several dermatomal regions. These symptoms are related in many cases to sclerodermal sources that do not follow customary dermatomal patterns.

According to Cailliet,[7] patients with sustained nerve root compression of 3 months' duration may not recover even after root compression is relieved.

Following are the more common causes of upper-extremity symptoms:

- Myofascial trigger points
  1. Pectoralis minor
  2. Scalenes
  3. Teres minor
  4. Levator scapulae
  5. Rhomboid
  6. Subscapular muscles
- Thoracic outlet syndrome
- Cervical disc protrusion
- Cervical nerve radicle/root
  1. Irritation/reduced set-point (threshold for firing)
  2. Ischemia
  3. Compression
- Multiple-lesion neuropathy–double crush
- Carpal tunnel syndromes

Cervical Radiculopathies/Root Pain

The pain in cervical radiculopathies is usually described by the patient as severe, shooting, gnawing, boring, nagging, sharp, or shocklike, moving distally in a narrow band.[115,147] Radicular pain usually is felt proximally and paresthesia is felt distally.[148] Radicular pain has also been described as similar to a toothache or a searing pain distributed in typical nerve root pattern, whereas muscle pain usually is dull and aching.[141]

The study by Williams[149] of 235 patients with intractable radicular pain found that trauma was the most common single initiating factor. Rockett,[145] in his traumatic cervical radiculopathy operative study, reported frequent scarring with attachment of the C-5 to C-6 nerve roots as they emerged from the vertebrae between the transverse processes to the anterior and medial scalene muscles. Small hemorrhages in these areas resulted in this scarring.[145] It was felt that any movement that caused the anterior and middle scalene muscles to tighten and compress the roots against the transverse processes would cause pain.[145] Animal studies have confirmed the tethered posttraumatic scarred nerve root.[150] Small mechanical motions on the nerve root result in 15 to 30 seconds of repetitive fiber firing, which in turn results in hypersensitivity and increased neural activity. In the absence of bulging discs or other objective findings, this scarring and tethering may explain why many patients develop chronic radicular symptoms.

Cervical radiculopathy has been shown in a study of 50 patients to correlate with abnormal coupling mechanisms of the cervical spine at the spinal level.[151] A surgical pathologic study found that most intractable radicular pain was due mainly to irritation of the cervical nerve root as it passes through the foramen.[149] This study of 235 patients with intractable radicular pain revealed that in patients having long-term root compression the perineural tissues changed from yellow to purplish; the root size decreased, and its normal wet and wrinkled appearance became withered, fibrous, dry, and discolored. Williams states that as the chronicity of clinical symptoms increases, so does the density with which the perineural tissue adheres to the foraminal wall.[149]

Provocative and Relief Tests for Nerve Root Lesions

There are several well-known methods of evaluating upper-extremity pain or paresthesias from various sources, including disc injury or adhesions. The first means is to conduct either provocative or relief tests that in effect either relieve or increase tension/compression on the cervical nerve roots. After these tests are done, other tests such as motor and sensory evaluation should be performed as indicated.

Arm Abduction Relief Test

This test[152] primarily evaluates compressive lesions affecting the C-5 nerve root. The patient sits, lifts the symptomatic arm, places the forearm on top of the head, and holds the position for 2 to 3 minutes. The examiner then asks whether the radicular symptoms improve. Lessening or elimination of upper-extremity paresthesia or pain is positive. Beatty et al.[152] found that shoulder abduction reduces nerve root pressure from cervical disc bulging. Fast et al.[153] found on X-ray films that arm abduction increases the distance between the coracoid process and the C-5 transverse process. Davidson et al.[154] tested 22 patients and found that symptom relief was associated with 73% of paresthesias and 100% of motor weakness of the upper extremity. They also found that 68% of patients with compressive radicular signs and symptoms noted pain relief after this procedure. Fast et al.,[153] as well as

the authors, feel that this test was earlier described by Spurling.[140]

Arm Abduction-Pull Relief Test

The patient abducts arms to head and the examiner pulls the symptomatic arm upward, reducing nerve root stretch. This action should relieve symptoms if root pressure exists. This is a method that looks for subtle disc lesions not found with arm abduction only.

Shoulder Flexion-Abduction, External Rotation Provocative Test

This rather complicated but useful test for C-5 root lesions was developed by Elvey[155] and is performed with the patient supine, with the symptomatic arm being flexed 90 degrees and abducted by the doctor until the painful range point is reached by the patient. The shoulder girdle is then slightly depressed. External rotation of the upper arm is done until pain is felt, followed by forearm supination to point of pain. The arm then is taken into flexion. Watch for reproduced arm pain or paresthesia at the level of the C-5 root. Quintner's use of this test[11] in 37 MVCI cases found positive results in 89% of the patients having arm pain; no false-positive results were noted.

Cervical Axial Compression Provocative Test

This test[136] is performed in neutral position first, lateral flexion next, and finally, in combination of lateral flexion with rotation on both sides of the neck, focusing on the symptomatic arm(s). The patient laterally flexes and rotates the head so as to narrow maximally the intervertebral foramen. The doctor then applies gentle axial loading to the head to reproduce the upper-extremity symptoms. Reproduction or increasing paresthesia or pain intensity typical for the patient is positive. The doctor should also note whether the test produces neck pain only. Neck pain intensification does not indicate nerve root compression. This test is not specific for the site of the lesion but it does verify compression from some source, i.e., edema, facet, capsule.

Manual Cervical Axial Distraction Test

This test[7] is done with the patient sitting. The doctor gently lifts the patient's head with both hands and asks the patient whether the neck pain is worse, stays the same, or is relieved. In acute patients increased pain indicates nonspecific injury to any number of soft tissues that stabilize the head or neck. If cervical distraction relieves neck pain or radicular pain, then root compression, joint adhesions, or other compressive lesions possibly are present. If distraction increases neck or radicular pain, the examiner may consider the presence of some tethering lesion such as scar tissue or adhesion.

Neck Flexion Provocative Test

This test can be performed with the patient sitting or supine and can be modified by various methods to verify compressive lesions. These maneuvers stretch the spinal cord, cervical rootlets and roots, and peripheral nerves. The test can be modified by having the patient straighten the lower leg and fully dorsiflex the foot and large toe at the same time. Further intensification can be done by having the patient take in a deep breath and bear down, as in a bowel movement, to see whether radicular symptoms are reproduced. Cailliet[7] describes the mechanisms for this maneuver, stating that many studies show cystic cavities containing cerebrospinal fluid, appearing to be diverticula of the arachnoid space, develop in nerve roots; when the patient coughs or sneezes, increased cerebrospinal fluid pressure increases radicular symptoms.

Ask the patient whether he or she notices reproduction or increase or decrease in arm or leg sensation when maximally flexing the neck while straightening the legs. If arm pain is reproduced, nerve root sleeve fibrosis or impingement may exist.

This test should be performed to rule out radiculopathy caused by disc fragmentation and/or slippage. If neck flexion causes electric

shocklike pain, then there may be a large disc fragment pressing on the cord.[145] This test yields positive results if the disc has bulged into the nerve root gutter.[7] Breig[156] proposes that if upon neck flexion the patient immediately feels "pain, paresthesia or stiffness of the neck, shoulder girdle or arms and if at the same time fibrillary twitching of the muscles is observed, the mechanical source of excitation will most probably be located in the vicinity of the cervical cord, or more accurately in the nerve-roots." Also ask the patient whether face (trigeminal) pain is reproduced with this procedure.[156]

Increased neck pain is not specific for source of pain. The doctor may be able to differentiate how extensive muscle involvement is by how far the head is able to flex before pain starts, and by how intense the pain response is.

Specific Findings Associated with Nerve Root Level

Common nerve root symptoms are discussed abundantly in the literature. Signs and symptoms of nerve root compression may include pain, paresthesia, muscle weakness, and loss of tendon reflexes. Henderson et al.,[157] in their study of 846 surgery patients with cervical root problems, found that there was a 73.8% correlation between subjective symptoms and the operation lesion. In 84.5% there was a correlation between motor deficit and operative lesion, and in 83.5% a correlation between tendon reflex and lesion. Another significant finding in this study was that in 53.9% of the patients paresthesia and pain were dermatomal, with 45.5% of the patients having nondermatomal or diffuse sensory findings.[157] This study also showed that some patients had no observable sensory, motor, or reflex changes.

Nerve root signs and symptoms specific to the nerve root indicated include the following:[11,141,158–160]

- *C-4 root (C-3 to C-4 level):* Pain and paresthesia in the neck, top of shoulder, and anterior chest area. Test for motor weakness by having the patient elevate shoulders against resistance.

- *C-5 root (C-4 to C-5 level):* Pain and paresthesia in lateral lower neck, into the top of the shoulder, and deltoid regions. Pain in the lateral aspect of the upper arm, thumb, ring finger, and index finger have been noted. May describe cervical angina also. Sensory changes occur in C-6 dermatome primarily and C-5 dermatome secondarily. Look for weakness in shoulder abduction. Test for motor deficits in biceps primarily and deltoid secondarily. Evaluate biceps reflexes for changes.

- *C-6 root (C-5 to C-6 level):* Pain and paresthesia in forearm, thumb, or thumb along with index and/or middle finger. Pain can be felt in the midscapular region and fingers as well. Sensory changes may occur in C-6 dermatome primarily and C-7 dermatome secondarily. Paresthesia occurs only in the index finger in about 18% of disc protrusions. To test motor strength, have the patient flex elbow and flex the wrist against resistance separately. May see decreases in biceps reflex primarily and triceps secondarily.

- *C-7 root (C-6 to C-7 level):* C-7 radiculopathy is not as well defined as C-6 radiculopathy. There may be pain and paresthesia into shoulder, forearm, elbow, and middle finger. Infrequent anterior chest wall pain has been noted in the pectoralis major region. Most frequently index finger pain was observed with pain in the middle finger, thumb, and ring finger, in that order. Sensory deficits are noted primarily in C-7 dermatome and secondarily in C-6 dermatome, with sensory loss mostly in the fingers. Motor strength is tested by having the patient extend the elbow and flex the wrist against resistance. There may also be some pectoralis major weakness. Decreased reflex occurs primarily in triceps

and secondarily in biceps.

- *C-8 root (C-7 to C-8 level):* Pain and paresthesia into medial forearm and fourth and fifth fingers or all fingers. Pain is often located predominantly in the medial scapular region, with radiation from the shoulder blade to the arm and fingers. Sensory deficits are almost equal for C-7 and C-8, with rare C-6 dermatome occurrence. Motor strength testing is done by having the patient extend the thumb and perform ulnar deviation against resistance. Generalized hand wasting and weakness occur in the triceps primarily, in the biceps rarely, and also in hand interosseous muscles. Deep tendon reflex is diminished primarily for triceps and secondarily for biceps. The teres minor trigger point may mimic C-8 radiculopathy as well.

Motor and Sensory Testing

Muscle Testing for Motor Weakness. One surgical finding concludes that about 50% of disc herniation cases will have single myotome deficits and 25% will have multiple myotome deficits.[139] Test specific muscles for each root level innervation while looking for comparative weakness. Sometimes the muscles will appear normal on the first try, but fatiguing the muscle with sustained stress over 15 to 30 seconds often will show weaknesses missed in brief examinations.

Deep Tendon Reflexes. Biceps (C-5), brachioradialis (C-6), and triceps (C-7) reflexes should be tested. Diminished reflexes may be due to alterations in motor fibers.[161] Normal reflexes were found in 35% to 47% of patients in one surgical study on cervical discogenic radiculopathy, and abnormal reflexes were found in 50% to 64%.[139]

Vibration Sensory Testing. The clinician should use a tuning fork on both upper and lower extremities with the patient's eyes closed. To differentiate pressure from vibration, the fork should be placed on an extremity with no vibration to validate sensory loss. A tuning fork of 256 cycles per second is used to evaluate peripheral nerve injury and compression neuropathy and has been found to correlate well with electrodiagnostic testing. Vibration tests the A-beta peripheral nerve fibers and their corresponding pacinian corpuscles.[162] Dellon,[163] in a study of 56 patients with peripheral nerve injuries, concluded that altered vibratory perception is possibly the first objective finding in injured nerve fibers. At the earliest onset of injury, slight hypersensitivity was perceived and diminished sensation was noted in chronic cases. Vibration tests the lateral spinal cord tract. Therefore, subtle changes in vibratory sense may pick up mild cord bruising caused by neck injury.

Sensory Dermatomal Evaluation. In one surgical study of cervical discogenic radiculopathy patients, 39% to 48% of patients were found to have single dermatome sensory deficits. Multiple dermatomes were involved in 24% to 30%.[139] When sensory deficits are found on more than one level this is typical of sclerogenous involvement, commonly ligaments or fasciae. Note that Benini's surgical research[158] shows that there are frequent variations of the sensory dermatomes and myotomes, due to anastomoses between anterior, posterior division and peripheral nerves.

Non–Root Differential Test: Trigger Point Testing

The doctor puts sustained digital pressure on known trigger points for 15 to 30 seconds and asks the patient whether the pressure reproduces the type and distribution of upper-extremity symptoms. The most common sites include the scalenes, pectoralis minor, levator scapulae, and subscapular muscles.

Neuroradiologic/Electrodiagnostic/ Physiologic Tests

The following tests are useful in diagnosing upper-extremity radiculopathies and neuropathies:

- magnetic resonance imaging[7]

- computed tomography (CT)[7]
- somatosensory evoked potential (SSEP)[164]
- H reflex[164]
- electromyography[136]
- nerve conduction velocity (NCV) for motor nerve damage[136]

Peripheral Neuropathies

Kopell and Thompson[142] believe that upper- and lower-extremity peripheral neuropathies are secondary to spinal myoligamentous derangement. This results in compensatory or secondary hypertonicity of primary muscle movers such as the scalenes, forming the basis for entrapment and thus symptom progression. Cailliet[1] concludes that pressure on a peripheral nerve causes only paresthesias, not pain. Therefore, if the primary radiating symptom of the patient is pain, the doctor needs to look for causes other than direct peripheral nerve irritation, such as myofascial adhesions.

Upper-Extremity Pain from Neuromyofascial Adhesions

Breig[156] refers to spinal pain originating from the formation of adhesions caused by either trauma or degeneration. Posttraumatic edema in and around the epidural sheath may cause scarring and, in the case of acute disc herniations, may cause anchoring of the dural root sheath to the disc. Breig also believes that if the nerve root retracts into the canal prior to the formation of adhesions the root may become fixed, leaving a permanent state of tension on the root. Teasell[165] feels that myofascial pain and sclerotomal pain offer the best explanation to pain referral after whiplash injuries.

Posttraumatic Thoracic Outlet Syndrome

The posttraumatic thoracic outlet syndrome (TOS) occurs more often than previously expected.[166] Sanders and Pearce[167] report that of

668 TOS surgeries, 86% had a trauma history, with 32% of the cases being involved in rear-end car crashes and 24% in frontal or side crashes. Richardson et al.[166] conducted a surgical study that summarizes this syndrome well, noting that even a minor crash can cause TOS. Postinjury epineural and vascular fibrosis and scarring around the lower brachial plexus region should be considered after any automobile-collision cervical injury. The most common muscles involved in TOS are the scalene muscles.

Most TOS cases involve rear-end or side collisions in which the anterolateral neck muscles are overstretched with resultant posttraumatic swelling and muscle spasm of the scalene musculature. Cailliet[1] describes a posttraumatic MVCI that causes thickening of the fasciae or fibrous bands of the anterior and/or middle scalenes, causing narrowing of the thoracic outlet. Pre-existing genetic variations of the neurovascular structures as they pass through or around the clavicle and muscles can make slight anatomic tension or structural changes more irritating to the contents of the thoracic outlet. "The pathophysiology of traumatic TOS is probably a combination of an anatomic predisposition to plexus pressure plus an injury to the scalene muscles."[168]

The majority of TOS cases are seen in women,[166] primarily those with upper-body weakness, weighty breasts, forward-rounded shoulders, and less-than-normal scapular muscle stabilization. The patient may have a history of occasional hand numbness during sleep. If so, it is usually experienced as an occasional annoyance. After trauma from a MVCI the patient notices nightly numbness of the arm(s), and even during the daytime the hands may fall asleep. Most TOS upper-extremity symptoms take 6 to 12 weeks to develop.

Common Symptoms of Posttraumatic TOS

Following are the common symptoms of posttraumatic TOS:

- upper-extremity sensory disturbances in 95%[1]
- ulnar paresthesia or pain in upper extremity in 90% of cases,[1] typically involving C-8 to T-1, and usually unilateral[140]
- headache[169]
- hand coldness and discoloration
- muscle-motor weakness of upper extremity in 10% of cases[1]
- usually intermittent pain; the ulnar nerve area or whole hand or arm may fall asleep.[170]

Aggravating/Perpetuating Factors in Posttraumatic TOS

Following are common aggravating or perpetuating conditions for posttraumatic TOS:

- activities that cause hyperabduction of arms[169]
- hands over the head or above 90 degrees while sleeping
- downward pull on the shoulders from carrying a purse, case, or objects
- droopy shoulder syndrome[7]
- weak shoulder girdle muscles, primarily muscles that hold the scapulae downwards and inward
- sustained forward head postures; rounded shoulders, causing contracture of pectoralis minor muscle
- sustained sitting postures such as sitting at a computer terminal
- excessive dorsal kyphosis

Diagnostic Stress Tests for Posttraumatic TOS

Upper-extremity symptom reproduction or intensification, including numbness, tingling, or pain is considered positive in the following tests. Neurogenic TOS symptoms are reproduced faster than vascular TOS symptoms. Tests that obliterate radial pulses are not *specifically diagnostic* of posttraumatic TOS. It is preferable for the clinician to use more accurate tests such as those described below.

Bilateral Arm Abduction-External Rotation Hand Opening-Closing Stamina Test. The patient sits in a chair, then raises both arms 90 degrees with external hand rotation, hands pointing toward the ceiling with shoulders maintained in a backward posture. In this position the patient is asked to open and close the fingers for 3 minutes rapidly while the doctor looks for symptom reproduction and early fatigue.[1] Results of this test are related in symptoms at various time intervals. For example, the patient has a left-sided TOS and when this test is performed the left hand goes numb at 20 seconds, the left forearm goes numb at 30 seconds, the left hand feels weak at 40 seconds, the patient has a difficult time closing left hand at 50 seconds, and at 60 seconds the patient has to drop the arm. Patient has no symptoms at 2 minutes in right hand. This test has good diagnostic value for TOS,[140] especially in unilateral cases when a normal side can be compared.

Digital Pressure Provocative Test. The doctor inserts a finger in the thoracic outlet, feels for ropy/tight texture, locates a tender spot, and sustains pressure for 15 to 45 seconds, looking for typical symptom reproduction.

Posterior Shoulder Provocative Test. The patient assumes a standing military posture with shoulders back and takes a deep breath while the doctor looks for symptom reproduction.

Hand Weight Provocative Test. The patient carries a 5-lb weight in each hand, both hands by the sides, for 3 minutes while the doctor looks for symptom reproduction or worsening of typical symptoms.

Pseudoangina-Cervical Angina

Anterior chest wall pain from sources other than the heart is called pseudoangina or, if originating from the neck, is termed cervical angina. Symptoms of cervical angina may include neck pain, stiffness, headache, shoulder, and arm pain. Other symptoms may encompass arm paresthesias related to neck motion and nonexertional activities.[171] Anterior chest wall pain may originate from C-5 to C-6 lesions, myofascial pain syndromes, disc lesions, thoracic outlet syndromes, rib trauma, shoulder disorders, and cervical degenerative arthritis. Less often it is from a C-6 to C-7 nerve root lesion.[148,171-174] Henderson et al.,[157] in their study of 846 patients with histories of cervical root compression surgeries, found that 50 had reported anterior chest wall pain.

If the patient's anterior chest wall pain is accentuated by neck and head rotation or motion while the torso is held stationary, the doctor should suspect cervical angina. Applying firm digital pressure in the deep pain-sensitive paraspinal areas from C-4 to C-7 on the same side as the patient's chest pain, separately or in combination with ipsilateral foraminal compression, may reproduce these symptoms. To isolate thoracic involvement, have the patient bend the torso and take in a deep breath without moving the neck and see whether pain is aggravated. Thoracic spine tenderness usually will be associated. Thoracic facet syndrome may also cause pseudoangina.

Other areas that may cause the pseudoangina symptoms include posttraumatic myofascial scar tissue areas that develop into chronic trigger points. These syndromes affect occupants having chest contusions by shoulder harness or steering wheel impacts. The examiner should try to reproduce the chest wall symptoms by goading deep pressure along the medial scapular border, subscapular muscles, teres minor, scalenes, intercostal, and pectoral muscles. The authors have found cases with single or multiple trigger point origins.

Factors To Rule Out in Diagnosing Upper-Extremity Disorders

Suspected cervical disc injuries causing neck and upper-extremity pain must be thoroughly evaluated, ruling out posttraumatic TOS, carpal tunnel compression, multiple-lesion neuropathies, myofascial pain syndrome, shoulder problems, radial head disorders, spinal stenosis, and amyotrophic lateral sclerosis. In addition, acute cervical disc herniation must be differentiated from heart attack, shoulder tendinitis or bursitis, acute arthritis, and thalamic ischemia, which may cause radicular sensory and motor symptoms with associated small areas of numbness around the face and mouth on the same side as the extremity pain.[77]

Spinal cord myelopathy, although uncommon in chiropractic practice, may be overlooked if special care is not taken. Breig[156] concluded that early in the extension phase of cervical motion a pinching effect on the cord may occur, especially if the canal is narrow or abnormally shaped resulting in spinal cord myelopathy. Cervical spondylotic myelopathy should be ruled out in older patients.[175] Look for the C-5 to C-6 reflex syndrome mentioned by Stewart,[77] in which the biceps and brachioradialis reflexes are depressed whereas hyper-reflexes are noted at the triceps and lower extremity. The C-8 to T-1 radiculopathies must be diagnosed differentially from Pancoast tumors and thoracic outlet syndromes.

SHOULDER, ELBOW, AND WRIST INJURIES

Shoulder, elbow, and wrist injuries are commonly seen in private practice after automobile crashes. These injuries most frequently occur to the driver holding onto the steering wheel in a frontal or rear-end crash or to the front passenger bracing against the dashboard or window in a frontal crash. These injuries may also occur when the occupant's arms flail about during the crash or in side crashes when an occupant's shoulder and arm are loaded by the crushing door panel. Rapid compressive and tension forces can occur to all three of these joints, depending on preimpact joint positioning, how tightly the hands are grasping the wheel, and the occupant's joint dynamics during the crash, such as wrist extension. For

example, if the occupant is aware of the impending impact, straightens the arms fully, and braces tightly against the steering wheel or dashboard, then there is a clear injury description.

Shoulder Injuries

The primary mechanism of shoulder injury is compression, although it may also have a tension or shearing component if the shoulder is moved laterally in a side crash or a tension component if the shoulder is pulled away from the steering wheel while grasping it in a rear-end car crash. In the frontal or rear-end crash the driver or front passenger is braced against the steering wheel or dashboard and, as the occupant's torso moves forward against a fixed shoulder and arm, posterior humerus motion occurs. The practitioner should try to determine how the arm was positioned at the time of collision and correlate this to the vector of impact. One of the most common complaints of shoulder injury is shoulder pain, which may be local or spread diffusely down the arm. Typically the patient will relate inability to sleep on the injured side, severe pain in all positions, or difficulty moving the arm on the injured side in certain directions or above a consistent height. The patient may state, "I can't lift my arm over the height of my shoulders," or "My shoulder locks when lifting my arm," or "My arm feels very weak."

Elbow and Wrist Injuries

The proposed mechanism of elbow and wrist injuries in a recent study of 157 MVCI patients diagnosed as having carpal tunnel syndrome (CTS), cubital tunnel syndrome, and radial sensory nerve entrapment[176] was found to include a direct blow or compressive force between the palmar aspect of the wrist and the steering wheel and/or dashboard, causing wrist hyperextension and median nerve stretch and trauma. This sequence causes an ulnar nerve traction injury within the postcondylar groove from elbow hyperflexion. Most patients developed symptoms within 1 week, were driving, and had use of a seat belt; almost equal numbers of patients had one or two entrapments. In cases in which the vector of the crash was correlated with the development of elbow or wrist peripheral nerve entrapment, 58% of patients were involved in rear-end crashes, 22% in frontal crashes, and 19% in side crashes.

The primary symptom of MVCI elbow and wrist peripheral nerve injury is numbness.[176] Patients with elbow joint injury will complain of radial head pain but may also have shoulder, hand, and finger pain and/or paresthesias. In chronic cases the application of deep digital pressure in the proximal lateral radial joint and adjacent myofascial structures may cause severe local pain or in more severe cases may reproduce typical hand and finger symptoms.

Most patients with wrist injury will have complaints of localized wrist pain that is intensified by certain motions. Other symptoms may include hand or finger paresthesias. Some patients having more severe injuries or having concomitant proximal nerve compression in lesser injuries may develop CTS.

Carpal Tunnel Syndrome

Some MVCI patients will develop CTS. Common symptoms of CTS include intermittent pain, primarily in the wrist, volar aspect of forearm, and the first three digits.[170] Usually mild, intermittent symptoms persist for some time before worsening. Many patients wake up at night, able to relieve pain and paresthesia only by shaking and massaging their arms and hands.[177] Sensory changes are usually seen before motor changes can be noted. Pain and paresthesia in the radial aspect of the third to fourth digits have also been noted.[178] Pain has been reported to be of a burning quality.[7] It may radiate up to the elbow and shoulder.[179] On the other hand, shoulder pain may be the only complaint.[180] One study of

1000 CTS cases found that 77% were women.[181]

Shoulder, Elbow, and Wrist Examination (Always Comparative)

The examiner should perform pertinent tests using references such as Magee.[159] The shoulder, elbow, and wrist examination should begin by palpating the patient's upper extremity for painful regions. Then active range-of-motion exercises should be performed by the patient, focusing on shoulder abduction and forward flexion, elbow and wrist flexion and extension, and other possible motions. Motion limitations should be measured in degrees and compared with normal side. The clinician needs to perform passive range-of-motion analysis of the joints, feeling for the ability to move through all motions. The examination should begin gently so that guarding can be noted and the examiner can modify the examination for the comfort of the patient. Joint play should be evaluated for normal motion, bony end-feel, or pathologic end-play. Joint crepitus is common during these examinations.

Motor and sensory testing should be performed to rule out tennis elbow syndrome and CTS. Fractures or grade I to grade III strain/sprains should be ruled out in higher-speed crashes in which the occupant was holding onto the steering wheel or dashboard and in cases where severe pain is noted with motion. In addition, the examiner should perform the following tests:

- Apply anterior-posterior glenohumeral gliding stress, looking for ligamentous laxity, and testing, looking for tendencies for dislocation and grade III ligament injuries.

- Pronate-supinate the forearm with the finger in the proximal radial-ulnar joint. Feel for swelling, joint restriction, joint lock, pathologic end-play, and tenderness.

- Feel for proximal and distal carpal row

mobility separately as the joint is flexed, extended, and laterally flexed. Feel for bogginess, pain, crepitus, joint restriction, joint locking, and pathologic end-play (usually sloppy motion).

MULTIPLE-LESION PERIPHERAL NERVE COMPRESSION SYNDROMES

Occasionally, after a MVCI, there are patients with coexisting cervical root lesion, thoracic outlet compression, pectoralis minor syndrome, radial or ulnar nerve compression at the elbow, and median nerve compression in the wrist. Such cases having several coexisting lesions are known as multiple-lesion peripheral nerve compression syndromes or, as referred to in the literature, as the *double-crush syndrome*. This complex neuropathy has been verified by several researchers,[177,181,182] who conclude that proximal lesions render the distal nerve less capable of withstanding entrapment.

In the multiple-lesion peripheral nerve compression syndrome, neural transmission and axoplasmic transport of nutrients is impaired by the proximal compression. One author feels that C-6 to C-7 radiculopathy is the most frequent entity that must be ruled out in CTS cases.[183] Breig[156] believes that peripheral nerve structures, as well as spinal cord lesions, can lead to distal nerve alterations. The proximal pressure may make a compressed median nerve symptomatic, whereas if the pressure proximally did not exist the patient would have little if any pain at the distal area in question. The clinician should approach all patients with chronic arm/hand pain and paresthesias as having multiple problems and diagnose them by reproducing symptoms and eliminating nonrelated areas. Treatment of multiple lesions must be done simultaneously if satisfactory results are to be achieved.

The coexistence of cervical radiculopathy and cervical arthritis with CTS has been established by several studies.[181,184] One study of 1000 CTS cases showed that the most commonly involved cervical root lesion was at C-6 with C-7 secondarily.[182]

THORACIC SPINE, CHEST WALL, AND LUMBAR SPINE INJURIES

Thoracic spine pain, chest wall pain, and lumbar pain are common complaints following car crashes.[165] Shoulder harness interaction with the chest wall, dorsal spine torsion/bending movements, and direct impacts with the car interior, such as the steering wheel, can cause thoracic spine and chest wall trauma. Other sources of injury occur from direct loading from the door in a side crash. These injuries can be complex in vehicles having armrests that protrude or angulate at angles sharp enough to induce injuries. If the occupant has the arm up, loading structures can impact directly with the chest wall. It is important for the physician to remember that in small, mid-sized, and some large passenger vehicles typically there are 6 to 10 inches of space between the occupant's torso/hip and the striking bumper in a side crash. There may be similar distances between the occupant's chest and the steering wheel in many instances as well. Occupants having higher risk of chest wall injury include those who move their seat to forward settings. Although frontal crashes account for the majority of these types of injuries, significant numbers also occur in side crashes, rear-end crashes, and rollovers. Taller and lighter-weight occupants are at higher risk of incurring chest wall injuries.

Occupants wearing only lap belts in a car crash are particularly vulnerable to low back injuries due to the focusing effect of the lap belt as the torso flexes forward and over the pelvis, which is being held against the seat. In particular, the rear-seat occupants can have significant low back pain because many current car models have only lap belts for rear-seat passengers. In most patients the neck pain and headaches initially are more intense but as the pain subsides the low back pain becomes more significant. However, experience has shown that if a patient having no prior history of low back pain complains of severe low back pain and sciatica within the first 24 to 48 hours, single or multiple disc protrusions should be suspected.

Thoracic Spine Injury

The primary mechanism of thoracic spine injury for the restrained occupant includes rapid deceleration as the rapidly forward-moving torso suddenly stops at the end of the shoulder strap, causing the side of the torso that does not have the shoulder strap to twist forward with flexion. If the occupant hits the torso on the steering wheel or dashboard, the spine is loaded indirectly, with the injury mainly due to bending movements and/or torsion.

Chest Wall Injury

Chest wall injury occurs frequently following car crashes and may include skin abrasions, contusions, bruising, intercostal strains, costochondral injuries, and fractures to the sternum or ribs. Belted occupants have been found to have twice the incidence of chest wall bruises, sternal fractures, and one to three rib fractures in frontal crashes than unbelted occupants.[185]

The occupant using the three-point seat belt system in a frontal or rear-end crash will usually have localized pain, palpable tenderness, and a feeling of being bruised along the entire length of the shoulder harness. More serious injuries may occur for occupants who tuck the shoulder harness under their arms, having the crash energy focusing on the lower ribs and abdominal region.

Be particularly aware of "seat belt sign" when visible bruising is present. Hayes et al.[186] report that if seat belt bruising is observed in the neck, chest, and abdomen, there is a 30% risk that the person has an internal injury. CT scans are indicated in recent injuries.

Major long-term pain and disability complications for the patient having chest wall injuries but not having any rib fracture is myofascial adhesion development beneath the pectoral muscles and subscapular muscle region, and within the intercostal muscles. A typical illustration is a male patient who was involved in a high-speed rear-end crash with sufficient force to cause his chest to impact the steering wheel. Every time this patient twisted his torso, bent forward, or lifted his left arm, his entire back would freeze or lock up with extremely severe pain. This patient was on complete disability for 1 year before entering an aggressive treatment program that emphasized subscapular motion and deep tissue myotherapy. After 2 months of therapy he was able to return to work full time.

Thoracic Spine and Chest Wall Examination

The examiner needs to begin by visually observing the patient for postural abnormalities such as scoliosis, kyphosis, and antalgic posture. Then, depending on the stage of injury, palpate for paraspinal muscle soreness, vertebral tenderness, spasm, and swelling. Test for prone dorsal spine spring or rebound motion quality when applying anterior vertebral motion. Be sure to note normal or bony end-feel. Conduct a comparative range-of-motion analysis, looking for limitation of motion with lateral bending, torsion, flexion, and extension. Notations about motion and pain intensification can be quantified as well.

When examining the chest wall the clinician needs to look for guarded breathing; sharp, localized rib pain when coughing or sneezing; forward and side antalgia (usually leaning toward fracture site); and hesistancy to sit or stand up straight. Focus attention on areas along the shoulder harness or lap belt path or impact points if the occupant hit any surface within the vehicle. If a rib fracture is suspected, a tuning fork can be used to rule it out. Place the vibrating tuning fork in a nonpainful site 3 to 4 inches away from the area having pain and ask the patient whether he or she feels an increase in pain at the painful site or at the tip of the tuning fork.

Lumbar Spine Injury

Lumbar spine injury and pain are common problems following MVCI.[187] The usual onset of low back pain associated with radiating symptoms into the buttocks and lower extremity follows from a variety of incidents. Incidents that can provoke these symptoms can vary from a mild bump (rear-end crash with the struck car being stopped), to a bus going over a pothole, to severe intersection collisions.[188]

The mechanisms of lumbar spine and disc injury are primarily due to restraint of the pelvis by a lap belt while the lumbar spine is flexed and stretched. In addition, if the lap belt compresses the abdomen 3 to 4 inches of the total abdominal depth, the belt may be in fact directly loading the anterior vertebral bodies because of the lumbar lordosis, depending on the anatomic characteristics of the occupant. The reviewed literature seems consistent in that about a 20-degree flexion angulation appears to be the tolerance limit for lumbar motion under dynamic flexion-shearing loading.[189]

Lap belt placement may focus energy forces on any of the lumbar, lumbosacral, or sacroiliac joints, depending on the anatomic shape of the occupant, belt placement, and the degree of lumbar flexion, with most forces focusing in the lower joint region. The anatomic position of the lap belt can vary in occupants who are obese, who fall outside normal for pelvic anatomy, and who are wearing heavy clothing.

Lumbar Spine Examination

The examiner needs to begin by observing the patient visually for postural abnormalities such as scoliosis, short leg syndrome, and antalgic posture. Then, depending on the stage of injury, palpate for paraspinal muscle soreness, vertebral tenderness, spasm, and swelling. The clinician can test the patient for lumbar vertebral motion with the patient in either a sitting or a standing position. Be sure to note normal or bony end-feel. Conduct a comparative range-of-motion analysis, looking for limitation of motion with lateral bending, torsion, flexion, and extension. Notations about motion and pain intensification can be quantified as well.

The examiner needs to perform pertinent orthopedic and neurologic tests, such as the Laseques and Kemps test, with notations being made if the stress testing causes localized low back pain or if radiating pain develops, indicating a positive test. Keep in mind that these tests are not specific for site of lesion but mainly give the clinician a better chance of narrowing down a diagnosis. Be sure to note when the straight-leg-raising test causes pain in degrees. This gives a baseline by which to determine response to treatment. Motor tests such as toe walk (L-5 to S-1), heel walk (L-4 to L-5), patellar reflex (L-4 root), and Achilles reflex (S-1 root) need to be performed. Tuning fork testing to detect cord involvement and pinwheel or pinprick testing to detect sensory abnormalities should be done.

HIP, KNEE, AND ANKLE/FOOT INJURIES

A recent report on lower-extremity injuries in occupants of frontal crashes concludes that about 12% have hip acetabulum fractures, 6% pubic ramus fractures, 19% femoral diaphysis fractures, 19% patellar fractures, 5% tibial diaphysis fractures, 21% distal tibia-fibula fractures, 8% talar or calcaneus fractures, 11% ankle sprains, and 10% metatarsal fractures.[190] Lateral ankle ligaments are implicated in most ankle sprains. Seat belt use does not appear to influence the risk of injury. This study also concluded that almost 45% of all lower leg injuries occur at delta V velocities between 15 and 28 mph. The risk of injury doubles if the impact is on the same side as the injured person in a side crash.

Hip Injury

Hip injuries, including sacroiliac joint injuries, may be seen in occupants using seat belts, having excessive flexion around a lap belt, or sliding under the seat belt (submarining). Hip injuries can occur from direct loading of the door in side impacts or indirectly when the femur impacts a knee bolster, steering wheel, or other occupant cage structure transmitting forces in a frontal or rear-end crash. Most commonly in private practice the patient will enter with complaints typical of a strain/sprain injury.

Knee Injury

Most knee injuries are due to direct impact with the knee bolster, dashboard, steering column, steering wheel, console, or side door structures. Knee injuries occur most commonly in frontal crashes but also occur frequently in side crashes and rear-end crashes in which the occupant rebounds from the elastic seat back, hitting interior surfaces. Several factors influence injury risk, such as vehicle interior contours, padding characteristics, and distance between knee and interior as determined by car size and the occupant's having the seat in the forward or backward position. Human risk factors may be affected by the length of the femur or lower leg or by the sitting profile, such as crossing the legs.

The physician must be alert to anterior superior tibial impact injuries and subsequent posterior cruciate injury. The posterior cruciate ligament has about 0.5-in motion tolerance. In a frontal car crash in which there was sufficient force to cause the occupant's knee to hit the dash, knee bolster, or other firm object and there is evidence that the anterior superior tibial region is contused, it is likely that posterior cruciate injury has occurred.

Ankle/Foot Injury

There appear to be several mechanisms of ankle/foot injury, including floor pan intrusion, which is the most common source of loading injury for the frontal-crash occupant;

the driver has a higher risk for floor pan intrusion due to pedal structures. Other injury mechanisms include direct inward or side-crushing forces, upper-leg-loading downward forces, and inversion/eversion loading.

Hip, Knee, and Ankle/Foot Examination (Always Comparative)

The clinician needs to begin by observing the patient visually for postural abnormalities in stance and gait. Palpate for joint muscle soreness, spasm, and swelling. Conduct a comparative range-of-motion analysis on any injured joint, looking for limitation of motion during all motions normal for the joint. Notations about motion and pain intensification can be quantified as well.

When examining hip regions, focus attention on areas along the lap belt path for signs of bruising, tenderness, and swelling. Include the quadratus lumborum, gluteal, and piriformis muscles. Also evaluate the thigh muscles and deep hip joint for tenderness. The examiner needs to perform pertinent orthopedic and neurologic tests along with motion analysis. Note any abnormalities in hip joint motion.

When evaluating the knee the clinician needs to correlate injury mechanism to the pain site. If the occupant is in a frontal or rear-end crash and has hit the knee on the dashboard or knee bolster, most of the forces will either involve the patella or move into the hip joint as forces move along the femur. If the occupant has a contusion to the anterior superior tibia, posterior cruciate ligament tearing needs to be ruled out. Anterior-posterior cruciate ligament stress testing is necessary to grade the severity. If the knee injury involved a side impact, the collateral ligaments and menisci must be evaluated closely.

Ankle and foot injuries require close examination for swelling and tenderness. The examiner should note swelling, pitting edema, bruising, and foot positions that increase pain. When evaluating joint motion note crepitus and pain, particularly in the subtalar region.

CHRONIC POSTTRAUMATIC NECK AND BACK PAIN

A significant number of people injured in collisions develop chronic neck and back pain, with some patients initiating health care several months after the accident. (See Chapter 11 on prognosis.) In the acute and subacute stages it is easier to locate causes of neck pain, but as the condition becomes more chronic it becomes more difficult to assess. "The most logical approach to investigating neck pain following whiplash injury is to provoke or eliminate the pain by stimulating or anesthetizing structures suspected of being symptomatic."[135] Most of the time the examiner can palpate these structures, but when the neck pain is originating from the zygapophyseal joints, anesthetic injections may be needed. Standard orthopedic and neurologic testing frequently is unremarkable in most patients having chronic neck pain. These tests include deep tendon reflexes, superficial sensation, and strength, as well as nerve root compression and stretch tests.

There are several current concepts as to the cause of chronic neck pain, including the conditions described below.

Myofascial Pain Syndrome

A study of 100 patients with chronic neck, shoulder, and upper and lower back pain concluded that tension myositis was the diagnosis in 18% of patients in whom a minor injury was the precipitant.[191] (See the section later in this chapter on posttraumatic myofascial pain syndrome.)

Cervical and Lumbar Zygapophyseal Joint Inclusions

Cervical and lumbar zygapophyseal joint inclusions or entrapment of the intra-articular synovial folds between the facets of zygapophyseal joints may cause pain.[119,135,192]

Chronic Neck and Back Deconditioning and Instability

Chronic neck pain may also lead to decrease in overall levels of function[193] and postural abnormalities, which may eventually lead to significant physical deconditioning. The decrease in activity levels, as well as development of poor postural and ergonomic habits in attempts to lessen pain, may have a significant effect on perpetuating and increasing overall neck and back pain levels in some patients over time.

Cervical and Lumbar Disc Pain

Cervical disc injuries to the outer pain-sensitive layers may result in chronic neck pain. Mendel et al.[194] found that nerve fibers, probably from the ventral primary rami, appeared to enter the cervical discs from the posterolateral direction and that these pain receptors may explain the occurrence of neck and shoulder pain after disc trauma. Panjabi et al.[146] report that disc injuries can affect spinal mechanics, which may lead to chronic neck pain.

Scarring around Nerve Roots

One of the newer concepts of chronic back pain development, and most certainly relevant to neck pain, is discussed in detail by Jayson et al.,[195] who suggest that vascular damage, fibrosis, and chronic inflammation occurring within the peridural soft tissues may be partly to blame. Defects in the normal enzymes present in the circulating blood of patients with spinal injury may cause excessive scar tissue around the spinal nerves.[196] Fibrinolysis is a normal process of dissolution of fibrin by enzymatic actions after injury. When low basal fibrinolytic activity is present in an individual, it may lead to nerve root disease.[196] Fibrous proliferation and nerve root injury may be associated with mechanical injury to vascular and other soft tissues.[195] Muscle nociception[197] may be modulated by any pathophysiologic alteration of muscle tissues, resulting in some dorsal horn neurons having long-term decreases in mechanical and chemical excitability threshold levels.

Denervation Supersensitivity

One plausible explanation for many cases of chronic neck and back pain is described by Gunn.[198,199] In the absence of ongoing injury or inflammation, he calls such pain neuropathic pain, and proposes that this neuropathic pain is responsible for a large percentage of chronic musculoskeletal syndromes. He notes that it is caused by a functional disturbance or pathologic changes in the peripheral nervous system or the nerve roots. This functional disturbance or pathologic change in the nervous system may also include perineural and intraneural fibrosis.[195]

The most common functional disturbance noted in patients with neuropathic pain is that the affected structures have increased sensitivity to circulating neurotransmitter agents.[199] This increased sensitivity in the peripheral nervous system is known as *denervation supersensitivity*. If the nerve root is involved, denervation supersensitivity is found in both the anterior and posterior primary rami. Denervation supersensitivity has both sensorimotor and sensoriautonomic manifestations.[198] Manifestations are subtle and therefore frequently overlooked or not evaluated by clinicians who do not understand these concepts. A summary of these manifestations follows:[198]

- *Pilomotor reflex:* As the patient undresses in cool air, there is a brief pilomotor effect, or "goose flesh," in the dermatomes of the affected segment.
- *Vasoconstrictor disturbances:* The skin in the affected region will have a lower temperature after exposure to cool air for 10 to 15 minutes. Objectification is improved with thermography.

- *Sudomotor reflex:* Noted by a regional increase in sweating.
- *Myalgic and cutaneous hyperesthesia:* The motor point on the skin and the neurovascular hilus point on the muscle become abnormally sensitive to pressure in the affected segments. The degree of sensitivity and the patient's progress can be quantified with the use of pressure-sensitive meters, such as described in Chapter 6.
- *Trophic disturbances:* There is a gradual fibrosis (cutaneous trophoedema) of the subcutaneous tissue in the affected segment. The skin becomes inelastic, fissured, and prone to have folds. Squeezing the skin together causes the peau d'orange effect. Indentations in the skin made with the end of a wooden matchstick are clear-cut and persist for several minutes, distinctly longer than those in normal skin.

The most frequent abnormality associated with denervation supersensitivity at the nerve root level is spondylosis. This spondylosis includes both the structural disintegration and morphologic alterations that occur in the disc and the pathoanatomic changes that occur in the surrounding tissues.[175]

POSTTRAUMATIC MYOFASCIAL PAIN SYNDROME

Myofascial pain, or fibromyalgia, is a common sequela of neck injury.[200,201] Myofascial pain is probably the most common source for chronic neck, head, and upper dorsal pain following the MVCI.[165] Myofascial pain syndrome (MPS), for the purposes of this chapter, includes chronic headaches, neck pain, back pain, extremity pain, auditory or visual symptoms, and other common MVCI symptoms that persist beyond 2 to 3 months and arise from painful stimuli from healed posttraumatic muscles or fascia. It excludes pain from nerve roots, discs, ligaments, and tendons.

MPS is a muscle fiber disorder.[202] Its source of pain is abnormally healed myofascial tissues that tether (attach and pull on other pain-sensitive structures), compress nerve structures that pass through them, or mechanically irritate peripheral nerves. MPS has several other descriptive terms in the literature, including myofascitis, myofibrositis, myalgia, and myofascial pain.

An understanding about the normal role of healthy fasciae will aid the doctor in understanding how trauma can dramatically change the quality of a person's life following MVCI. Healthy, functional fasciae in the neck have a significant role in normal movement patterns and motion quality. After minor to moderate car accident trauma, alterations in the complex interaction of these structures may occur. Note that the neck fasciae are slow to heal because of their poor blood supply.[203] Normally, fasciae provide support and cohesion for the body.[204] Specifically, they do the following:[205]

- Have an extensive sensory network, providing input to the central nervous system.

- Produce, assist, control, limit, and interrelate various moving parts. They are vitally involved in all aspects of motion.[204]

- Provide support and stabilization for many tissues.[204]

- Have extensive attachment sites for deep and superficial muscles. Maintain muscular force by controlling muscle pressure and volume.[203]

- Include a pathway for nerves and lymphatic vessels, thus regulating venous and lymphatic circulation and nutritional function.[204]

- Provide means for fluids (e.g., lymph, blood, and cerebrospinal fluid) to travel along fascial planes.

- Provide means for muscles to glide over each other.

- Are essential for support, metabolism, and defense of the body.[206]

- Are part of the reticuloendothelial system.[204]

- Aid in injury repair by fibroblastic activity by deposition of scar tissue.[204]

Myofascial Trauma

In car accidents, very rapid, high-acceleration, overstretching forces often injure normal myofascial tissues with any number of the following consequences:

- Burning pain occurs after sudden injury.

- Abnormal fascial tension is present on attaching tissues. Injured fasciae can tether, catch, irritate, and inflame other soft tissues in close proximity.

- Fascial attachments shorten, thicken, calcify, erode, and become less elastic with trauma, age, and inactivity.[207] Short and contracted fasciae cause abnormal or unequal tension on other fasciae, attaching muscles, and vascular structures. This tension causes symptoms to develop. Fascial thickening results in passive vascular congestion.

- Entrapment neuropathies may develop as a result of nerve compression as they traverse an affected muscle or pass between a taut band or an unyielding structure such as a ligament. The most common entrapments are said to involve the brachial plexus (from the scalenus), radial nerve (from the supinator, triceps, or brachialis), ulnar nerve (from the flexor carpi ulnaris), or sciatic nerve (from the piriformis).[8]

Trigger Points

Trigger points can be described in two categories: latent and active. The following information will help the doctor to evaluate both types of trigger points. Generally, trigger points are self-sustaining, hyperirritable sites located in myofascial tissue[208] that are tender and extremely sensitive. They may be superficial or deep and are usually areas about 1 cm in diameter.[8] Trigger points have an abnormal palpable consistency, sometimes described as being ropy, fibrotic, hard, nodular, or having a taut band. Trigger points usually develop in areas of greatest biomechanical stress. Many trigger points will show evidence of local vasoconstriction, pilomotor erection, or cutaneous erythema.[8]

Trigger points may be evaluated by briskly snapping the taut fiber transversely at its most tender point. There will usually be an immediate jump sign reaction in the immediate tissue, and the patient's underlying muscles may flinch as they react to the snapping pressure. Another method is to apply sustained digital pressure for 5 to 20 seconds. If a trigger point site exists, it will cause referral of pain. Figure 1–10 illustrates common referring pathways for many of the common trigger points.[209] Pressure on a trigger point may also cause muscle twitching and fasciculation.[204]

Most trigger points begin to develop 4 to 6 weeks after neck injury. At first these tissues may start as tender points and as time passes added trauma and perpetuating factors may occur, causing them to develop into latent trigger points. Under digital pressure, latent trigger points will refer pain but will not produce pain at rest or with muscle activity.[210] Occasionally they may refer pain when palpated, but the pain usually is local. As these latent trigger points progress to more pathologic and ischemic states they become active, referring pain even at rest.

Physiology of Myofascial Trigger Points

Travell and Simons[211] have hypothesized that myofascial trigger points are dysfunctional areas, producing continuous focal neurologic irritability that may maintain persistent neural activity. Some authors feel that trigger points are ischemic and as a result have excessive metabolite accumulation.

Bennett[212] proposes that muscle injury traumatizes the sarcolemmal membrane, resulting in increased membrane permeability to calcium. This causes localized muscle contraction that stimulates nociception. If the intrafusal fibers of the muscle spindles are affected, they will reset at a higher sensitivity level, increasing muscle reaction. Subsequently the fibers never reach full resting length.

As discussed earlier, trigger points are hypersensitive or hyperirritable to mechanical and sensory input[88] and painful on compression. Furthermore, trigger points also react to emotional stress.[213] With tension and stress, shoulders are often drawn upward in response to increased neurologic activity, resulting in decreased blood flow.[214]

Diagnosis of Posttraumatic MPS Trigger Points following MVCI

Any MVCI, including the low-speed crash, can transform the occupant's nonsymptomatic tender muscles and latent trigger points into active trigger points. Once activated, these trigger points will refer symptoms with many activities of living and even with normal posture. This process usually takes 2 to 6 months to develop following MVCI. Trigger points are part of the MPS diagnosis that can be made by attention to standard diagnostic tools.

History of Trauma

The patient's history is extremely important in diagnosing posttraumatic MPS. In one MPS study 95% of the patients cited some event that triggered onset, such as stress, trauma, or overactivity.[215] As many as 17% to 50% of MVCI cases may develop chronic MPS.[216,217] MPS may even be precipitated by slight trauma.[207,218,219]

Lifestyle History

The patient with an active MPS will describe certain activities that seem to aggravate

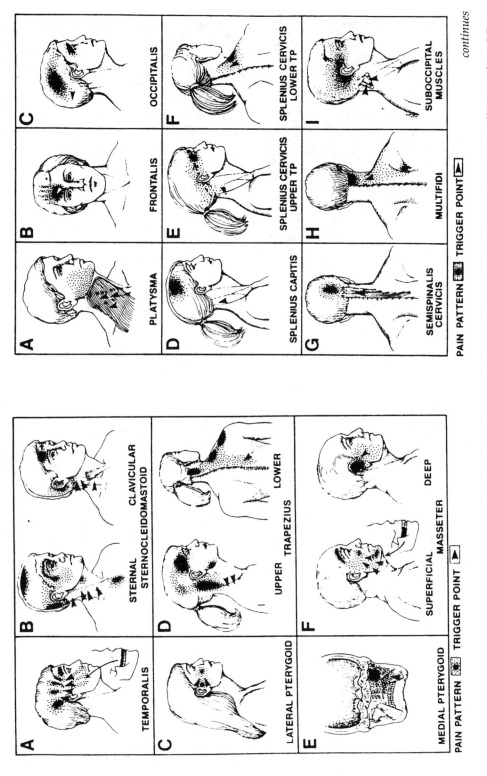

Figure 1-10 Common trigger points that cause head, neck, and arm pain. *Source:* Reprinted from Simons D., and Travell J., Myofascial Pain Syndromes, in *Textbook of Pain*, 2nd ed., P.D. Wall and R. Melzack, eds., pp. 371–375, with permission of Churchill Livingstone, © 1989.

Figure 1-10 continued

ARM

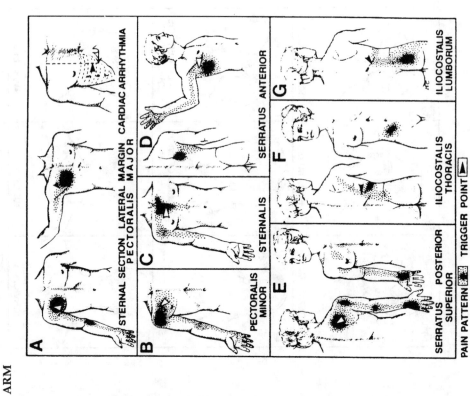

symptoms, restrict certain activities, or describe activities that have to be avoided completely. MPS is often associated with tiredness, poor sleep, morning stiffness, and chronic headaches.[213] Symptoms are worsened by modulating effects of poor posture, overwork, fatigue, exposure to cold, and sleep disorders.[143,213] Symptoms are worsened by a sedentary lifestyle.[220]

Symptom Description

Pain, stiffness, and fatigue are the three primary symptoms in MPS.[221] The quality of pain in one study was described by patients as follows: 47.5% pressure, 27% dull, 25% throbbing, 18% sharp, 16% burning, and 14% heavy.[217] In this same study of 164 head and neck MPS patients, 20% had additional symptoms of tingling, numbness, nausea, fatigue, tension, tinnitus, ear pain, dizziness, depression, anxiety, temporomandibular joint dysfunction, poor sleep, and poor dietary habits.[217]

Pain Drawings/Anatomic Illustrations

Use pain drawings or anatomic illustrations to aid diagnosis. The patient can fill out a pain drawing or be shown trigger point illustrations (artwork). The clinician can then correlate these findings to those found in the literature.

Muscle Motion Characteristics

There will always be some degree of loss of muscle motion in these cases.[210]

Tissue Texture

Digital soft tissue examination should reveal myofascial tissue texture abnormalities such as nodular, hard, indurated, ropy, or tender areas. Trigger points are usually located within a taut band of skeletal muscle or muscle fascia.[88]

Widespread areas of involvement, usually five[222] to seven[223] trigger points, should exist to confirm diagnosis. Tender-point maps have been developed by several authors and are consistent among different patients.[217,223] A lo-

cal twitch response of the brisk rolling action or the "jump sign" is pathognomonic of a trigger point.[88,210,224]

Symptom Reproduction

Reproduction of patient symptoms that are similar in distribution and characteristics will identify the area in question as a trigger point.[210] Direct finger pressure on anatomically known trigger point areas will reproduce the patient's usual referred symptom characteristics and location if it is active.

Postural Evaluation

Of those MPS patients evaluated, 96% had poor sitting or standing posture, 84% had forward head tilt, 82% had rounded shoulders, and 46% had abnormal cervical lordosis.[217] Poor head and neck posture results in localized ischemia, and metabolite buildup in these already highly sensitized abnormal tissues is responsible for perpetuating some of the patients' pain.

Strength and Fatigue Examination

When affected muscle tissue is tested for strength by an examiner, the involved muscle will give way short of its normal strength to avoid painful contraction.[208] A trigger point fatigues more easily and may need to be tested several times to detect it accurately. Although electromyography shows that trigger points are essentially normal at rest, they show abnormal reflex hyperirritability when stressed.[8]

Pressure Algometry

Various instruments have been designed to document myofascial pain and texture. An algometer can be used to quantify the amount of force that will induce pain. The findings can then be compared with normal population values.[225] See Chapter 6 for more details.

Reactive Cutaneous Hyperthermia or Hyperemia

Reactive cutaneous hyperthermia or hyperemia[215] should be looked for after the foci are palpated deeply. It then becomes hyperemic and then erythematous.[226] After the examiner has finished the palpation examination, he or she needs to examine the skin surface to check for prolonged reddening in the suspected areas. This is compared with areas not affected. This effect can be seen in the neck, middle back, and low back regions and explains why thermography may be helpful in detecting these cases.

Disorders That Mimic or Perpetuate Myofascial Syndrome

The symptom complex of myofascial pain may be mimicked by underlying systemic, metabolic, or endocrine disorders as well as by drug reactions, allergies, neoplasm, sleep disorders, or connective tissue disease. Articular dysfunction may confuse the doctor because MPS may be coupled with it. Other disorders that may cause similar symptoms include hepatitis; infectious mononucleosis; and endocrinopathies such as hypothyroidism, polymyositis, and polymyalgia rheumatica. Referral to a rheumatologist may be indicated in further diagnosis and multispecialist management.

Endocrine and nutritional[208] disorders such as hypothyroidism and deficiencies in calcium, iron, and folic acid can perpetuate MPS. These conditions result in an inability of muscles to relax fully and maintain full resting length, causing localized ischemia.

TEMPOROMANDIBULAR JOINT INJURY

Temporomandibular joint (TMJ) pain and associated pain syndromes are frequent sequelae of MVCIs. Several studies find that TMJ problems arise specifically from MVCIs.[60,227] Other reports also confirm that the most problematic initiating factor for temporomandibular joint disorders is trauma.[228,229] These posttraumatic TMJ figures are higher than those for the normal general population.[230] Although the insurance industry frequently challenges the etiology and even the existence of TMJ problems, recent literature has many claims to its frequent posttraumatic existence.

Typical History

TMJ disorders frequently follow rear-end collisions[231,232] in which the occupant is unaware of the impending collision.[233] Direct blows to the jaw from the occupant's hitting the car interior or another occupant's body may also produce this disorder. Masseter muscles are fully capable of withstanding most inertial forces but only if pretensed. In general, the TMJ dysfunctional syndrome seems to be tied intimately with cervical spine problems, forward-head tilt, and tight shoulder girdle.[234]

Mechanics of TMJ Injury

The TMJ is particularly vulnerable to rear-end collisions[235] or direct blows. The anatomy of the TMJ includes a loose joint capsule and nonlimiting bony shape.[235] As the head hyperextends backward in a rear-end collision, the jaw opens on its hinge joint. The jaw rapidly reaches maximal extension and rapidly closes, causing localized joint soft tissue tearing and anterior meniscus dislocation. One recent study on computer-simulated models evaluated the kinematic and dynamic responses to 15- and 30-mph rear-collision forces. It concluded that at 15 mph the jaw opens 63.5 degrees and at 30 mph it opens 67.1 degrees. Peak opening of the jaw occurred at 0.10 seconds, which is at the end of the typical rear-end collision time sequence.

TMJ injuries primarily occur from two types of MVCIs: (1) inertial loading in a rear-end crash in which the jaw lags behind the rearward skull motion, then rapidly closes as the head moves in flexion; and (2) by direct impact from being hit by an interior vehicle structure or another occupant. At higher-speed rear-end collisions, those over 10 mph, occupant bracing has little mitigating benefit. If the vehicle has headrests above the mid-skull level of the occupant, a TMJ injury is unlikely because the head will not hyperextend far enough. In rear-end low-speed collisions in which the occupant braces prior to the crash, the occurrence of TMJ injuries is uncommon. Frontal and side collisions typically do not cause TMJ inertial loading unless the person is completely facing the opposite impact direction.

Lader[236] reports that neck spasms from MVCI may create a pathologic occlusal TMJ dysfunction directly. He also shows that a sequence of events takes place with initial injury to the neck, causing muscle spasm and reflexive alterations in the normal cranioverteberal posture in response to the injury. This increases the muscular demands and tone on the suprahyoid muscles, which in turn pulls the mandible inferior and posterior. This secondary abnormal occlusive relationship then stimulates neural input from the central nervous system, resulting in muscle compensation. The sustained muscle contraction may result in ischemia, localized myofascial pain, and referred pain. One arthrographic investigation of 28 whiplash patients continuing to have jaw symptoms for an average of 126 days showed that 22 out of 25 postwhiplash patients had TMJ disc derangements postwhiplash.[237]

TMJ disorders may also have delays in onset due to secondary posttraumatic biomechanical or postural changes in the cervical spine. If there are changes in the anteroposterior position of the head because of loss or reversal of cervical curvature, the distance between the teeth can change and alterations can occur in the jaw musculature. This may result in pain developing 4 to 6 weeks after injury; by 3 to 4 months the alterations may develop into trigger points that lead to headaches and vertigo.

Common Posttraumatic TMJ Symptoms

TMJ symptoms may include the following:

- Jaw pain or discomfort when talking, chewing, or opening mouth. Approximately 70% to 90% of patients have jaw pain as a primary complaint; most are unilateral.[238] Weinberg and Lager[229] suggest that trismus (loss of motion), chewing pain, and pain when opening the mouth classically are the symptoms that are pathognomonic for TMJ dysfunction. Pain during sleep may occur.

- Headaches. Headaches frequently follow the MVCI, often with the patient waking up with one. About 30% of rear-end collision female patients with headaches develop trigger points in the jaw. TMJ headaches typically are unilateral, over the temporalis or the maxillary sinus area.

- Joint popping, difficulty opening the mouth, trismus, jaw locking, and jaw clicking. Weinberg and Lager[229] conclude that TMJ crepitus is caused by one of three things: disc perforation, dry synovial cavities, or roughened bony surfaces due to degenerative joint disease.

- Joint noise. Joint noise is unilateral in 40% to 60% of all cases.[238] Jaw popping and clicking are seen frequently in the normal population and are significant only if no prior history of joint noise exists.

- Jaw deviation when opening and closing or change in occlusion.

- Neck pain/shoulder pain. Neck pain in 39% and shoulder pain in 32% have been reported in TMJ cases.[229]

- Grinding (bruxism) of teeth during the day or night, which may cause teeth, gums, and jaw to be sore. When bruxism occurs at night the patient may wake up in the morning with soreness. Confirmation may also be obtained by inspecting the inside of the mouth for "bite lines" on the inside of the cheek and also by asking the spouse about grinding noises at night.

- Palpable muscle spasm or fibrotic texture about the TMJ.
- Ear and eye symptoms. Ear symptoms such as ear pain, ear popping, tinnitus, buzzing, or fullness, vertigo, and dizziness[239-241] were reported in 48% of patients.[229] Eye symptoms may include nystagmus, tearing, blurry vision, and double vision.[239]

Diagnosis of TMJ Disorder

A typical diagnosis of posttraumatic TMJ disorder would include reviewing the mechanism of injury, symptoms the patient exhibits, diagnostic testing, and evaluating the following:

- Changed bite or teeth not meeting together properly.
- New muscle spasms in pterygoid, masseter, and/or temporalis.
- Jaw clicking of recent onset.
- Grinding of teeth (bruxism).
- Patient being unable to open mouth 35 to 40 mm from tips of the front teeth, considered the normal range.[240]
- Clicking manifested immediately upon opening or closing of the jaw, indicating a posterior condylar displacement.[240]
- Lateral jaw deviation toward the involved side upon opening and closing.[240]
- Changes in patient's head posture. If the patient's normal head posture changes anteriorly or posteriorly, bite alterations may result.

Diagnostic Testing

Using latex gloves, the doctor should hold the patient's mandible, firmly taking the jaw to tension and gently evaluating joint play. During examination the doctor should check for boggy or bony end-point feel, crepitus, laxity, and tension.[242] Do not force the mandible when testing. Evaluate for jaw popping, which indicates disc derangement.[229] Palpable findings should confirm muscle spasm, tenderness, and fibrosis in the lateral and medial pterygoid muscles, masseter muscles, and temporal muscles. Rule out sinus infection and prior TMJ disorders before making this diagnosis and relating it to a MVCI.

Double-contrast arthrotomography for disc alignment has a diagnostic accuracy of 85%.[243] Mandibular kinesiography and myomonitoring also are useful.[244] TMJ X-rays should be done by a specialist who has equipment designed especially for this purpose. MRI can be used to detect position of the articular discs.[245] Doppler ultrasound or digital ultrasonography can be used to hear TMJ noises. Computed mandibular tracking can be useful as well. Electromyography is sometimes used, but with low accuracy.[245]

Factors To Rule Out When Diagnosing TMJ Disorder

Cervical spine disorders or myofascial pain syndromes that may refer pain into the jaw area, infection, tooth disorders, and hysterical trismus should be ruled out, as well as other neuropathies. Numerous diseases may affect the TMJ, such as lupus, Reiter's syndrome, temporal arteritis, acromegaly, and hyperparathyroidism and gout.[245]

Aggravating/Perpetuating Factors in TMJ Disorder

Common aggravating factors in TMJ disorders include poor posture, forward-head posture, carrying purse on shoulders, chewing gum, biting hard objects or food, scoliosis, short leg, hypothyroidism, bruxism, and malocclusion.

POSTTRAUMATIC STRESS DISORDER

No text about MVCI would be complete without discussing posttraumatic stress disorder (PTSD). It occurs occasionally after an individual has gone through a highly stressful event outside the normal range of human experience. Several studies have found that PTSD may occur following either neck or head injury from car crashes.[43,246–248]

The prevalence of PTSD is 11.3% in women and 6% for men overall.[249] One Kansas study concluded that postaccident psychiatric disorders were less likely to occur in individuals having extensive tissue damage; it appears that serious physical damage neutralizes the reactive psychologic problems.[250] Patients having visible outward indicators of injury fare better. Those who have cervical collar, wound bandage, or tangible evidence of injury have something real to cope with,[250] inhibiting neuroticism. One author suggests that over 40% of postaccident psychologic problems should be diagnosed as PTSD.[250] An accident may disrupt travel, work schedules, child care, appointments, and finances. Additional inconveniences may involve dealing with doctors, insurance companies, car repair shops, and attorneys.

The majority of people experiencing PTSD after head injuries in motor vehicle collisions have a true organic basis for their disorder, sometimes called an *organic personality syndrome*. One postconcussion study found that 43% of cases had PTSD.[251] Scrignar[248] concludes that some PTSD patients are predisposed or vulnerable to these exposures and may have a history of hyperactivity or anxiety disorders. Additionally, these patients may have poor coping skills and lack good social support groups. A recent study on survivors in a hotel that was hit by a plane found that of those who had postdisaster psychopathology, 72% had a history of predisaster disorder with a specificity of 90%.[252] A small study of 36 patients having chronic PTSD concluded that 66% had a positive history of familial psychopathology such as drug and alcohol abuse (60%), depression, and anxiety disorders.[253]

Posttraumatic stress disorder syndrome is said to occur if characteristic symptoms last more than 1[246] to 3 months. Diagnostic criteria for PTSD should include at least three of the following primary symptoms:[250,254]

- an extreme stressor event such as a car crash
- persisting re-experiencing or reliving trauma, i.e., nightmares
- numbing of responsiveness to other people and environment
- exaggerated startle reaction/reflexes
- abnormal anxiety

In addition, the patient should have two of the following symptoms that were not present before the injury:[247,255]

- flashbacks
- apathy
- irritability
- difficulty falling asleep
- fatigue
- memory impairment
- hypervigilance
- feeling detached from others or social withdrawal
- loss of concentration
- persistent avoidance of anything that is associated with the trauma
- guilt about surviving and intensification of symptoms when exposed to situations similar to the traumatic event

The doctor should beware of misdiagnosing PTSD as alcoholism, drug abuse, schizophrenia, or phobic and depressive states.[256] It is also important for the doctor, attorney, and insurance carrier to realize that individuals' personalities vary greatly in their strengths and weaknesses and that each individual's tolerance levels are unique. Sometimes a MVCI happens to someone who is near the breaking point,[250] and PTSD subsequently occurs. These patients may have persistent PTSD symptoms that need help, and the attending physician should refer them to an appropriate specialist.

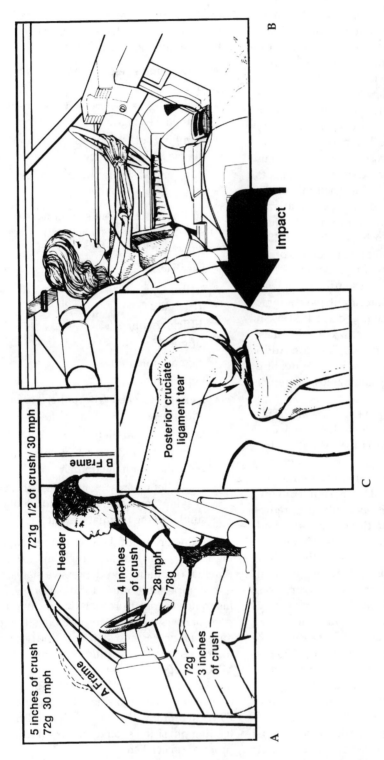

Figure 1–11 Potential head, shoulder, elbow, wrist, chest, and knee injury in a frontal collision of 30 mph. A, estimates of crush distance and acceleration levels in a 30-mph frontal collision for a belted driver. B, illustration of potential elbow injury. C, posterior cruciate ligament tears if the anterior tibia is sheared backward as it hits the knee bolster in a frontal collision. *Source:* Data from Mackay, M., An Historical Perspective on Impact Biomechanics and Some Basic Kinematics, in *Biomechanics of Impact Trauma,* B. Aldman and A. Chapon, eds., ICTS, 1984; from *Handbook of Road Safety Research* by G. Grime, Butterworth-Heinemann, 1987; and from Mackay, M., Kinematics of Vehicle Crashes, *Advances in Trauma,* Vol. 2, pp. 21–42, Mosby-Year Book, Inc., 1987.

Table 1–5 Use of Diagnostic Procedures in California and New York

| | California | | New York | | | |
| | BI | | BI | | PIP | |
Diagnostic Procedure	No. of BI Claimants	% of BI Claimants	No. of BI Claimants	% of BI Claimants	No. of PIP Claimants	% of PIP Claimants
X-Ray	4,121	57%	781	72%	1,204	61%
MRI	419	6	261	24	260	13
Muscle Strength Evaluation	342	5	57	5	61	3
Neuropsychologic Evaluation	198	3	50	5	61	3
CT	164	2	161	15	171	9
EMG	84	1	133	12	113	6
EEG	77	1	99	9	100	5
Sonogram	54	1	15	1	26	1
Bone Scan	49	1	17	2	21	1
Discogram	20	*	4	*	9	*
At Least One Procedure	4,293	60%	864	79%	1,284	65
None of These Procedures	2,887	40%	226	21%	687	35
Total Claimants	7,180	100%	1,090	100%	1,971	100%

*Percentage lower than 0.5%.

Source: Reprinted from *Auto Injuries: Claiming Behavior and Its Impact on Insurance Costs* with permission of the Insurance Research Council, © 1994.

USE OF DIAGNOSTIC PROCEDURES FOR MVCI

A recent insurance claims study has looked at two states, New York and California, and evaluated diagnostic tests used by physicians for MVCIs. Table 1–5 outlines the various types used and the frequency used. These two states do not represent the entire nation, as many states do not use these procedures as frequently.

CONCLUSION

We have discussed briefly the diagnosis of patients involved in motor vehicle collisions.

We have seen clearly that these injuries are complex and frequently multiple. Occupants have the potential for many types of injuries, as illustrated in Figure 1–11.[257–259] Figure 1–11 outlines the potential for occupant injury in a 30-mph frontal crash with acceleration levels, the amount of crush typical for a passenger car, and hopefully will leave the reader with a visual representation of the tremendous forces seen in auto crashes. Our ultimate goal is to assist the treating doctor in establishing an accurate diagnosis that will in turn provide for more effective patient management and improved treatment outcomes.

REFERENCES

1. Cailliet R. *Soft Tissue Pain and Disability.* 2nd ed. Philadelphia: FA Davis Co; 1988.

2. Hyde AS. *Crash Injuries: How and Why They Happen.* Key Biscayne, Fla: Hyde Associates; 1992.

3. Jensen MC, Brant-Zawadzki MN, Obuchowski N, et al. Magnetic resonance imaging of the lumbar spine in people without back pain. *N Engl J Med.* 1994;331(2):69–73.

4. Luchter S. Multiple injuries in motor vehicle crashes. In: Program of the 34th Proceedings of the Association for the Advancement of Automotive Medicine; Scottsdale, Ariz; 1990:111–126.

5. Foret-Bruno JY, Tarriere C, Le Coz JY, et al. Risk of cervical lesions in real-world and simulated collisions. In: Program of the 34th Proceedings of the Association for the Advancement of Automotive Medicine; Scottsdale, Ariz; 1990:373–389.

6. Insurance Research Council. *Auto Injuries: Claiming Behavior and Its Impact on Insurance Costs*. Oak Brook, Ill: IRC; 1994.

7. Cailliet R. *Neck and Arm Pain*. 3rd ed. Philadelphia: FA Davis; 1991.

8. Campbell SM. Regional myofascial pain syndromes. *Rheum Dis Clin North Am*. 1989;15(1):31–43.

9. Jeffreys E, McSweeney T. *Disorders of the Cervical Spine*. London: Butterworth; 1980.

10. Aldman B. *Injury Biomechanics*. Government/Industry Meeting and Exposition. Washington, DC: Society of Automotive Engineers; 1987;SP-731:85.

11. Quintner JL. A study of upper limb pain and paraesthesiae following neck injury in motor vehicle accidents: assessment of the brachial plexus tension test of Elvey. *Br J Rheumatol*. 1989;28:528–533.

12. Balla JI. The late whiplash syndrome. *Aust N Z J Surg*. 1980;50(6):610–614.

13. Petrucelli E, States JD, Hames LN. The Abbreviated Injury Scale: evolution, usage, and future adaptability. *Accid Anal Prev*. 1981;13:29–35.

14. Petrucelli E, States JD, Hames LN. The Abbreviated Injury Scale: evolution, usage, and future adaptability. In: International Conference of the Association for Accident and Traffic Medicine (IAATM); Copenhagen, Denmark; 1980:163.

15. Pike JA. *Automotive Safety: Anatomy, Injury, Testing, and Regulation*. Warrendale, Pa: Society of Automotive Engineers; 1990.

16. Association for the Advancement of Automotive Medicine. *The Abbreviated Injury Scale*. 1990 rev. Des Plaines, Ill: AAAM; 1990.

17. Luchter S. *Injury Biomechanics*. Government/Industry Meeting and Exposition. Washington, DC: Society of Automotive Engineers; 1987; SP-731:123–129.

18. Frazee JG. Head trauma. *Emerg Med Clin North Am*. 1986;4(4):859–875.

19. Sances A Jr, Yoganandan N. Human head injury tolerance. In: Sances A Jr, Thomas DJ, Ewing CL, et al., eds. *Mechanisms of Head and Spine Trauma*. Goshen, NY: Aloray Publisher; 1986:189–218.

20. Rimel RW, Giordani B, Barth JT, et al. Disability caused by minor head injuries. *Neurosurgery*. 1981;9:221–228.

21. Levine AM. Minor head injury: a not so minor problem. *J Neurol Orthop Med Surg*. 1987;8(4):242–282.

22. MacLennon C, Ommaya AK. Head injury and outcome: a critical review of methodology. In: *Crash Injury Impairment and Disability: Long Term Effects*. International Congress and Exposition; paper 860425. Detroit, Mich: Society of Automotive Engineers; 1986; SP-661:9–29.

23. Salerno G, Bleicher JN, Fruin A, et al. Head injury in traffic accidents. In: *Crash Injury Impairment and Disability: Long Term Effects*. International Congress and Exposition; paper 860504. Detroit, Mich: Society of Automotive Engineers; 1986:87–91.

24. Alves WM. Motor vehicle head injury: damage and outcome. In: *Crash Injury Impairment and Disability: Long Term Effects*. International Congress and Exposition; paper 860423. Detroit, Mich: Society of Automotive Engineers; 1986;SP-661:167–176.

25. Fan WRS, Jettner E. Light vehicle occupant protection: top and rear structures and interiors. In: *Crash Protection*. International Congress and Exposition; paper 820244. Detroit, Mich: Society of Automotive Engineers; 1982; SP-513:52–63.

26. Malliaris AC, Hitchcock R, Hedlund J. *A Search for Priorities in Crash Protection*. International Congress and Exposition; paper 820242. Detroit, Mich: Society of Automotive Engineers; 1982;SP-513:1–33.

27. Ommaya AK. The head: kinematics and brain injury mechanisms. In: Aldman B, Chapon A, eds. *The Biomechanics of Impact Trauma. ICTS*. New York: Elsevier Science Publishing Co; 1984:117–126.

28. Strub RL, Black FW. *Organic Brain Syndromes: An Introduction to Neurobehavioral Disorders*. Philadelphia: FA Davis Co; 1981.

29. Scott WE. *Epidemiology of Head and Neck Trauma in Victims of Motor Vehicle Accidents, Head and Neck Injury Criteria, A Consensus Workshop*. Washington, DC: US Government Printing Office; July 1983:1–6.

30. Rutherford WH, Merrett JD, McDonald JR. Symptoms at one year following concussion from minor head injuries. *Injury*. 1978;10:225–230.

31. Evans RW. Postconcussive syndrome: an overview. *Tex Med*. 1987;83:49–53.

32. Lishman WA. Physiogenesis and psychogenesis in the "post-concussional syndrome." *Br J Psychiatry*. 1988;153:460–469.

33. Mandel S. Minor head injury may not be "minor." *Postgrad Med*. 1989;85(6):213–225.

34. Kelly R. Headache after cranial trauma. In: Hopkins A, ed. *Headache: Problems in Diagnosis and Management*. Philadelphia: WB Saunders; 1988.

35. Robertson A. The post-concussional syndrome: then and now. *Aust N Z J Psychiatry*. 1988;22:396–403.

36. Gronwall D, Wrightson P. Duration of post-traumatic amnesia after mild head injury. *J Clin Neuropsychol.* 1980;2(1):51–60.

37. Jennett B, Teasdale G. *Management of Head Injuries.* Philadelphia: FA Davis Co; 1981.

38. Biary N, Cleeves L, Findley L, et al. Post-traumatic tremor. *Neurology.* 1989;39:103–106.

39. Reik L Jr. Cluster headache after head injury. *Headache.* 1987;27:509–510.

40. Bullock R, Teasdale G. Head injuries, I, ABC of major trauma. *Br Med J.* 1990;300:1515–1518.

41. Immordino FM. Management of minor head trauma. *Bull Clin Neurosci.* 1986;51:81–88.

42. Wagner MB, Winfield JA. Head trauma. *Patient Care.* 1990:96–113.

43. Masters SJ, McClean PM, Arcarese JS, et al. Skull X-ray examinations after mild head trauma: recommendations by a multidisciplinary panel and validation study. *New Engl J Med.* 1987;316(2):84–91.

44. Thornbury JR, Campbell JA, Masters SJ, et al. Skull fracture and the low risk of intracranial sequelae in minor head trauma. *AJR.* 1984;143:661–664.

45. Cook WI. Mathematical models of head injury: a ranking experiment. *J Safety Res.* 1980;12(3):127–137.

46. Adams JH, Graham DI, Murray LS, et al. Diffuse axonal injury due to nonmissile head injury in humans: an analysis of 45 cases. *Ann Neurol.* 1982;12:557–563.

47. Cawing LY, Rifai S, Khatua T, et al. Finite element analysis of diffuse axonal injury. In: *Vehicle Crashworthiness and Occupant Protection in Frontal Collisions.* Warrendale, Pa: American Society of Engineers; February 1990; SP-807:141–154.

48. Blumbergs PC, Jones NR, North JB. Diffuse axonal injury in head trauma. *J Neurol Neurosurg Psychiatry.* 1989;52:838–841.

49. Gennarelli TA. Mechanisms and pathophysiology of cerebral concussion. *J Head Trauma Rehabil.* 1986;1(2):23–29.

50. Speed WG III. Closed head injury sequelae: changing concepts. *Headache.* 1989;29:643–647.

51. Gronwall D, Wrightson P. Cumulative effect of concussion. *Lancet.* 1975;2:995–997.

52. Alves WM, Colohan ART, O'Leary TJ, et al. Understanding posttraumatic symptoms after minor head injury. *J Head Trauma Rehabil.* 1986;1(2):1–12.

53. Boismare F, Boquet J, Moore N, et al. Hemodynamic, behavioral and biochemical disturbances induced by an experimental cranio-cervical injury (whiplash) in rats. *J Auton Nerv Syst.* 1985;13:137–147.

54. Kay T. *Minor Head Injury: An Introduction for Professionals.* Framingham, Mass: National Head Injury Foundation; December 1986:1–12.

55. Leininger BE, Gramling SE, Farrell AD, et al. Neuropsychological deficits in symptomatic minor head injury patients after concussion and mild concussion. *J Neurol Neurosurg Psychiatry.* 1990;53:293–296.

56. Ewing R, McCarthy D, Gronwall D, et al. Persisting effects of minor head injury observable during hypoxic stress. *J Clin Neuropsychol.* 1980; 2(2):147–155.

57. Tamura T. Cranial symptoms after cervical injury: aetiology and treatment of the Barré-Lieou syndrome. *J Bone Joint Surg [Br].* 1989;71(2):283–287.

58. Toglia JU. Acute flexion-extension injury of the neck: electronystagmographic study of 309 patients. *Neurology.* 1976;26:808–814.

59. Svensson MY, Aldman B, Hansson HA, et al. Pressure effects in the spinal canal during whiplash extension motion: a possible cause of injury to the cervical spinal ganglia. In: International Conference on the Biomechanics of Impacts; Eindhoven, Netherlands; 1993.

60. Baker BA. The muscle trigger: evidence of overload injury. *J Neurol Orthop Med Surg.* 1986; 7(1):35–44.

61. Behrman S. Traumatic neuropathy of second cervical spinal nerves. *Br Med J.* 1983;286:1312–1313.

62. Hinoki M. Vertigo due to whiplash injury: a neurotological approach. *Acta Otolaryngol Suppl (Stockh).* 1985;419:9–29.

63. Hülse M. Disequilibrium, caused by a functional disturbance of the upper cervical spine: clinical aspects and differential diagnosis. *Manual Med.* 1983;1:18–22.

64. Rowe MJ III, Carlson C. Brainstem auditory evoked potentials in postconcussion dizziness. *Arch Neurol.* 1980;37:679–683.

65. Lund L. Dizziness and vertigo in the posttraumatic syndrome: a physiological background. *Acta Neurochir Suppl.* 1986;36:118–120.

66. Revel M, Andre-Deshays C, Minguet M. Cervicocephalic kinesthetic sensibility in patients with cervical pain. *Arch Phys Med Rehabil.* 1991;72:288–292.

67. Hildingsson C, Wenngren BI, Bring G, et al. Oculomotor problems after cervical spine injury. *Acta Orthop Scand.* 1989;60(5):513–516.

68. House JW, Schleuning AJ II, Shea JJ. Help for the patient with tinnitus. *Patient Care.* October 15, 1987;89–104.

69. Fitz-Ritson D. Assessment of cervicogenic vertigo. *J Manipulative Physiol Ther.* 1991;14(3):193–198.

70. Fioravanti M, Napoleoni A, Thorel M, et al. Post-traumatic headache: a comparative assessment of headache, vertigo, and other subjective complaints. *Cephalalgia.* 1985;5(S3):320.

71. Jaeger B, Reeves JL, Graff-Radford SB. A psychophysiological investigation of myofascial trigger point sensitivity vs EMG activity and tension headache. *Cephalalgia.* 1985;5(S3):68–69.

72. Welch KMA. Migraine: a biobehavioral disorder. *Arch Neurol.* 1987;44:323–327.

73. Kidd RF, Nelson R. Musculoskeletal dysfunction of the neck in migraine and tension headache. *Headache.* 1993;33:566–569.

74. Sluijter ME, Rohof OJJM, Vervest ACM. Cervical headache: diagnosis with the aid of computerised analysis of cervical mobility. *Cephalalgia.* 1989; 9(S10):199–200.

75. Weiss HD, Stern BJ, Goldberg J. Minor head or neck trauma, post-traumatic migraine: chronic migraine precipitated. *Headache.* 1991;31:451–456.

76. Saper JR. Chronic headache syndromes. *Neurol Clin.* 1989;7(2):387–412.

77. Stewart JD. *Focal Peripheral Neuropathies.* New York: Elsevier Science Publishing Co; 1987.

78. Bogduk N. Cervical causes of headache and dizziness. In: Grieve GP, ed. *Modern Manual Therapy of the Vertebral Column.* Edinburgh: Churchill Livingstone; 1986.

79. Bogduk N. The anatomical basis for cervicogenic headache. *J Manipulative Physical Ther.* 1992; 15(1):67–70.

80. Seletz E. Whiplash injuries: neurophysiological basis for pain and methods used for rehabilitation. *JAMA.* 1958; November 29:1750.

81. Wilson PR. Chronic neck pain and cervicogenic headache. *Clin J Pain.* 1991;7:5–11.

82. Babur H. Occipital neuralgia alias C2-3 radiculopathy. *J Neurol Orthop Med Surg.* 1989; 10(2):133–139.

83. Bogduk N, Marsland A. On the concept of third occipital headache. *J Neurol Neurosurg Psychiatry.* 1986;49:775–780.

84. Jaeger B. Cervicogenic headache: relationship to cervical spine dysfunction and myofascial trigger points. *Cephalalgia.* 1987;7(S6):398–399.

85. Ebelin M, Furno P, Patel A. Functional sequelae of benign cervical spine sprains from whiplash injuries: report on 61 cases. *J Traumatol.* 1981;2(2):77–81.

86. Schellhas KP, Wilkes CH, Baker CC. Facial pain, headache, and temporomandibular joint inflammation. *Headache.* 1989;29(4):229–232.

87. Rapoport AM, Weeks RE. Characteristics and treatment of analgesic rebound headache. In:

Diener H-C, Wilkinson M, eds. *Drug-Induced Headache.* Berlin: Springer-Verlag; 1988:162–168.

88. DeMar E. Treatment of myofascial pain and dysfunction. In: Gerhardt JJ, et al., eds. *Interdisciplinary Rehabilitation in Trauma.* Baltimore: Williams & Wilkins; 1987.

89. Snell RS. *Clinical Anatomy for Medical Students.* 3rd ed. Boston: Little, Brown, and Co; 1986.

90. Orsay EM, Dunne M, Turnbull TL, et al. Prospective study of the effect of safety belts in motor vehicle crashes. *Ann Emerg Med.* 1990;19:258–261.

91. Otremski I, Marsh JL, Wilde BR, et al. Soft tissue cervical spinal injuries in motor vehicle accidents. *Injury.* 1989;20:349–351.

92. Tsuchisashi M, Nishikawa S, Mii K, et al. Road traffic accidents and the abbreviated injury scale (AIS) in Japan. *Accid Anal Prev.* 1981; 13:37–42.

93. Maag U, Desjardins D, Bourbeau R, et al. In: Seat belts and neck injuries. Program of the International Research Committee on the Biomechanics of Impacts; Bron, France; 1990:1–13.

94. Olney DB, Marsen AK. The effect of head restraints and seat belts on the incidence of neck injury in car accidents. *Injury.* 1986;17:365–367.

95. Lövsund P, Nygren Å, Salen B, et al. Neck injuries in rear end collisions among front and rear seat occupants. In: Program of the International Research Committee on the Biomechanics of Impacts; Bergisch-Gladbach, Germany; 1988.

96. Larder DR, Twiss MK, Mackay GM. Neck injury to car occupants using seat belts. In: Proceedings of the 29th Annual Conference of the Association for the Advancement of Automotive Medicine. Washington, DC; 1985:153–165.

97. Tarriere C. *Risk of Head and Neck Injury If There Is No Direct Head Impact, Head and Neck Injury Criteria, A Consensus Workshop*, Washington, DC: US Government Printing Office; July 1983:13–15.

98. Goldsmith W, Ommaya AK. Head and neck injury criteria and tolerance levels. In: Aldman B, Chapon A, eds. *The Biomechanics of Impact Trauma.* ICTS. Amsterdam: Elsevier Science Publishing Co; 1984:149–180.

99. Yoganandan N, Pintar FA, Haffner M, et al. Epidemiology and injury biomechanics of motor vehicle related trauma to the human spine. In: Proceedings of the 33rd Stapp Car Crash Conference, P-227, 892438, p223-242, Washington, DC, 1989, SAE.

100. Mackay M. Biomechanics and the regulation of vehicle crash performance. In: Proceedings of the 33rd Annual Conference of the Association for the Advancement of Automotive Medicine; Baltimore; 1989:323–336.

101. Patrick LM. Neck injury incidence, mechanisms and protection. In: Proceedings of the 31st annual

conference of the Association for the Advancement of Automotive Medicine; New Orleans; 1987:409–431.

102. Winters JM, Peles JD. Neck muscle activity and 3-D head kinematics during quasi-static and dynamic tracking movements. In: Winters JM, Woo SL-Y, eds. *Multiple Muscle Systems: Biomechanics and Movement Organization.* New York: Springer-Verlag; 1990.

103. Deans GT, Magalliard JN, Kerr M, et al. Neck sprain: a major cause of disability following car accidents. *Injury.* 1987;18:10–12.

104. Kahane CJ. *Evaluation of Head Restraints: Federal Motor Vehicle Safety Standard 202.* Washington, DC: National Highway Traffic Safety Administration Agency, Department of Transportation; 1982: HS 806 108.

105. Dunn EJ, Blazar S. Soft-tissue injuries of the lower cervical spine, instructional course lectures. Griffin PP, ed. *Am Acad Orthop Surgeons.* 1987; 36:499–512.

106. Trimble MR. *Post-Traumatic Neurosis: From Railway Spine to Whiplash.* Chichester, England: John Wiley & Sons; 1981.

107. Pintar FA, Yoganandan N, Sances A Jr, et al. Kinematic and anatomical analysis of the human cervical spinal column under axial loading. In: Proceedings of the 33rd Stapp Car Crash Conference, P-227, 892436. Washington, DC: Society of Automotive Engineers; 1989:191–214.

108. MacNab I. The "whiplash syndrome." *Orthop Clin North Am.* 1971;2(2):389–403.

109. Deng Y-C, Goldsmith W. Response of a human head/neck/upper-torso replica to dynamic loading, I: physical model. *J Biomechanics.* 1987; 20(5):471–486.

110. Unterharnscheidt F. Pathological and neuropathological findings in rhesus monkeys subjected to –Gx and +Gx indirect impact acceleration. In: Sances A Jr, Thomas DJ, Ewing CL, et al., eds. *Mechanisms of Head and Spine Trauma.* Goshen, NY: Aloray Publisher; 1986;565–663.

111. Jónsson H Jr, Bring G, Rauschning W, et al. Hidden cervical spine injuries in traffic accident victims with skull fractures. *J Spinal Disord.* 1991; 4(3):251–263.

112. Nusholtz GS, Huelke DE, Lux P, et al. Cervical spine injury mechanisms. In: 27th Stapp Car Crash Conference Proceedings with International Research Committee on Biokinetics of Impacts (IRCOBI); paper 831616. San Diego, Calif: Society of Automotive Engineers; 1983:179–198.

113. Roaf R. *Spinal Deformities.* Philadelphia: JB Lippincott Co; 1977.

114. Kallieris D, Mattern R, Miltner E, et al. *Considerations for a Neck Injury Criterion.* SAE paper 912916. Warrendale, Pa: Society of Automotive Engineers; 1991.

115. Bland JH. The cervical spine: from anatomy to clinical care. *Med Times.* 1989;117(9):15–33.

116. National Safety Council. *Accident Facts.* ed 1994. Chicago: NSC; 1994.

117. Janda V. Muscle spasm: a proposed procedure for differential diagnosis. *J Manual Med.* 1991;6:136–139.

118. Aprill C, Bogduk N. The prevalence of cervical zygapophyseal joint pain: a first approximation. *Spine.* 1992;17:744–747.

119. Lord S, Barnsley L, Bogduk N. Cervical zygapophyseal joint pain in whiplash. *Spine State Art Rev.* 1993;7:355–372.

120. Dwyer A, Aprill C, Bogduk N. Cervical zygapophyseal joint pain patterns, 1: a study in normal volunteers. *Spine.* 1990;15(6):456.

121. Lantz SA, Adams KM, King AI. Experimental determination of cervical facet joint capsule stretch. In: *Advances in Bioengineering.* Program of the winter annual meeting of the American Society of Mechanical Engineers; San Francisco; 1989.

122. Zimmerman M. Components of pain and pain-associated phenomena in the musculoskeletal system. In: Roland MO, Jenner JR, eds. *Back Pain: New Approaches to Rehabilitation and Education.* Manchester, England: Manchester University Press; 1989.

123. Allen WMC. After the head injury. *Practitioner.* 1986;230:155–158.

124. Bayless P, Ray VG. Incidence of cervical spine injuries in association with blunt head trauma. *Am J Emerg Med.* 1989;7:139–142.

125. Krantz KPG, Löwenhielm CGP. Head and neck injuries. *Acta Neurochir Suppl.* 1986;36:47–50.

126. Michael DB, Guyot DR, Darmody WR. Coincidence of Head and Cervical Spine Injury. *J Neurotrauma.* 1989;6(3):177–189.

127. Yoganandan N, Haffner M, Maiman DJ, et al. Epidemiology and injury biomechanics of motor vehicle related trauma to the human spine. *Soc Automotive Eng Trans.* 1990;98(6):1790–1807.

128. Steudel WI, Rosenthal D, Lorenz R, et al. Prognosis and treatment of cervical spine injuries with associated head trauma. *Acta Neurochir Suppl.* 1988;43:85–90.

129. Liu YK. Problems in the mathematical and physical modeling of head and neck injury. In: *Head and Neck Injury Criteria, A Consensus Workshop.* Washington, DC: US Government Printing Office; 1983:125–132.

130. Yoganandan N, Pintar FA, Sances A Jr, et al. Strength and kinematic response of dynamic cervical spine injuries. *Spine.* 1991;16(10):S511–S517.

131. Emori RI, Horigruchi J. *Whiplash in Low-Speed Vehicle Collisions.* Warrendale, Pa: Society of Automotive Engineers; 1990: paper 900542.

132. McConnell WE, Howard RP, Guzman HM, et al. *Analysis of Human Test Subject Kinematic Responses to Low Velocity Rear End Impacts,* paper 930889. Society of Automotive Engineers; 1993.

133. Scott MW, McConnell WE, Guzman HM, et al. *Comparison of Human and ATD Head Kinematics During Low-Speed Rearend Impacts.* paper 930094. Society of Automotive Engineers; 1993.

134. McElhaney JH, Paver JG, McCrackin HJ, et al. Cervical spine compression responses. In: 27th Stapp Car Crash Conference Proceedings with International Research Committee on Biokinetics of Impacts (IRCOBI); paper 831615. San Diego, Calif: Society of Automotive Engineers; 1983:163–178.

135. Barnsley L, Lord S, Bogduk N. The pathophysiology of whiplash. *Spine State Art Rev.* 1993;7:329–353.

136. Eliyahu DJB. Disc herniations of the cervical spine. *Am J Chiro Med.* 1989;2(3):93–100.

137. Sances A Jr, Maiman DJ, Myklebust JB, et al. Biodynamics of vehicular injuries. In: Peters GA, Peters BJ, eds. *Automotive Engineering and Litigation.* vol 1. New York: Garland Law Publishing; 1984:449–550.

138. Hammer AJ, Gargan MF, Bannister GC, et al. Whiplash injury and surgically treated cervical disc disease. *Injury.* 1993;24(8):549–550.

139. Lunsford LD, Bissonette DJ, Jannetta PJ, et al. Anterior surgery for cervical disc disease, I: treatment of lateral cervical disc herniation in 253 cases. *J Neurosurg.* 1980;53:1–11.

140. Spurling RG. *Lesions of Cervical Disc.* Springfield, Ill: CC Thomas; 1956.

141. Batzdorf U. Differential diagnosis of arm and thoracic radicular pain and sensory disturbance. *Spine State Art Rev.* 1988;2(4):565–583.

142. Kopell HP, Thompson WA. *Peripheral Entrapment Neuropathies.* Malabar, Fla: Krieger Publishing Co; 1976.

143. Maiman D, Yoganandan N, Weinshel S, et al. Epidemiology of motor vehicle related cervical spine injuries. In: *Crashworthiness and Occupant Protection in Transportation Systems.* Program of the winter annual meeting of the American Society of Mechanical Engineers. San Francisco; 1989:121–122.

144. Proano FA, Morgan PJ, Hymes JA, et al. Cervical steroid epidural block for treatment of cervical herniated intervertebral discs, pain (suppl 5). In:

Abstracts of the Sixth World Congress on Pain; Adelaide, Australia: Elsevier Science Publishers BV, 1990:S87.

145. Rockett FX. Observations on the "burner": traumatic cervical radiculopathy. *Clin Orthop.* 1982;164:18–19.

146. Panjabi MM, Krag MH, Chung TO. Effects of disc injury on mechanical behavior of the human spine. *Spine.* 1984;9(7):707–713.

147. Wells P. Cervical dysfunction and shoulder problems. *Physiotherapy.* 1982;68(3):66–73.

148. Brodsky AE. Cervical angina: a correlative study with emphasis on the use of coronary arteriography. *Spine.* 1985;10(8):699–708.

149. Williams RW. Microcervical foraminotomy: a surgical alternative for intractable radicular pain. *Spine.* 1983;8(7):708–716.

150. Howe JF, Loeser JD, Calvin WH. Mechanosensitivity of dorsal root ganglia and chronically injured axons: a physiological basis for the radicular pain of nerve root compression. *Pain.* 1977;3:25–41.

151. Carrick FR. Cervical radiculopathy: the diagnosis and treatment of pathomechanics in the cervical spine. *J Manipulative Physiol Ther.* 1983;6(3):129–137.

152. Beatty RM, Fowler FD, Hanson EJ Jr. The abducted arm as a sign of ruptured cervical disc. *Neurosurgery.* 1987;21(5):731–732.

153. Fast A, Parikh S, Marin EL. The shoulder abduction relief sign in cervical radiculopathy. *Arch Phys Med Rehabil.* 1989;70(5):402–403.

154. Davidson RI, Dunn EJ, Metzmaker JN. The shoulder abduction test in the diagnosis of radicular pain in cervical extradural compressive monoradiculopathies. *Spine.* 1981;6(5):441–446.

155. Elvey RL. Brachial plexus tension tests and the pathoanatomical origin of arm pain. In: Idczak RM, ed. *Biomechanical Aspects of Manipulative Therapy.* Carlton, Australia: Lincoln Institute of Health Sciences; 1981.

156. Breig A. *Adverse Mechanical Tension in the Central Nervous System: An Analysis of Cause and Effect.* Stockholm and New York: Almqvist and Wiksell and John Wiley & Sons, Inc; 1978.

157. Henderson CM, Hennessy RG, Shuey HM Jr, et al. Posterior-lateral foraminotomy as an exclusive operative technique for cervical radiculopathy: a review of 846 consecutively operated cases. *Neurosurgery.* 1983;13(5):504–512.

158. Benini A. Clinical features of cervical root compression C5-C8 and their variations. *Neuro-orthopedics.* 1987;4:74–88.

159. Magee DJ. *Orthopedic Physical Assessment.* Philadelphia: WB Saunders; 1987.

160. Post M. *Physical Examination of the Musculoskeletal System*. Chicago: Year Book Medical Publishers, Inc; 1987.

161. Wienir MA. Limb radicular pain and sensory disturbance. *Spine State Art Rev*. 1988;2(4):533–564.

162. Szabo R, Gelberman RH, Williamson RV, et al. Vibratory sensory testing in acute peripheral nerve compression. *J Hand Surg*. 1984;9A:104–108.

163. Dellon AL. Clinical use of vibratory stimuli to evaluate peripheral nerve injury and compression neuropathy. *Plast Reconstr Surg*. 1980; 65(4):466–476.

164. Schimsheimer RJ, Ongerboer de Visser BW, Bour LJ, et al. Digital nerve somatosensory evoked potentials and flexor carpi radialis H reflexes in cervical disc protrusion and involvement of the sixth or seventh cervical root: relations to clinical and myelographic findings. *Electroencephalogr Clin Neurophysiol*. 1988;70:313–324.

165. Teasell RW. The clinical picture of whiplash injuries: an overview. *Spine State Art Rev*. 1993;7:373–389.

166. Richardson RR, Torres H, Analitis S, et al. Traumatic thoracic outlet syndrome: a six case report. *J Neurol Orthop Surg*. 1983;4(4):327–337.

167. Sanders RJ, Pearce WH. The treatment of thoracic outlet syndrome: a comparison of different operations. *J Vasc Surg*. 1989;10:626–634.

168. Sanders RJ, Haug CE. *Thoracic Outlet Syndrome: A Common Sequela of Neck Injuries*. Philadelphia: JB Lippincott; 1991.

169. Smith KF. The thoracic outlet syndrome: a protocol for treatment. *JOSPT*. 1979;1(2):89–99.

170. Roos DB. Thoracic outlet and carpal tunnel syndromes. In: Rutherford RB, ed. *Vascular Surgery*. 2nd ed. Philadelphia: WB Saunders; 1984:708–724.

171. Jacobs B. Cervical angina. *NY State J Med*. 1990;90(1):8–11.

172. Booth RE Jr, Rothman RH. Cervical angina. *Spine*. 1976;1(1):29–32.

173. Fam AG. Chest wall pain: if not cardiac disease, then what?, I. *J Musculoskel Med*. 1987;4(2):65–74.

174. Mitchell LC, Schafermeyer RW. Herniated cervical disk presenting as ischemic chest pain. *Am J Emerg Med*. 1991;9:343–346.

175. Clark CR. Cervical spondylotic myelopathy: history and physical findings. *Spine*. 1988;13(7):847–849.

176. Coert JH, Dellon AL. Peripheral nerve entrapment caused by motor vehicle crashes. *J Trauma*. 1994;37(2):191–194.

177. Osterman AL. The double crush syndrome. *Orthop Clin North Am*. 1988;19(1):147–155.

178. Hirsh LF, Thanki A. Carpal tunnel syndrome: avoiding poor treatment results. *Postgrad Med*. 1985;77(1):185–191.

179. Gerstner DL, Omer GE Jr. Peripheral entrapment neuropathies in the upper extremity, I: key differential findings, median nerve syndromes. *J Musculoskel Med*. 1988;5(3):14–29.

180. Kummel BM, Zazanis GA. Shoulder pain as the presenting complaint in carpal tunnel syndrome. *Clin Orthop*. 1973;92:227–230.

181. Hurst LC, Weissberg D, Carroll RE. The relationship of the double crush to carpal tunnel syndrome: an analysis of 1,000 cases of carpal tunnel syndrome. *J Hand Surg [Br]*. 1985;10:202–204.

182. Massey EW, Rilery TL, Pleet AB. Coexistent carpal tunnel syndrome and cervical radiculopathy (double crush syndrome). *South Med J*. 1981; 74(8):957–959.

183. Beydoun SR. Focal entrapment neuropathies of the arm: signs, symptoms, electrodiagnosis, and etiologic considerations. *Spine State Art Rev*. 1988;2(4):627–668.

184. Carroll RE, Hurst LC. The relationship of thoracic outlet syndrome and carpal tunnel syndrome. *Clin Orthop*. 1982;164:149–153.

185. Newman RJ. Chest wall injuries and the seat belt syndrome. *Injury*. 1984;16:110–113.

186. Hayes CW, Conway WF, Walsh JW, et al. Seat belt injuries: radiologic findings and clinical correlation. *Radiographics*. 1991;11:23–36.

187. Walsh K, Cruddas M, Coggon D. Risk of low back pain in people admitted to hospital for traffic accidents and falls. *J Epidiol Community Health*. 1992;46(3):231–233.

188. King AI. Injury to the thoraco-lumbar spine and pelvis. In: Nahum AM, Melvin JW, eds. *Accidental Injury: Biomechanics and Prevention*. New York: Springer-Verlag; 1993.

189. Osvalder A-L, Neumann P, Lövsund P, et al. Dynamic load response of the in vitro lumbar spine in flexion. In: Conference of the International Research Committee on the Biomechanics of Impacts. Verona, Italy; 1992.

190. Portier L, Trosseille X, Le Coz J-Y, et al. Lower leg injuries in real-world frontal accidents. In Conference of the International Research Committee on the Biomechanics of Impacts. Eindhoven, Netherlands; 1993.

191. Sarno JE. Etiology of neck and back pain: an autonomic myoneuralgia? *J Nerv Ment Dis*. 1981; 169(1):55–59.

192. Giles LGF. Lumbo-sacral and cervical zygapophyseal joint inclusions. *Manual Med*. 2:89–92, 1986.

193. Soric RJ. Selected physical medicine modalities. In: Tollison CD, Satterthwaite JR, eds. *Painful Cervical Trauma: Diagnosis and Rehabilitative Treatment of Musculoskeletal Injuries.* Baltimore, Md: Williams & Wilkins; 1992.

194. Mendel T, Wink CS, Zimny ML. Neural elements in human cervical intervertebral discs. *Spine.* 1992;17:132–135.

195. Jayson MIV. General aspects of back pain: an overview. In: Jayson MIV, Swezey RL, Knoplich J, et al., eds. *Back Pain, Painful Syndromes and Muscle Spasms: Current Concepts and Recent Advances.* London: Parthenon Publishing Group; 1990.

196. Hurri HO, Patäjä JM, Alaranta HT, et al. Fibrinolytic defect in chronic back pain: a controlled study of plasminogen activator activity in 20 patients. *Acta Orthop Scand.* 1991;62(5):407–409.

197. Mense S. Physiology of nociception in muscles. *J Manual Med.* 1991;6:24–33.

198. Gunn CC. Early and subtle signs in low-back sprain. *Spine.* 1978;3:267–281.

199. Gunn CC. "Prespondylosis" and some pain syndromes following denervation supersensitivity. *Spine.* 1980;5(2):185–192.

200. Fricton JR. Myofascial pain and whiplash. *Spine State Art Rev.* 1993;7:403–422.

201. Wolfe F. Fibromyalgia and cervical pain. In: Tollison CD, Satterthwaite JR, eds. *Painful Cervical Trauma: Diagnosis and Rehabilitative Treatment of Neuromusculoskeletal Injuries.* Baltimore: Williams & Wilkins; 1992.

202. Danneskiold-Samsøe B, Christiansen E, Lund B, et al. Regional muscle tension and pain ("fibrositis"): effect of massage on myoglobin in plasma. *Scand J Rehabil Med.* 1982;15:17–20.

203. Manheim CJ, Lavett DK. *The Myofascial Release Manual.* Thorofare, NJ: Slack, Inc; 1989.

204. Chaitow L. *Soft-Tissue Manipulation: A Practitioner's Guide to the Diagnosis and Treatment of Soft Tissue Dysfunction and Reflex Activity.* Wellingborough, Northamptonshire: Thorsons Publishing Group; 1987.

205. Cathie A. The fascia of the body in relation to function and manipulative therapy. In: *American Academy of Osteopathy.* Chicago: Year Book Medical Publishers, Inc; 1974;81–84.

206. Hoag JM, Cole WV, Bradford SG. *Osteopathic Medicine.* New York: Blakiston Div McGraw-Hill Publishing Co; 1969.

207. Bonica JJ. Management of myofascial pain syndromes in general practice. *JAMA.* 1957;164:732–738.

208. Simons DG. Myofascial pain syndromes due to trigger points, 1: principles, diagnosis, and perpetuating factors. *Manual Med.* 1985;1:67–71.

209. Simons D, Travell J. Myofacial Pain Syndrome. In: Wall PD, Melzak R, eds. *Textbook of Pain,* 2nd ed. Edinburgh: Churchill Livingstone; 1989.

210. Simons DG. Fibrositis/fibromyalgia: a form of myofascial trigger points? *Am J Med.* 1986; 81(suppl 3A):93–98.

211. Travell JG, Simons DG. *Myofascial Pain and Dysfunction, The Trigger Point Manual.* Baltimore: Williams & Wilkins; 1983.

212. Bennett RM. Myofascial pain syndromes and the fibromyalgia syndrome: a comparative analysis. *J Manual Med.* 1991;6:34–45.

213. Taylor MR. Fibromyalgia syndrome: literature review. *Am J Chiro Med.* 1990;3(3):118–126.

214. Sandman KB, Backstrom CJ. Psychophysiological factors in myofascial pain. *J Manipulative Physiol Ther.* 1984;7(4):237–242.

215. Wolfe F. The clinical syndrome of fibrositis. *Am J Med.* 1986;81(suppl 3A):7–14.

216. Chester JB Jr. Whiplash, postural control, and the inner ear. *Spine.* 1991;16(7):716–720.

217. Fricton JR, Kroening R, Haley D, et al. Myofascial pain syndrome of the head and neck: a review of clinical characteristics of 164 patients. *Oral Surg Oral Med Oral Pathol.* 1985;60(10):615–623.

218. Hench PK. Secondary fibrositis. *Am J Med.* 1986;81(suppl 3A):60–62.

219. Loane SR. Cryotherapy, using cold to treat injuries. In: Appenzeller O, ed. *Sports Medicine, Fitness, Training, Injuries.* 3rd ed. Baltimore: Urban & Schwarzenberg; 1988.

220. Graff-Radford SB, Reeves JL, Jaeger B. Management of chronic head and neck pain: effectiveness of altering factors perpetuating myofascial pain. *Headache.* April 1987:186–190.

221. Bennett RM. Current issues concerning management of the fibrositis/fibromyalgia syndrome. *Am J Med.* 1986;81(suppl 3A):15–18.

222. Russell IJ, Vipraio GA, Morgan WW, et al. Is there a metabolic basis for the fibrositis syndrome? *Am J Med.* 1986;81(suppl 3A):50–54.

223. Smythe H. Tender points: evolution of concepts of the fibrositis/fibromyalgia syndrome. *Am J Med.* 1986;81(suppl 3A):2–6.

224. Cooper BC, Lucente FE. *Management of Facial, Head, and Neck Pain.* Philadelphia: WB Saunders Co; 1989.

225. Fischer AA. Pressure algometry over normal muscles: standard values, validity, and reproducibility of pressure threshold. *Pain.* 1987;30:115–126.

226. Yunus MB, Kalyan-Raman UP, Kalyan-Raman K, et al. Pathologic changes in muscle in primary fibromyalgia syndrome. *Am J Med.* 1986;81(suppl 3A):38–42.

227. Roydhouse RH. Torquing of neck and jaw due to belt restraint in whiplash-type accidents. *Lancet.* June 8, 1985:1341.

228. Graff-Radford SB. Oromandibular disorders and headache: a critical appraisal. *Neurol Clin.* 1990;8(4):929–945.

229. Weinberg LA, Lager LA. Clinical report on the etiology and diagnosis of TMJ dysfunction-pain syndrome. *J Prosthet Dent.* 1980;44:642–653.

230. Schneider K, Zernicke RF, Clark G. Modeling of jaw-head-neck dynamics during whiplash. *J Dent Res.* 1989;68(9):1360–1365.

231. Hodge CJ. Vehicular impact and its relationship to TMJ dysfunction syndrome. *Med Trial Tech Q.* 1990;36:230–234.

232. Moles RC. *Ending Head and Neck Pain: The TMJ Connection.* Racine, Wis: CGM Publications; 1989.

233. Nassif NJ. A brief questionnaire for craniomandibular disorders, II: etiology. *J Craniomandib Pract.* 1989;7(2):154–161.

234. Makofsky HW, August BF, Ellis JJ. A multidisciplinary approach to the evaluation and treatment of temporomandibular joint and cervical spine dysfunction. *J Craniomandib Pract.* 1989; 7(3):205–213.

235. Friedman MH. The temporomandibular joint. In: Gould JA III, Davies GJ, eds. *Orthopaedic and Sports Physical Therapy.* St Louis, Mo: CV Mosby Co; 1985.

236. Lader E. Cervical trauma as a factor in the development of TMJ dysfunction and facial pain. *J Craniomandib Pract.* 1983;1(2):85–90.

237. Weinberg S, LaPointe H. Cervical extension-flexion injury (whiplash) and internal derangement of the temporomandibular joint. *J Oral Maxillofac Surg.* 1987;45:653–656.

238. Chase DC, Hendler BH, Kraus SL. Spelling relief for TMJ troubles. *Patient Care.* 1988;158–161.

239. Royder JO. Structural influences in temporomandibular joint pain and dysfunction. *J Am Osteopath Assoc.* 1981;80(7):460–467.

240. Weinberg LA. Temporomandibular joint injuries. In: Foreman SM, Croft AC, eds. *Whiplash Injuries: The Cervical Acceleration/Deceleration Syndrome.* Baltimore: Williams & Wilkins; 1988:347–383.

241. Williamson EH. The interrelationship of internal derangements of the temporomandibular joint, headache, vertigo, and tinnitus: a survey of 25 patients. *J Craniomandib Pract.* 1990;8(4):301–306.

242. Gillespie BR. Assessment and treatment of TMJ muscles, fascia, ligaments, and associated structures. *J Craniomandib Pract.* 1990;8(1):51–55.

243. Westesson PL, Rohlin M. Diagnostic accuracy of double-contrast arthrotomography of the temporomandibular joint: correlation with postmortem morphology. *AJR.* 1984;143:655–660.

244. Moses AJ, Skoog GS. Cervical whiplash and TMJ: similarities in symptoms. *Trial.* 1986;22(3):63–64.

245. Talley RL, Murphy GJ, Smith SD, et al. Standards for the history, examination, diagnosis, and treatment of temporomandibular disorders (TMD): a position paper. *J Craniomandib Pract.* 1990;8(1): 60–71.

246. Figley CR, Scrignar CB, Smith WH. PTSD: the aftershocks of trauma. *Patient Care.* May 15, 1988:111–127.

247. Modlin HC. Posttraumatic stress disorder: no longer just for war veterans. *Postgrad Med.* 1986;79(3):26–44.

248. Scrignar CB. *Post-Traumatic Stress Disorder: Diagnosis, Treatment, and Legal Issues.* 2nd ed. New Orleans: Bruno Press; 1988.

249. Breslau N, Davis GC, Andreski P, et al. Traumatic events and posttraumatic stress disorder in an urban population of young adults. *Arch Gen Psychiatry.* 1991;48:216–222.

250. Modlin HC. Traumatic neurosis and other injuries. *Psychiatr Clin North Am.* 1983;6(4):661–683.

251. Keshavan MS, Channabasavanna SM, Reddy GN. Post-traumatic psychiatric disturbances: patterns and predictors of outcome. *Br J Psychiatry.* 1981;138:157–160.

252. Smith EM, North CS, McCool RE, et al. Acute postdisaster psychiatric disorders: identification of persons at risk. *Am J Psychiatry.* 1990;147:202–206.

253. Davidson J, Swartz M, Storck M, et al. A diagnostic and family study of posttraumatic stress disorder. *Am J Psychiatry.* 1985;142:90–93.

254. Breslau N, Davis GC. Posttraumatic stress disorder: the stressor criterion. *J Nerv Ment Dis.* 1987;175:255–264.

255. McDaniel E, McClelland P. Posttraumatic stress disorder. *Am Fam Physician.* 1986;34(2):180–189.

256. Sierles FS, Chen J-J, McFarland RE, et al. Posttraumatic stress disorder and concurrent psychiatric illness: a preliminary report. *Am J Psychiatry.* 1983;140:1177–1179.

257. Grime G. *Handbook of Road Safety Research.* London: Butterworth; 1987.

258. Mackay M. An historical perspective on impact biomechanics and some basic kinematics. In: Aldman B, Chapon A, eds. *The Biomechanics of Impact Trauma.* Amsterdam: ICTS; 1984.

259. Mackay M. Kinematics of vehicle crashes. *Adv Trauma.* 1987;2:21–42.

Chapter 2

History and Physical Examination Forms

Lawrence S. Nordhoff, Jr.

INTRODUCTION

This chapter provides the doctor with examples of the forms necessary to collect pertinent historical data and examination findings. Ways in which to make this process more effective are also discussed. Specific tests and their significance are discussed in Chapter 1. Obtaining a complete history and physical examination is important for patients with motor vehicle collision injuries (MVCIs). The objectives of properly obtaining and then documenting the history and examination data are fourfold, as follows:

1. to provide the clinician with one or more diagnostic impressions based on the mechanisms of the injury and its signs and symptoms, and the tolerance of the individual, providing the basis for developing a management plan and reimbursement

2. to set the stage for diagnostic tests that might be indicated immediately or in the future

3. to alert the doctor if the patient needs to be referred for further testing or evaluation

4. to provide future documentation for other physicians, the patient's lawyer, or the insurance carrier

Collecting pertinent information close to the time of the crash and most certainly at the time of the consultation is important because the occupant and the doctor may forget details relevant to the injury or prognosis. The MVCI is unique in the United States in that almost half of all these cases have legal representation, and the doctor must be able to provide data. Many patient intake forms currently used are too generalized, too outdated, or too brief. The detailed questionnaires presented in this chapter cover almost every aspect of the car accident case.

PATIENT HISTORY FORMS

The history paperwork starts when the patient shows up at the doctor's office, before the patient interview. The doctor's staff person who sets up the initial appointment needs to inform the incoming patient about the need to bring along any pertinent documentation, such as police reports and insurance company

70

information, and to allow about 15 to 20 minutes to complete the necessary preconsultation questionnaires. The patient should be carefully instructed in the purpose and importance of doing this paperwork. The forms should be filled out by the patient, returned to the front desk receptionist, and looked over to be certain that they have been completed and then given to the doctor to review on the first visit. Patients may overlook or forget to fill out questionnaire sections, and if located by the receptionist, should be completed before seeing the doctor. Next, the patient should be sent to the room in which the doctor will do the history interview and examination. The doctor should be given the information sheets prior to seeing the patient, so that the data can be previewed. The doctor should go over areas of question and expand on areas not clearly understood.

The main purpose for obtaining a detailed crash history and other patient questionnaires for the doctor in the MVCI case is to determine the mechanism of injury, the extent of injury, the types of tissues involved, and the appropriate examination or radiographic protocol. Exhibits 2–1, 2–2, 2–3, and 2–4 illustrate head injury, concussion, and post-traumatic symptom questionnaires, and a questionnaire that documents any prior treatment. These forms have been included for the reader's benefit as options, and the author does not imply that these are the standards for the industry.

In MVCI cases that do not resolve and instead develop the chronic pain syndromes common with car crashes, the initial questionnaire can become the focal point in determining factors that influenced the prognosis. Keep in mind that many patients who are represented by an attorney do not have their cases settled for more than 2 years. Most victims cannot remember details about the crash, their head restraints, bruises, severity of pain, and all the complex aspects of the injury. Although time consuming, the use of specific questionnaires is a must.

The initial office questionnaire needs to be tailored to the patient's injury location and presenting symptoms. The doctor's office should have available the following forms:

- automotive crash form
- patient introduction form
- general health history form
- head injury form (if head injury occurred)
- symptom chart that monitors progression
- forms that address specific complaints, such as headaches, neck pain, middle back pain, and low back pain—all in detail
- previous treatment forms

AUTOMOTIVE CRASH FORM

One of the most important medicolegal aspects to a personal injury case is obtaining a complete history of the crash, subsequent injury and/or symptoms, and any previous treatment. Exhibit 2–5 outlines a questionnaire that covers most car crashes seen in practice.

Specific literature on the appropriate history-taking techniques for the doctor is limited in personal injury. Controlled, randomized, clinical trials measuring the reliability and validity of specific history-taking procedures are absent in the MVCI as well. The intent of this chapter is to provide the practitioner with up-to-date forms that relate specifically to the MVCI. Regardless of the history-taking technique used, it is essential that the doctor spend adequate time and use appropriate forms to obtain the patient's account of the clinical problem and the nature of the crash.

In the MVCI case it is essential that the doctor obtain a copy of the police report and records of treatment by any emergency departments or other doctors seen. The doctor must review these records as soon as they are available. Reviewing the nature of the crash may save the

Exhibit 2–1 Head Injury Questionnaire

HOW DID YOU INJURE YOUR HEAD?

AUTO COLLISION

(Check what your head hit or what hit your head)

❏ Windshield   ❏ Steering wheel
❏ Dashboard   ❏ Side car window
❏ Other passenger   ❏ Mirror
❏ Other _____

WHAT PART OF YOUR HEAD WAS HIT?

❏ Front   ❏ Back
❏ Left side   ❏ Right side
❏ Top   ❏ Other

HISTORY

Yes No

❏ ❏   Did you lose consciousness or black out for any time (seconds or minutes) after the head injury? How long? _____

❏ ❏   Have you lost any memory before the head injury?

❏ ❏   Have you lost any memory or has your memory been different since the head injury?

❏ ❏   Did you have a lump or bruise after the head injury? Where? _____

❏ ❏   Have you had any head injuries in your past (include childhood)?

❏ ❏   Have you seen other doctors for this head injury?

❏ ❏   Have you had any X-rays taken?

❏ ❏   Have you had a computed tomography (CT) or magnetic resonance imaging (MRI) scan taken of your head?

doctor from an embarrassing situation. For example, the patient might lie as to how the injury occurred. The patient may have told the doctor that he or she was rear-ended at an intersection when in fact the patient was being chased by a tow truck driver who rammed the vehicle from the rear because the patient did not pay for gasoline at the gas station. Fault or criminal acts may be at issue. The emergency department may provide clues as to the types of injuries that the patient did not mention. Patients' recollections about the injury, what X-rays were done, and what the doctor told them may not be clear, especially recollections of patients with head injuries or those who were dazed after the injury.

Exhibit 2–2 Concussion Questionnaire

Please check the following boxes that correspond to any symptoms that you have had recently since your neck or head injury.

YES SYMPTOM
- ❑   Headaches
- ❑   Loss of coordination
- ❑   Reduced drive/motivation
- ❑   Poor memory
- ❑   Difficulty finishing tasks
- ❑   Sleep disorders
- ❑   Abnormal levels of anxiety
- ❑   Reduced tolerance to alcohol
- ❑   More assertive
- ❑   Forgetful
- ❑   Anger outbursts
- ❑   Depression
- ❑   Fatigue
- ❑   Absence of ability to anticipate
- ❑   Inflexibility
- ❑   Impaired sexual function
- ❑   Language difficulty
- ❑   Impaired judgment
- ❑   Need day-timer to remember home and/or work activities
- ❑   Blurry vision
- ❑   Loss of balance
- ❑   Difficulty handling multiple tasks
- ❑   Dizziness/lightheadedness
- ❑   Irritability
- ❑   Personality change
- ❑   Hand tremors
- ❑   Ringing in ears
- ❑   Less diplomatic than normal
- ❑   Mood swings
- ❑   Reduced attention span
- ❑   Blackouts
- ❑   Indifference to other people
- ❑   More shallow relationships
- ❑   Difficulty with problem solving
- ❑   Less mental stamina
- ❑   Performance inconsistencies
- ❑   Verbal learning problems
- ❑   Slower reaction times

Exhibit 2–3 Symptom Questionnaire

PATIENT INSTRUCTIONS: It is important for this section to be filled out in detail. CHECK if you have had any single or multiple symptom(s) listed below. Leave row blank if the symptom listed does not apply to you.

Symptom List	Felt Right after Injury	Felt 24–48 Hours Later	Have Symptoms Now	Had Similar Symptoms 1–3 Months before This Injury
Headache				
Dizziness				
Tinnitus (ear ringing)				
Blurry vision				
Memory problems				
Poor concentration				
Irritability				
Balance problems				
Loss of coordination				
Sensitivity to sound				
Sensitivity to light				
Fatigue				
Anxiety				
Pain/difficulty swallowing				
Jaw pain				
Neck pain/soreness				
Neck stiffness				
Shoulder pain/stiffness				
Arm pain/tingling/numbness				
Wrist/hand/finger pain/numbness				
Weakness in arms/legs				
Upper/mid back pain				
Chest wall pain (rib)				
Low back pain/soreness				
Hip pain				
Leg pain				
Leg numbness/tingling				
Pain shoots down legs				
Knee pain				
Ankle/foot pain				
Other				

Exhibit 2–4 Prior Treatment Questionnaire

LIST ALL DOCTORS, TESTS, AND TREATMENT SINCE INJURY

Start with the first doctor/office/hospital you saw after your injury and check all that apply:

---

(1)

Name hospital/doctor/therapist/center: _____

Address: _____ Date: _____

Indicate what was done:

- ❑ Exam-consultation
- ❑ X-ray of neck
- ❑ X-ray of low back
- ❑ Other X-rays
- ❑ MRI/CT scan
- ❑ Other diagnostic test
- ❑ Rehabilitation
- ❑ Physical therapy
- ❑ Exercises recommended

- ❑ Medications prescribed
- ❑ Neck collar
- ❑ Spinal manipulation/adjustments
- ❑ Muscle massage/myotherapy
- ❑ Low back brace
- ❑ Heat packs
- ❑ Cold/ice packs
- ❑ Ultrasound
- ❑ Other

Indicate if treatment: ❑ Made condition worse   ❑ Did not help   ❑ Helped

---

(2)

Name hospital/doctor/therapist/center seen: _____

Address: _____ Date: _____

Indicate what was done:

- ❑ Exam-consultation
- ❑ X-ray of neck
- ❑ X-ray of low back
- ❑ Other X-rays
- ❑ MRI/CT scan
- ❑ Other diagnostic test
- ❑ Rehabilitation
- ❑ Physical therapy
- ❑ Exercises recommended

- ❑ Medications prescribed
- ❑ Neck collar
- ❑ Spinal manipulation/adjustments
- ❑ Muscle massage/myotherapy
- ❑ Low back brace
- ❑ Heat packs
- ❑ Cold/ice packs
- ❑ Ultrasound
- ❑ Other

Indicate if treatment: ❑ Made condition worse   ❑ Did not help   ❑ Helped

continues

Exhibit 2–4 continued

---

(3)

Name hospital/doctor/therapist/center seen: _____

Address: _____ Date: _____

Indicate what was done:

- ❑ Exam-consultation
- ❑ X-ray of neck
- ❑ X-ray of low back
- ❑ Other X-rays
- ❑ MRI/CT scan
- ❑ Other diagnostic test
- ❑ Rehabilitation
- ❑ Physical therapy
- ❑ Exercises/stretching

- ❑ Medications prescribed
- ❑ Neck collar
- ❑ Spinal manipulation/adjustments
- ❑ Muscle massage/myotherapy
- ❑ Low back brace
- ❑ Heat packs
- ❑ Cold/ice packs
- ❑ Ultrasound
- ❑ Other

Indicate if treatment: ❑ Made condition worse   ❑ Did not help   ❑ Helped

---

PATIENT INTERVIEW

After the history forms are completed and the doctor has had time to review the records, the patient interview begins with an introduction. The doctor should introduce himself or herself to the patient and attempt to create a relaxed atmosphere. Some patients may deny or avoid discussion of previous pain or injuries because of fears about insurance or legal system ramifications. The patient needs to be encouraged that full disclosure of his or her past history relating to this injury is important. It is relatively easy to document intensity and frequency of previous problems. If the patient persists in not wanting the doctor to document previous injuries, a decision then must be made about the credibility of the patient and whether the patient was coaxed by an attorney or a friend.

During the interview process, be alert to discrepancies in the history. Although uncommon, a patient may be exaggerating facts about the injury, may be distorting the truth about how the accident occurred, or may have

monetary motivations. One particular case emphasizes the need to read police reports and compare what they say with what the patient says in the history. For example, Stacie was 21 years old and was driving a new Toyota truck; she states in the history that she was making a U-turn on a road when another truck rear-ended her truck, probably because the other truck could not stop soon enough. The police report showed that in fact she was playing a prank on a friend whereby she went to a gas station, filled her tank, and left without paying the bill. The gas station attendant chased her in a tow truck, not wanting her to escape, and deliberately rammed the back of her truck. This case ended up as a civil suit that became very complicated.

If the patient personally brings in any records or the doctor receives any records in the mail, it is important that the doctor read them. Inconsistencies may be found that could ultimately damage the credibility of the doctor. The defense attorney could ask the doctor on the stand a question such as: "Doctor, is it customary for you to request records from

Exhibit 2–5 Automotive Crash Form

BILLING INFORMATION

Patient name: _____

Date of injury: _____ Time of injury:_____ ❏ AM ❏ PM

City and street where crash occurred: _____

What is the estimated damage to your vehicle? $ _____

❏ Yes ❏ No   Do you have automobile medical insurance coverage?

Name/address/phone _____

_____

What is your car insurance medical coverage limit? $ _____

What is the claim number? _____

❏ Yes ❏ No   Do you know the claims adjuster's name? _____

❏ Yes ❏ No   Have you reported this injury to your car insurance company?

❏ Yes ❏ No   Did the police come to the accident scene and make a report?

❏ Yes ❏ No   Is an attorney representing you? Name/address/phone: _____

_____

AUTO ACCIDENT DESCRIPTION

Describe how the crash happened

_____

_____

_____

_____

_____

_____

_____

_____

_____

_____

Collision Description

Check all that apply to you:

❏ Single-car crash   ❏ Two-vehicle crash   ❏ More than three vehicles

❏ Rear-end crash   ❏ Side crash   ❏ Rollover

❏ Head-on crash   ❏ Hit guardrail/tree   ❏ Ran off road

You were the

❏ Driver   ❏ Front passenger   ❏ Rear passenger

Describe the vehicle you were in

Model year and make:

❏ Subcompact car   ❏ Compact car   ❏ Mid-sized car

❏ Full-sized car   ❏ Pickup truck   ❏ Larger than 1 ton vehicle

continues

Exhibit 2–5 continued

Describe the other vehicle
Model year and make:
❑ Subcompact car   ❑ Compact car   ❑ Mid-sized car
❑ Full-sized car   ❑ Pickup truck   ❑ Larger than 1 ton vehicle

Estimated crash speeds
Estimate how fast your vehicle was moving at time of crash.   _____ mph
Estimate how fast the other vehicle was moving at time of crash.   _____ mph

At the time of impact your vehicle was
❑ Slowing down ❑ Stopped   ❑ Gaining speed   ❑ Moving at steady speed

At the time of impact the other vehicle was
❑ Slowing down ❑ Stopped   ❑ Gaining speed   ❑ Moving at steady speed

During and after the crash, your vehicle
❑ Kept going straight, not hitting anything ❑ Spun around, not hitting anything
❑ Kept going straight, hitting car in front ❑ Spun around, hitting another car
❑ Was hit by another vehicle ❑ Spun around, hitting object other than car

Describe yourself during the crash
Check only the areas that apply to you:
❑ You were unaware of the impending collision.
❑ You were aware of the impending crash and relaxed before the collision.
❑ You were aware of the impending crash and braced yourself.
❑ Your body, torso, and head were facing straight ahead.
❑ You had your head and/or torso turned at the time of collision:
    ❑ Turned to left   ❑ Turned to right
❑ You were intoxicated (alcohol) at the time of crash.
❑ You were wearing a seat belt.
    If yes, does your seat belt have a shoulder harness?   ❑ Yes   ❑ No
❑ You were holding onto the steering wheel at the time of impact.

Indicate if your body hit something or was hit by any of the following
Please draw lines and match the left side to the right side.

Head	Windshield
Face	Steering wheel
Shoulder	Side door
Neck	Dashboard
Chest	Car frame
Hip	Another occupant
Knee	Seat
Foot	Seat belt

Check if any of the following vehicle parts broke, bent, or were damaged in your car
❑ Windshield   ❑ Seat frame   ❑ Knee bolster
❑ Steering wheel   ❑ Side/rear window   ❑ Other _____
❑ Dash   ❑ Mirror   ❑ Other _____

continues

Exhibit 2–5 continued

Rear-end collisions only

Answer this section only if you were hit from the rear.

Does your vehicle have

❑ Movable head restraints

❑ Fixed, nonmovable head restraints

❑ No head restraints

Please indicate how your head restraint was positioned at the time of crash.*

❑ At the top of the back of your head

❑ Midway height of the back of your head

❑ Lower height of the back of your head

❑ Located at the level of your neck

❑ Located at the level of your shoulder blades (upper back) below neck

*Estimate the distance between the back of your head and the front of the head restraint. _____ inches

All types of collisions

Answer this section regardless of the type of crash, indicating those relevant to your case.

Yes	No	
❑	❑	Did any of the front or side structures, such as the side door, dashboard, or floorboard of your car, dent inward during the crash?
❑	❑	Did the side door touch your body during the crash?
❑	❑	Was your hand(s) on the steering wheel or dash during the crash?
❑	❑	Did your body slide under the seat belt?
❑	❑	Was the door(s) of your vehicle damaged to the point where you could not open the door?

Emergency department

Yes	No	
❑	❑	Did you go to the emergency department after the accident? What is name of the emergency department? _____ When did you go (date and time)? _____
❑	❑	Did you go to the emergency department in an ambulance?
❑	❑	Did you or another person drive you to the emergency department?
❑	❑	Were you hospitalized overnight?
❑	❑	Did the emergency department doctor take X-rays? Check what was taken: ❑ Skull ❑ Neck ❑ Low back ❑ Arm or leg
❑	❑	Did the emergency department doctor give you pain medications?
❑	❑	Did the emergency department doctor give you muscle relaxants?
❑	❑	Did you have any cuts or lacerations?
❑	❑	Did you require any stitching for cuts?
❑	❑	Were you given a neck collar or back brace to wear?

continues

Exhibit 2–5 continued

When did you first notice any pain after injury?
❑ Immediately   ❑ _____ Hours after injury   ❑ _____ Days after injury

If you did not see a doctor for the first time within the first week, indicate why
Check all that apply
❑ No pain was noticed   ❑ No appointment schedule available
❑ No transportation   ❑ Work/home schedule conflicts

If you did not see a doctor for the first time within the first month after injury, indicate why
Check all that apply
❑ No pain was noticed   ❑ No appointment schedule available
❑ No transportation   ❑ Work/home schedule conflicts
❑ I thought pain would go away   ❑ I had no insurance or money
❑ I self-treated with over-the-counter drugs   ❑ I took hot showers, used ice, heat

Have you been unable to work since injury?
❑ Yes   ❑ No   If yes, you were off work ❑ partially or ❑ completely
Please list dates off work: _____ to _____.

---

other treating doctors and, if so, is it also reasonable that you would read them over?"

Some represented MVCI cases that are attempting to settle may be argued by plaintiff and defense sides. This is especially true for cases requiring extensive treatment or having questionable merit and when the defense or the plaintiff is considering going to court. The truth about the victim's injury severity may be difficult to discern in some cases; therefore, the doctor's notes may provide the necessary information to substantiate the injury levels and the disability associated with the injury. When the physician writes a narrative report at the close of the case, an impartial opinion should be given as to any conclusions regarding apportionment issues (pre-existing problems) and any future care needed.

Any notes taken during the interview should be recorded in the descriptions used by the patient. Quotation marks can be used to document accurate descriptions.

Defense lawyers may take the position that the doctor or the patient deliberately hides relevant injuries or pain. The defense may con-tend that old injuries and degenerative changes are responsible for the present symptoms. The plaintiff's attorney in a legal case will take the position that the patient was asymptomatic before this injury, and that all current symptoms are solely due to this injury and apportionment is not an issue.

PHYSICAL EXAMINATION FORMS

In the current medicolegal environment, the doctor should use forms that show the customary examinations that every personal injury patient undergoes. If 10 to 20 orthopedic and neurologic tests on the office form were not performed and spaces on the form were left blank, the doctor's testimony in a deposition or trial probably will not be considered valid. The examination form should include all tests that are standard in the doctor's community, according to professional degree and specialty. Exhibit 2–6 illustrates a sample form that would allow a clinician to document many injuries. Additional tests should be

Exhibit 2–6 Examination Form

❑ New Examination   ❑ Comparative Examination   ❑ IME/AME

Patient Name: _____   Date: _____

This patient appears: ❑ Alert and oriented to time, place, and person   ❑ Confused

Postural evaluation: ❑ Normal erect posture   ❑ Torticollis/antalgia to L/R side

Height: _____ inches   Weight: _____ pounds   B/P _____/_____ mm Hg

HEAD INJURY/CONCUSSION EXAMINATION

Exam	WNL	Abnormal Findings
Pupillary checks (PERRLA)		
Cranial nerve exam		
Romberg's test—feet together (eyes open) cerebellar		
Romberg's test—feet together (eyes closed) posterior column		
Tandem Romberg's test—(eyes open) (heel-to-toe)		
Tandem Romberg's test—(eyes closed) (heel-to-toe)		
Standing heel-to-shin balance testing—posterior column		
Finger-to-nose testing (note accuracy and speed)		
Have patient count from 100 backward in 3s		
Short-term memory (ask patient to repeat complex sentence)		
Long-term memory		
Amnesia (retrograde or anterograde)		

PATHOLOGIC TESTS

Test	WNL	Abnormal Findings
Pathologic or clonic reflexes (upper motor)		
Vibratory testing for lateral tract involvement		
Babinski reflexes (upper motor)		
Vertebral artery ischemia testing (George's test)		

EXTERNAL/INTERNAL INJURY SIGNS

Signs	Not Present/Normal	Present/Abnormal
Abrasions/lacerations/bruising		
Suturing/casting/bracing		
Neck measurement (C-5 level)		
Supraclavicular notch swelling		
Patient has difficulty or unable to ❑ lift head ❑ sit		
Seat belt sign: ❑ neck ❑ chest ❑ abdomen-hip		

REFLEXES (MOTOR)

Nerve Level	Left Side	Right Side
Biceps (C-5 to C-6) axillary nerve		
Triceps (C-7 to C-8) radial nerve		
Radial (C-6) musculocutaneous nerve		
Patellar (L-3 to L-4) L-4 root		
Achilles (L-5 to S-1) S-1 root		

Explanation

0 = Absent

1 = Needs facilitation

2 = Normal

3 = Hyperactive

4 = Clonus

continues

Exhibit 2–6 continued

MUSCLE STRENGTH TESTING

	Normal Strength	Weakens Early with Repeated Testing	Weakness Noted on First Test (Note Grade)
Shoulder abduction—deltoid muscle (C-5)		L R	L R
Elbow flexion—biceps muscle (C-6)		L R	L R
Elbow extension—triceps muscle (C-7)		L R	L R
Wrist flexors (C-8)		L R	L R
Finger interossi (T-1)		L R	L R
Quadriceps and psoas muscles (L-2 & L-3 nerve roots)		L R	L R
Tibialis anterior muscle (L-4 nerve root)		L R	L R
Extensor hallucis muscle (L-5 nerve root)		L R	L R
Gastronemius/hamstring muscles (S-1/S-2 nerve roots)		L R	L R

DYNAMOMETER GRIP TESTING

Grip tested in pounds. Indicate dominant hand.	Test 1	Test 2	Test 3
Left hand			
Right hand			

ORTHOPEDIC TESTING

Region	Test Procedure Name	Normal	Local Pain Only	Radiating Pain
Cervical	Shoulder distraction testing			
	Forminal compression testing:			
	Neutral position			
	Left lateral flexion			
	Right lateral flexion			
	Left lateral flexion with rotation			
	Right lateral flexion with rotation			
	Neck flexion stress test (Soto Hall)			
	Valsalva neck maneuver			
Lumbar	Lasegue's test sitting and supine. The pain intensifies at ____° left, ____° right leg		L R B	L R B
	Kemp's test		L R B	L R B
	Valsalva sit test (head flexed, legs extended)			
	Heel walk (L-4 to L-5)		❏ Weak	N/A
	Toe walk (L-5 to S-1)		❏ Weak	N/A
	SI joint stress testing (Yeoman's, Ely's)		❏ SI pain	❏ LBP

L = Left   R = Right   B = Bilateral   LBP = Low back pain   SI = Sacroiliac

EXTREMITY MEASUREMENTS

Region	Left Side (cm)	Right Side (cm)
Middle biceps muscle		
Middle forearm		
Thigh (6 inches above patella)		
Calf (at thickest portion)		

continues

Exhibit 2–6 continued

SENSORY EXAMINATION

☐ Sensory exam for cervical and lumbar regions is normal.

Left Side		*Dermatome*	*Right Side*	
Hyperesthesia	*Hypoesthesia*		*Hypoesthesia*	*Hyperesthesia*
		C-3		
		C-4		
		C-5		
		C-6		
		C-7		
		T-1		
		L-3		
		L-4		
		L-5		
		S-1		
		S-2		

DIGITAL PALPATION FINDINGS

Mark as follows: + = Slight, ++ = Moderate, +++ = Severe

Left Side				*Spine Level*		*Right Side*		
Fibrotic Texture	*Boggy Edema*	*Muscle Spasm*	*Pain Level*		*Pain Level*	*Muscle Spasm*	*Boggy Edema*	*Fibrotic Texture*
				Occ				
				C-1				
				C-2				
				C-3				
				C-4				
				C-5				
				C-6				
				C-7				
				T-1				
				T-2				
				T-3				
				T-4				
				T-5				
				T-6				
				T-7				
				T-8				
				T-9				
				T-10				
				T-11				
				T-12				
				L-1				
				L-2				
				L-3				
				L-4				
				L-5				
				S-1				

continues

Exhibit 2–6 continued

RANGE-OF-MOTION (ROM) ASSESSMENT

Cervical ROM ROM done in degrees using digital inclinometer	Active ROM (Patient performs)	Pain Intensifies at Middle and End Range	Pain Intensifies Only at End Range
Flexion	60/		
Extension	50/		
Left lateral flexion	40/		
Right lateral flexion	40/		
Left rotation	80/		
Right rotation	80/		

Lumbar ROM			
Flexion. Distance floor to finger tip	inches		
Extension	30/		
Left lateral flexion	20/		
Right lateral flexion	20/		
Left rotation	30/		
Right rotation	30/		

Passive cervical lateral bending (doctor) shows:

Left: ❑ Normal   ❑ Bony end-feel   ❑ Boggy end-feel
Right: ❑ Normal   ❑ Bony end-feel   ❑ Boggy end-feel

Thoracic ROM (Passive spring testing):   ❑ WNL   ❑ Bony end-feel   ❑ Boggy end-feel
                                                              limited motion   limited motion

MYOFASCIAL EVALUATION

Muscle or Muscle Groups Palpated	Tender to Touch	Boggy and Swollen	Fibrotic and Tender	Trigger Point	Side of Body
Scalp adhesions (posttraumatic)					L R B
Temporalis					L R B
Masseter					L R B
Sternocleidomastoid					L R B
Trapezius					L R B
Scalenes					L R B
Teres minor					L R B
Levator scapulae					L R B
Pectoralis major/minor					L R B
Rhomboids					L R B
Intercostals					L R B
Quadratus lumborum					L R B
Piriformis					L R B
Other					L R B

C-5 Nerve root/thoracic outlet syndrome tests	WNL	Positive
Arm abduction relief test (C-5 root)		
Shoulder flexion/abduction, external rotation provocative test (C-5 root)		
Bilateral arm abduction/external rotation, hand opening/closing stamina test (thoracic outlet syndrome test). How many minutes before arm drop?		

done when indicated and added to the examination form. The form should include a glossary of abbreviations if the doctor uses nonstandard terminology. There should be some notation as to who did the examination. It is not advised that an intern or another doctor do these examinations. Several suggestions that will aid the doctor doing the various types of examinations are given below.

External Body Injury Evaluation

Looking at the outer body of the crash occupant can give clues to injury extent, injury sites, and potential complications. The first area of concern is evaluation of contusions and lacerations and descriptions of their location, size, and severity. Second, if the occupant was wearing a seat belt, looking for obvious or subtle bruising along the belt line is extremely important. Bruising should be looked for along the neck, anterior chest wall, abdomen, and pelvic areas. The "seat belt sign" has a notable risk of internal complications such as cardiac contusion or visceral ruptures. If known, the doctor should note how the external body injuries occurred. Ask the patient whether he or she hit the windshield or metal car frame or was hit by another occupant, as may be the case. The more rigid the object the more potentially harmful the injury.

Another area of interest is visually examining the supraclavicular notch for unilateral or bilateral swelling, primarily in rear-end collisions in which the scalene and sternocleidomastoid muscles are traumatized. In moderate to severe injuries the notch may be absent as a result of bleeding caused by injury to the sternocleidomastoid and scalene muscles. Gravitational forces will cause the inflammatory exudates to migrate below the clavicle and under the pectoral muscles. These fluids move between the fascial planes.

Photographs should be taken of every MVCI bruise or laceration and kept in the patient's records.

Orthopedic/Neurologic Testing

When performing orthopedic and neurologic tests, it is important for the doctor to take the time briefly to describe to the patient what is going to be done and what verbal responses the patient is being tested for, if any. The patient needs to understand that many of these tests are provocative and need to be performed to establish the degree of injury and the types of tissues injured, to determine the diagnosis, and to differentiate complicating factors. For example, when doing the cervical foraminal compression test, the doctor needs to tell the patient that he or she is going to push down gently on the patient's head in several positions. The patient is instructed to tell the doctor immediately if there is any increase in neck pain or any pain or numbness in the upper extremity occurring as a result of the hand pressure. The patient is not told of the significance of the results until the time a report is given, to ensure that the patient is not exaggerating responses.

Range-of-motion evaluations should be performed on all areas injured. Notations should be made as to when the patient notes increased pain, as muscle injuries will cause pain before the ligaments are stretched. The type of end-feel should be noted as well. In the acutely injured patient the end-feel is usually boggy or mushy because of the edema around the joint capsular tissues. In the chronically injured patient a bony or abrupt end-feel in the cervical spine joints is frequently noted on the injured side. When doing range-of-motion testing it is not as important to compare the patient's measurements with normalized standards as it is to note asymmetric loss of motion. Normalized standards do not take into account the patient's age, pre-existing stiffness, or degenerative joint diseases that may limit motion. For example, patients with cervical spondylosis will have reduced extension and lateral flexion.[1] If the examiner suspects the patient of deliberately limiting his or her range of motion, the doctor later during the exam can ask the patient to look at an anatomic chart of some type. The doctor holds the chart at a position that requires the patient to rotate the head about 70 to 80 degrees. If the patient is able to do this on one side, the other side can be tested later.

Motor Testing

When doing motor evaluation,[2] weakness may be difficult to discern when the patient is exaggerating responses or is inattentive, and when pain interferes with ability. During extremity muscle (motor) testing[3] the doctor is advised to use comparative active resistance techniques. The patient should perform the action requested by the doctor to his or her limits (push, pull, grip, etc.) but never to the point of causing severe pain. The action then should be repeated or sustained to see whether the muscle being stressed fatigues early or gives way. Stressing the muscle for 15 to 20 seconds may detect subtle weakness not observed in single maximal resistance moves. The doctor may use variable resistance in patients who are suspected of exaggerating weakness, i.e., rapidly vary the amount of resistance faster than the patient can respond to it. The threshold for overcoming resistance should be consistent. It is important to consider the patient's age, severity of pain, and physical condition when doing this testing, and then test the patient accordingly.

Dynamometer grip testing is a useful technique for evaluation of upper-extremity weakness, keeping in mind that the dominant side usually has about 10% more strength.

The acutely injured patient should have extremity girth measurements taken initially. These measurements can then be compared with those of chronically injured patients who develop neuropathies and subsequent muscle atrophy.

When performing deep tendon reflex testing it is advised that the reflex hammer be appropriate for the area being tested. Small hammers work well in the upper extremity and jaw regions. Larger, heavier, circular hammers work well on the lower extremities. If reflexes are absent or very sluggish, the doctor can use a facilitative reflex maneuver to heighten the normal reflex responses. For example, if attempting to establish an Achilles tendon reflex, have the patient sit in a chair with feet off the floor. Have the patient very gently push the toes down against the doctor's hand as the doctor simultaneously strikes the Achilles tendon with the reflex hammer. This technique works better than the distractive maneuvers. By using the facilitative reflex maneuver the author has observed several cases of clonic reflexes that were missed when doing the reflex by traditional methods. These cases usually involve subtle spinal cord bruising from high neck injury forces. Upper motor lesions can be confirmed by pathologic jaw reflexes.

Sensory Examinations

Sensory examinations of the extremities and neck and back frequently are performed with a pin or brush. Pinwheels, if used, need to be sterilized between patients and should be pretested for jamming before use. One medical roundtable[3] suggests that when performing an extremity sensory examination, the doctor should ask the patient whether the sensation produced by the pin on the skin is sharp, and whether it is as sharp as on the other side. If the patient says no, the doctor should try putting more pressure with the pin on the extremity that is symptomatic and less pressure on the opposite extremity to see whether the patient notices differences in sensation.

Sensory examinations on upper and lower extremities should be done on both sides at the same time. This allows the patient an easier comparison. The doctor needs to be sure that the pressure was exerted equally during the examination and should repeat the test once or twice when a patient is not sure of any discrepancies.

When testing for vibration loss, it is suggested that the examiner have the patient close the eyes when the test is performed. Test both sides with the tuning fork both vibrating and not vibrating to determine whether the patient actually is able to differentiate. Vibration testing using a 256-Hz tuning fork will pick up more subtle deficits. As the cord is pushed posterior from an anterior lesion, vibration may be altered in legs and feet from long tract compression. Posterior column lesions may decrease vibration, tactile sense, and position sense.[4] Vibration testing also is accurate for testing acute peripheral nerve compression.[5]

Palpation Evaluation

When doing the myofascial palpation examination, it is important for the doctor to look at the pain drawing (if used in his or her office) that was filled out by the patient and to be attentive to patient feedback during the examination. It is suggested that the palpation examination start in the noninjured or less painful areas first. The pain drawing can assist the doctor in locating sites. Attempting to get a sense of what the normal soft tissue consistency and texture are prior to palpating the injured area will help the examiner differentiate injury-related problems from the pre-existing problems. Some MVCI patients have pre-existing myofascial problems such as fibrotic muscles from previous tension, injury, or ergonomic stresses. As these patients should be treated to preinjury status, the doctor has to determine or estimate the patient's status just prior to the car crash.

In the patient with acute pain, begin the palpation examination by gently feeling larger painful areas for warmth comparisons between sides and various spinal areas. Then begin the evaluation of the underlying muscles. The doctor should gently probe and feel for texture and tone. Findings such as edema, bogginess, muscle spasm, and patient response to pressure should be noted. Deeper pressure should locate any pre-existing fibrotic texture abnormalities. In the patient with chronic pain, muscle consistency findings such as fibrotic, ropy muscles; adhesions; and trigger points are noted. Figure 2–1 illustrates one method to document chronic soft tissue abnormalities, such as myofascial adhesions and trigger points. Other methods to document soft tissue abnormalities are discussed in Chapter 6, Part 2. Tissue compliance meters may objectively measure muscle spasm and muscle tone abnormalities.[6] If the doctor uses the various pressure threshold and tissue compliance meters to validate injury and response to treatment, appropriate forms need to be utilized so that comparisons may be made over time.

When palpating for joint motion or joint play in the neck or extremities, the doctor should describe the end-feel, as these notations verify the extent of soft tissue injury and what tissues are involved. For example, if bony end-play is noted between two spinal joints when laterally bending the neck, then articular fixation from some mechanism is apparent. If bogginess is felt in the end-range, then capsular swelling is present.

Pathologic end-feel is most useful for extremity injuries and may be detected in shoulder, elbow, knee, or ankle injuries following MVCI. The pathologic end-feel may feel as though the joint is going to dislocate. The author has found that pathologic end-feel results most commonly in the frontal crash driver who was holding onto the steering wheel and the humerus was rammed posteriorly, causing severe ligament and/or osseous injury. Another common antecedent of pathologic end-feel is the posterior cruciate ligament injury in which the front-seat occupant's knee, specifically the anterior-superior tibial surface, strikes the knee bolster, causing posterior motion and ligament rupture.

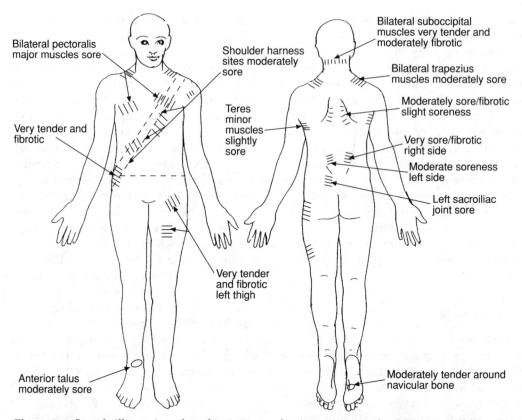

Bilateral pectoralis major muscles sore

Shoulder harness sites moderately sore

Bilateral suboccipital muscles very tender and moderately fibrotic

Bilateral trapezius muscles moderately sore

Moderately sore/fibrotic slight soreness

Teres minor muscles slightly sore

Very tender and fibrotic

Very sore/fibrotic right side

Moderate soreness left side

Left sacroiliac joint sore

Very tender and fibrotic left thigh

Anterior talus moderately sore

Moderately tender around navicular bone

Figure 2–1 Sample illustration of a palpation exam from a patient involved in a 30-mph frontal crash with significant chest wall pain, middle back pain, low back pain, and left leg pain at 4 months.

REFERENCES

1. Batzdorf U. Differential diagnosis of arm and thoracic radicular pain and sensory disturbance. *Spine State Art Rev.* 1988;2(4):565–583.

2. Stewart JD. *Focal Peripheral Neuropathies.* New York: Elsevier Science Publishing Co; 1987.

3. Asbury AK, Dyck PJ, Johnson AC, et al. A focused workup for neuropathy, a patient care roundtable. *Patient Care.* April 15, 1985:136–151.

4. Goodman BW Jr. Neck pain. *Prim Care.* 1988; 15(44):689–707.

5. Szabo R, Gelberman RH, Williamson RV, et al. Vibratory sensory testing in acute peripheral nerve compressions. *J Hand Surg (Am).* 1984;9:104–108.

6. Fischer AA. Objective measurement of muscle spasms, and pressure algometry in evaluation of myofascial trigger points, fibromyalgia, and arthritis. In: Roland MO, Jenner JR, eds. *Back Pain: New Approaches to Rehabilitation and Education.* Manchester, England: Manchester University Press; 1989:chap 6.

SUGGESTED READINGS

Cailliet R. *Neck and Arm Pain.* 3rd ed. Philadelphia: FA Davis Co; 1991.

Cailliet R. *Soft Tissue Pain and Disability.* 2nd ed. Philadelphia: FA Davis Co; 1988.

Chase DC, Hendler BH, Kraus SL. Spelling relief for TMJ troubles. *Patient Care.* 1988;158–161.

Diamond S, Dalessio DJ. *The Practicing Physician's Approach to Headache.* 4th ed. Baltimore: Williams & Wilkins; 1986.

Eliyahu DJB. Disc herniations of the cervical spine. *Am J Chir Med*. 1989;2(3):93–100.

Fitz-Ritson D. Assessment of cervicogenic vertigo. *J Manipulative Physiol Ther*. 1991;14(3):193–198.

Gerstner DL, Omer GE Jr. Peripheral entrapment neuropathies in the upper extremity, part I: key differential findings, median nerve syndromes. *J Musculoskel Med*. 1988;5(3):14–29.

Gillespie BR. Assessment and treatment of TMJ muscles, fascia, ligaments, and associated structures. *J Craniomandibular Pract*. 1990;8(1):51–55.

Goldstein J. Posttraumatic headache and the postconcussion syndrome. *Med Clin North Am*. 1991;75(3):641–651.

Hodge CJ. Vehicular impact and its relationship to TMJ dysfunction syndrome. *Med Trial Tech Q*. 1990;36:230–234.

Janda V. Muscle spasm: a proposed procedure for differential diagnosis. *J Manual Med*. 1991;6:136–139.

Kunkel RS. Diagnosis and treatment of muscle contraction (tension-type) headaches. *Med Clin North Am*. 1991;75(3):595–603.

Magee DJ. *Orthopedic Physical Assessment*. Philadelphia: WB Saunders Co; 1987.

Mondell BE. Evaluation of the patient presenting with headache. *Med Clin North Am*. 1991;75(3):521–525.

Nassif NJ. A brief self-administered questionnaire for craniomandibular disorders (CMD): rationale, patient complaints, and craniomandibular symptoms. *J Craniomandibular Pract*. 1989;7(1):63–69.

Post M. *Physical Examination of the Musculoskeletal System*. Chicago: Year Book Medical Publishers; 1987.

Speed WG III. Posttraumatic headache. In: Diamond S, Dalessio DJ, eds. *The Practicing Physician's Approach to Headache*. 4th ed. Baltimore: Williams & Wilkins; 1986:113–119.

Ziegler DK, Hassanein RS, Couch JR. Headache syndromes suggested by statistical analysis of headache symptoms. *Cephalalgia*. 1982;2:125–134.

Chapter 3

Radiologic Evaluation of Cervical Spine Trauma

Tyrone Wei and Timothy Sellers

INTRODUCTION

Radiologic evaluation has long been considered an integral part of the diagnostic work-up of any patient who has experienced trauma to the cervical spine.[1–12] This is particularly important to doctors and therapists who utilize spinal manipulation as part of their therapeutic regimen. Plain film studies are relatively inexpensive and provide essential information about the skeletal structures as well as the surrounding soft tissues, including the paraspinal ligaments, intervertebral disc spaces, and cervical musculature. While these studies are much less sensitive than special imaging procedures such as computed tomography (CT) and magnetic resonance imaging (MRI), their accessibility and affordability make them the initial procedure of choice in the diagnostic work-up.[1,2,12,13] In cases in which radiographs fail to provide the necessary structural information, follow-up special imaging studies relevant to the patient's suspected injury should be obtained.[1,2,4,14,15]

Following a thorough history and physical or regional examination, plain film studies should be obtained prior to manipulation of the patient.[8,10,11] The importance of obtaining a high-quality series appropriate to the type of injury cannot be overemphasized.[3,9,12,15]

Although the patient has a history of trauma and the initial concern is with abnormalities that may be the result of this trauma, it is important for the evaluator to take note of any nontraumatic abnormalities, such as underlying pathology or congenital anomalies. Minor injuries might not be detected radiographically,[1,16–18] and it has been well documented that many patients continue to have symptoms despite the absence of abnormal radiographic signs.[3,17,18] If the physical examination results and radiographs fail to demonstrate any abnormalities that would contraindicate the desired form of therapy, treatment may be initiated at that time.

RADIOGRAPHIC PROJECTIONS EMPLOYED IN ACUTE CERVICAL SPINE INJURY

Limited radiographic examination of the cervical spine should include a minimum of three projections: the anteroposterior (AP) open mouth (APOM), anteroposterior lower cervical, and lateral cervical. Often the APOM projection is neglected, but since the upper cervical projection cannot be visualized adequately in the AP lower cervical projection, the APOM projection should be regarded as essential. Ligamentous injury with laterolisthesis creating asymmetry of the periodontoid space can be viewed only in this projection.

Evaluation of the intervertebral foramina requires additional oblique projections. These projections should be included in the initial study in patients presenting with upper-extremity radicular symptoms and those with signs of nerve root compression. Patients with significant degenerative hypertrophic changes should also be evaluated with these projections in order to demonstrate the extent of the resulting stenosis. Segmental motion can be further studied by including flexion and extension lateral projections. These projections may not be appropriate during the initial study, however, unless there is absence of severe splinting muscle spasm, as this type of hypertonicity will often mask an area of instability. In this case, these stress views may be better deferred for 2 to 3 weeks posttrauma until the acute spasm subsides.

Swimmer's lateral projection is employed when the lower cervical spine cannot be visualized adequately in the routine lateral projection or when the upper thoracic spine needs to be evaluated. It has been found that there is an increased incidence of fracture at T-1 to T-4 when the head hits the windshield or header while the neck is in a flexed position. This occurs because much of the kinetic energy is focused at these levels during impact. Proper evaluation of this area with the swimmer's lateral projection should be included in the initial study in patients presenting with such a history. Pillar views are occasionally employed to demonstrate the posterior structures of the cervical spine.

Fracture of the inferior occiput may occur in hyperextension injuries. Skull study should be considered if there are persistent symptoms in this area. Routine skull study, however, provides less than 10% yield in detecting fractures.[19] This number would be even lower for ambulatory patients. It is one author's opinion that skull study be entertained only in patients with persistent symptomatology or in the presence of a normal cervical spine study in patients with severe symptoms. Furthermore, any persistent neurologic deficits can be better assessed by CT and MRI.

Guidelines for Initial and Follow-Up Procedures in Acute Cervical Spine Injury

There is little doubt that radiographic analysis of the cervical spine following hyperflexion and hyperextension injury plays a vital role in the initial work-up, facilitating a complete diagnosis and proper management; however, there is a lack of established standards regarding the makeup, that is, the types of projections necessary for an adequate study. Figure 3–1 is an algorithm illustrating a general guide for radiographic procedures in acute cervical spine injury. It is the intention that this guideline be used as a basis for ordering radiographic studies but not serve as a rigid rule. Follow-up radiographic studies should vary from the initial work-up. For example, AP projections are seldom necessary unless there is evidence of new pain or new trauma. The most useful comparison is the flexion-extension stress study, particularly in patients with a second flare-up, since many practitioners consider that the occurrence of two or more flare-ups during the course of treatment leads to a poorer prognosis. A comparison flexion-extension study may also be considered for evaluation of permanent impairment and disability. Patients with persistent symptoms of a severe nature, including neurologic deficits, should be followed with CT and MRI studies.

Anteroposterior Open Mouth Projection

The frontal projection of the upper cervical complex, referred to as the AP open mouth projection (APOM), is taken to demonstrate the occipital condyles, C-1 and C-2 (including

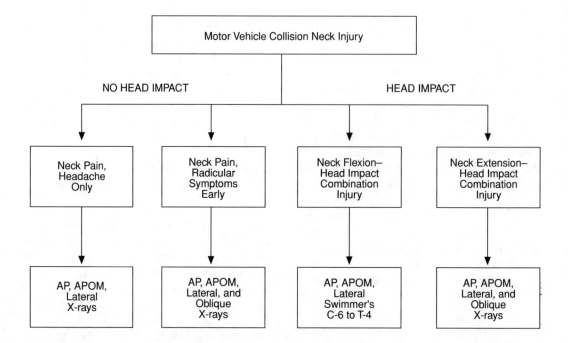

Note: For the patient who has initial radiographs more than 2 weeks after injury, flexion-extension stress views are indicated, unless severe splinting muscle spasm still exists.

Figure 3–1 Initial radiographic algorithm for acute cervical spine injury.

their articulations), and the odontoid process. Proper patient positioning is essential to avoid undesirable superimposition of the teeth over the occipitoaxial joints. The best method is to line up the corners of the patient's mouth with the transverse processes of C-1, which are found just inferior to the mastoid processes along the horizontal plane of the central ray. If visualization of the upper half of the odontoid process is still poor, Fuchs' method (AP projection) or Judd's method (PA projection)[20] can be entertained. These methods require that the head be placed in extension and projections of the odontoid process made through the foramen magnum. This position should not be attempted if fracture is suspected. In these cases, linear tomography is the procedure of choice. To avoid superimposition of the tongue, Ballinger[20] suggests instructing the patient to phonate softly "ah" during the exposure. Proper collimation is also essential to avoid

unnecessary exposure of the orbits and to reduce scattered irradiation.

Anteroposterior Lower Cervical Projection

Segments C-3 to C-7 and often the first two thoracic segments are included in the AP lower cervical projection. A 15° to 20° cephalad central ray angulation is essential to visualize optimally the uncovertebral joints and disc spaces of the lower cervical spine.[20]

Neutral Lateral Projection

All seven cervical vertebral segments, including the lower portion of the occiput and the atlanto-occipital articulation, should be demonstrated in the neutral lateral projection. Care should be taken to ensure that the midsagittal plane is parallel to the plane of the film in order to avoid rotation that may simulate abnormal alignment that is not actually present. The mandibular rami should be superimposed or at least in close approximation to each other. Often C-7 is obscured by the shoulder girdle in patients with short necks or in those unable to relax because of muscular hypertonicity. A supplementary study of the cervicothoracic junction (swimmer's lateral projection) is recommended for these patients.

Flexion and Extension Lateral Projections

As in the neutral lateral projection, care must be taken to avoid rotation in the flexion and extension lateral views. It is very important to instruct the patient to draw the chin in as close as possible before flexing the head forward, and to elevate the chin before extending the head backward.[20] This will help eliminate the undesirable paradoxical motion of the upper cervical spine in hyperflexion, as discussed later in this chapter on motion analysis of the cervical spine.

Oblique Projections

Oblique projections are taken to demonstrate the intervertebral foramina and the surrounding anatomic structures such as the uncovertebral joints, pedicles, and facet joints. It is essential that complementary oblique studies be performed either in the right anterior oblique and left anterior oblique or right posterior and left posterior oblique positions to ensure proper evaluation of both sides of the spine. A 15° caudad angulation for the anterior oblique or 15° cephalad angulation for the posterior oblique positions should be used. The mid-sagittal plane of the body is placed at 45° to the plane of the film. The upper cervical intervertebral foramina can be better demonstrated by further rotating the head so that the mid-sagittal plane of the head is parallel to the plane of the film.[20]

Pillar Projections

The articular pillars should be scrutinized carefully in order to rule out fracture, especially in patients with hyperextension injuries. These structures can be demonstrated easily by angling the central ray along the plane of the facet joints (35° caudad for AP projections or 35° cephalad for PA projections). Both sides can be demonstrated at the same time with the head maintained in the neutral position, or the left and right sides may be demonstrated separately by rotating the head in each direction.[20]

Swimmer's Lateral Projection

Often the lower cervical spine cannot be visualized completely in the routine lateral cervical projection because of superimposition of the shoulder girdle. In the swimmer's lateral projection, the shoulders are separated by elevating the arm next to the grid device and dropping the other shoulder and arm down. The central ray is angled 5° caudad if the shoulder away from the film cannot be sufficiently depressed.[20] This projection should also be included in the examination of any patient presenting with upper thoracic complaints, as the routine lateral thoracic projection does not include the upper thoracic segments.

STABLE VS. UNSTABLE SPINAL INJURIES

Throughout history, numerous attempts have been made to define and classify stable and unstable spinal injuries.[21-25] Systems have been devised that classify these injuries according to location,[21] mechanism of injury,[15,22,26,27] extent of bony and/or soft tissue damage,[9,24,28] presence or absence of neurological injury,[24,29] and resulting biomechanical aberrations.[30]

Injuries that are considered stable according to some classification systems may be considered unstable according to others. From an orthopedic/neurologic standpoint, many authors feel that unstable injuries of the spine result in neurologic damage either at the time of the trauma, or may occur at some later date because of the damage incurred.[24,28,31,32] While many of these injuries should be treated surgically, some (e.g., C-1 neural arch fractures, types I and III odontoid fractures, and unilateral facet dislocation) may be treated conservatively via traction and/or immobilization.[24,31,32] As a result of the lack of neurologic or significant ligamentous damage at the time of the trauma, and the nonsurgical approach to treatment, these injuries are considered by some authors to be stable.[23,33]

The following is a list of motor vehicle collision injuries (MVCIs) that may be seen by chiropractors and general practitioners:

- soft tissue injuries (e.g., ligaments, muscles, etc.)
- disc herniations
- other disc injuries (e.g., lucent clefts)
- subluxation (due to ligamentous injury)
- delayed instability
- unilateral facet dislocations
- compression fractures
- Clayshoveler's fractures
- pillar fractures
- end-plate avulsion fractures
- odontoid fractures
- Jefferson and C-1 posterior arch fractures
- hangman's fractures

While many of these injuries would be considered stable according to the various definitions and classification systems available, any of these injuries could be made worse by injudicious manipulation of the injured area. As a result, manual manipulation of the injured area should be avoided until adequate healing of the osseous structures and the soft tissues has taken place. Obviously, the amount of time necessary for this healing will vary, depending on the nature of the injury.

RADIOLOGIC EVALUATION OF SPINAL INJURIES COMMONLY SEEN BY CHIROPRACTORS

Numerous textbooks and articles have been written describing the radiographic appearance of spinal fractures and dislocations.[9,12,13,23,26,28,33] It is beyond the scope of this text to cover that subject in its entirety. Instead, we will discuss some of the important general radiologic concerns that are often ignored or neglected. As with other chapters of this text, these concerns will focus on patients with mild to moderate traumatic injuries.

Film analysis should include an organized, comprehensive search pattern that evaluates osseous alignment, the skeletal structures, articular spacing, and soft tissues.[12,23] It should be noted by the reader that there is some overlap of these various areas.

Over the years, much has been written about the sagittal plane curvature of the cervical spine. Some authors feel that the normal cervical curve is lordotic, and that any variation from this presentation (straightening or, especially, reversal of the curve) is abnormal, possibly as a result of trauma.[7,34,35] Others believe that there is a wide variation of normal, and that a straight curve, or even kyphosis, can be found in normal individuals.[4,5,15,36-38] Unfortunately, at this point in time there are no available large-scale, controlled studies that take into consideration all related factors, including age, gender, body type, and patient history in determining normative values for the cervical curve. Only with studies that consider these factors will it be possible to determine whether there is a significant difference between the cervical curves found in asymptomatic patients with no history of flexion/extension injuries and those found in patients with this history.

There is conflicting evidence regarding the significance of angular kyphosis in the cervical spine. Although several early studies suggested that the presence of a posttraumatic kyphosis indicates a poor prognosis,[7,37] more recent studies do not support this conclusion.[5,6]

In addition to the postural aberrations that can be detected on plain films, segmental dysrelations should also be recognized. Cervical spine spondylolisthesis, while commonly seen as a result of degenerative disease, is found as a result of trauma only when there is associated fracture, facet dislocation, or significant injury of the posterior ligamentous complex.[24,28,38–40] Laterolisthesis in the cervical spine is a rare development, and when present, almost always indicates significant soft tissue and/or bony injury.[22] Abnormal separation or "fanning" of the spinous processes is commonly seen in patients with damage to the posterior ligamentous structures.[22,25,39] Conversely, approximation of the spinous processes, with widening of the anterior disc space, is often found in patients who have sustained injury to the anterior longitudinal ligament and/or intervertebral disc.[16,22] It is important to understand that posttrauma film studies demonstrate only residual displacement that may be present, without showing any gross displacement that may have spontaneously reduced.[9,24,26,29]

Rotational malpositions are frequently seen in patients with no history of trauma. An area of the cervical spine where nontraumatic rotational malpositions may cause undue clinical concern is the upper cervical complex. Rotation of the atlas relative to the axis creates asymmetry of the paraodontoid space, as well as in the appearance of the lateral masses of C-1.[23,39,41,42] This should not be mistaken for traumatic injury (e.g., Jefferson fracture). Close analysis of the surrounding structures should prevent this error. With rotation of the atlas, there is often overhanging of the inferior articular facet of C-1 relative to the superior articular facet of C-2 on the side of posteriority.[39,43] There is also widening of the paraodontoid space on this side. The opposite side, which moves anteriorly, exhibits medial migration of the C-1 articular process and narrowing of the paraodontoid space.[39,41,42]

Abrupt or isolated segmental rotation is also seen in patients with unilateral facet dislocations,[39,44] and this finding may be the most useful clue as to the nature of the injury.

Evaluation of the skeletal structures should detect any variations from normal. Osseous findings resulting from trauma include changes in contour or disruption of the cortex,

along with changes in the internal architecture of the vertebrae. Focal areas of increased bone density due to condensation of the bony trabeculae are commonly seen with compression fractures, especially in the thorax and lumbar spine, but they are less frequently seen in the cervicals. Pre-existing degenerative changes have been shown to have an effect on trauma patients' symptomatology as well as their prognosis for recovery.[1,5–7,45] In these patients, degenerative spurring reduces the area of the lateral recesses, intervertebral foramina, and spinal canal, thus predisposing them to neurologic injury.[1,18] It has also been shown that the elastic limits of the ligamentous structures are reached earlier in these patients than in normal patients, thus compounding the problem.[1,18]

Normal variants should be recognized when present. One such variant that can create an abnormal postural appearance is hyperplasia of the articular pillars.[46] In most lower cervical vertebrae, there is convergence of the articular facet planes posteriorly.[46,47] This arrangement allows the osseous structures to form a "normal" lordotic curve. In some people, however, the facet planes at one or more cervical levels are found to diverge posteriorly. This condition has been termed hyperplasia of the articular pillars.[46] Since this arrangement may be found in articular pillars of normal height, a more appropriate term might therefore be anomalous development of the articular facets. Divergence of the articular facet planes, especially when present at more than one level, can create a structural reduction or reversal of the cervical lordosis.[46]

Os odontoideum is usually described as a congenital anomaly that may simulate an odontoid fracture.[12,42] Some authors believe that this anomaly is the result of an early nonunion fracture of the odontoid process.[48,49] Since both os odontoideum and odontoid fractures are potentially unstable, surgical fusion of the C-1 and C-2 segments is considered by many to be the treatment of choice.[50,51]

Congenital synostosis of the cervical vertebrae (Klippel-Feil syndrome) is a relatively common condition. The most frequently affected segments are C-2 to C-3 and C-5 to C-6, but any segments may be involved.[12,52] Hypermobility of the segments above and below the vertebral block is not unusual.[15,53] Consequently, these patients are at increased risk for neurologic injury as a result of flexion/extension trauma, and there are several reported cases documenting this development.[15,53] Obviously, the greater the number of segments involved in the synostosis, the greater is the risk of injury.

Soft-tissue injury to the cervical spine is often difficult to detect.[17,38] In fact, it is not uncommon for patients with substantial soft tissue injuries to have no abnormal radiographic findings.[4,25,54] Swelling of the prevertebral soft tissues is not often seen in ambulatory patients, but when present, is considered to be a reliable sign of hemorrhage or edema.[1,9,16,55] This finding is also seen with fractures and may indicate biomechanical instability.[1,3,55,56]

There are a variety of radiographic signs indicative of injury to the intervertebral disc. Widening of the anterior disc space is often seen in patients with tears of the annulus fibrosus and anterior longitudinal ligament.[16,55] Narrowing of the disc space also can be a sign of disc injury, although it is more commonly associated with degenerative disease.[9,24] Comparison to the discs above and below may be useful in this regard. Lucent clefts are small, gas-filled defects located in the intervertebral disc space, adjacent to the vertebral end-plate.[12,57] They are best demonstrated on extension radiographs, and may not be visible on the neutral lateral or flexion studies.[16] In the cervical spine, they have been associated with acute hyperextension injuries to the disc.[16] Because of the ligamentous damage implied by these injuries, spinal manipulation of the area is contraindicated.[12] Although most soft tissue injuries heal relatively quickly, due to the deficient vascular supply to the intervertebral disc, these injuries heal slowly or not at all.[1,58] In some patients, lucent clefts may persist unchanged over an extended period of time.

Although cervical disc herniations may occur as a result of a single macrotrauma (including spinal manipulation),[2,59] many of these injuries develop without any history of a precipitating event.[60] Plain film findings of traumatic disc herniations may be normal, or there may be a loss of disc height at the involved level.[9,58] MRI or contrast-enhanced CT is the procedure of choice for optimal visualization of the lesion.[1,2] Forceful manipulation of acute cervical disc herniations is contraindicated.[14,61,62]

LINES AND ANGLES COMMONLY USED TO EVALUATE OR SUPPORT EVIDENCE OF ACUTE CERVICAL SPINE TRAUMA

Utilization of radiographic mensuration (lines and angles) may be extremely useful in evaluation of the relationship between anatomic structures. When using lines and angles, several considerations must be taken into account by the observer in order to ensure the accuracy of the interpretation. The correct location of the radiographic landmarks used is of utmost importance. Certainly observer error is possible, particularly when working with radiographs of suboptimal quality. Common problems include blurry image due to patient motion and projectional distortion secondary to patient positioning and poor exposure technique. Another important but often overlooked factor is the anatomic variation between individuals that may simulate an abnormality.[12] Following are some of the measurements commonly used in the evaluation of the cervical spine.

Chamberlain's Line

Chamberlain's line is constructed on the lateral projection of the cervical spine from the posterior margin of the hard palate to the posterior aspect of the foramen magnum (Figure 3–2). If the apex of the odontoid process projects above this line, basilar impression or

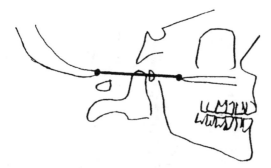

Figure 3–2 Chamberlain's line.

invagination should be considered. A normal variation of up to 3 mm may be present in certain individuals.[63] This line is also very useful in analysis of the cervical curvature. When the head is in the neutral position, Chamberlain's line should be parallel to the horizon. Any variation from this may accentuate or diminish the cervical curve.

Atlantodental Interspace

The atlantodental interspace (ADI) demarcates the median atlantoaxial joint measured between the posterior margin of the anterior tubercle of C-1 and the anterior margin of the odontoid process (Figure 3–3). The ADI should not exceed 3 mm in adults and 5 mm in children.[12] Because of the normal posterior slanting of the odontoid process, a V-shaped ADI is not necessarily indicative of ligamen-

tous injury.[64] Bohrer et al.[65] report that V-shaped widening of the ADI with widening of the C-1 to C-2 interspinous distance in a flexion study may be a "worrisome" finding in trauma patients, representing injury to the transverse ligament. According to Resnick and Niwayama,[66] traumatic subluxation of C-1 to C-2 is almost always accompanied by a fracture of the odontoid process. Traumatically induced subluxation without fracture is usually associated with abnormalities of the underlying bone or ligament, as seen in patients with Down syndrome and the inflammatory arthropathies.

Atlantoaxial Alignment

In atlantoaxial alignment, the lateral margins of the lateral masses of C-1 are usually aligned vertically with the articular pillars of C-2 when there is no head rotation or tilt (Figure 3–4). Offset of these landmarks may be indicative of injury of the transverse ligament, Jefferson fracture, or odontoid fracture.[42]

George's Line

George's line is a continuous line drawn along the posterior vertebral body margins (Figure 3–5). Disruption of the continuity of this line is seen when there is anterior or posterior displacement of a vertebral body relative to the segment below.[67,68] Disruption of

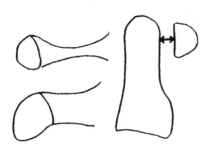

Figure 3–3 Atlantodental interspace.

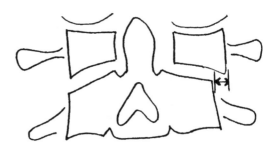

Figure 3–4 Abnormal atlantoaxial alignment.

this line may be indicative of fracture, ligamentous injury, or degenerative disease involving the intervertebral disc and/or facet
joints. Flexion/extension radiographs are
valuable in confirming the presence of instability of the vertebral motion segments. Care
should be taken to avoid misinterpreting segmental rotation for anterolisthesis or
retrolisthesis.

Posterior Cervical Line

The posterior cervical line is a continuous
line formed by connecting the cortical margins
of the spinolaminar junctions of the cervical
segments (Figure 3–6). Disruption of this line
is suggestive of fracture, ligamentous injury,
or degenerative disease.[12]

Prevertebral Soft Tissues

The prevertebral soft tissues are those structures that lie posterior to the pharynx and trachea and anterior to the cervical spine (Figure
3–7). The space occupied by these tissues
should not exceed 6 mm at the level of C-2 and
20 mm at the level of C-6. Widening of this distance due to hemorrhage or edema is often
seen in trauma patients. Nontraumatic condi-

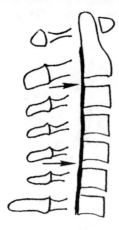

Figure 3–5 George's line.

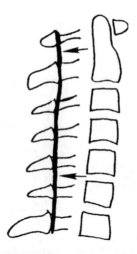

Figure 3–6 Posterior cervical line.

tions such as retropharyngeal abscess, cyst, or
neoplasm may also widen this soft-tissue
space.[12]

RADIOGRAPHIC EVALUATION AND ANALYSIS OF CERVICAL SPINE JOINT DYSFUNCTION WITH FLEXION/EXTENSION MOTION STUDIES

Ligamentous injury of the cervical spine following whiplash trauma is commonly evaluated by flexion and extension studies. These
stress views are simple to perform and still remain the preferred method for evaluating
intersegmental sagittal motion,[69] although
other, more complex methods such as cineradiography and stereoradiography have also
been described.[70] Some investigators have
demonstrated a slight increase in accuracy in
these more complex studies; however, this is
offset by their increased radiation and the
need for special equipment.[71]

The analysis of the flexion and extension
studies is usually made by overlay template
tracings comparing the flexion and extension
radiographs only, or including the neutral projection as well. A transparent medium such as
clear plastic or tracing paper is placed over the

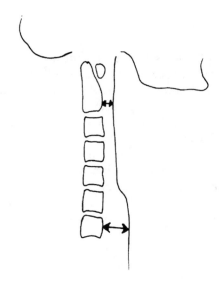

Figure 3–7 Prevertebral soft tissues.

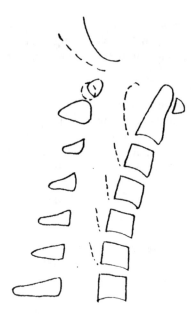

Figure 3–8 Flexion-extension template.

flexion radiograph. The vertebral landmarks are traced onto this plastic or paper. This tracing is then placed over the extension radiograph. The tracing of C-7 in the flexion radiograph is superimposed over C-7 in the extension radiograph. With a different color pencil, C-6 in the extension radiograph is traced.[72,73] The entire cervical spine is traced accordingly. If the neutral projection is used, then this radiograph is traced first. The flexion and extension radiographs are then subsequently superimposed and traced one segment at a time as described earlier (Figure 3–8).

Numerous investigators have developed varying methods of interpreting these studies.[71-77] Some measure the angle made between the selected reference point such as one of the vertebral body margins in flexion and the same point in extension. Others measure the sagittal excursion distance between the vertebral body margins from flexion to extension, or from neutral to flexion and from neutral to extension. It is the opinion of the authors that measuring the sagittal excursion distance between the posterior vertebral body margin in flexion and extension is the most practical method of choice. A greater margin

of error is present when the neutral projection is included in the analysis, as the findings are directly influenced by the placement of the cervical spine in this neutral position. If the patient is slightly flexed in the neutral projection, a normal vertebral motion segment may simulate hypomobility upon flexion and hypermobility upon extension in this analysis. Similarly, if the patient is slightly extended in the presumed neutral position, hypermobility upon flexion and hypomobility upon extension may be simulated. Other factors, such as muscle spasm or degenerative disease, that result in changes of the cervical lordosis in the neutral position incorrectly interpreted may mimic articular or ligamentous abnormality.

Sagittal motion of the cervical spine comprises both pivotal tilting and translation in the form of glide.[47] The gliding motion is greater in the upper cervical spine, whereas the lower cervical spine demonstrates more tilting motion. A paradoxical tilt occurs between the occiput, C-1, and C-2 in flexion.[73] This motion is accentuated if the chin is not drawn in prior to flexion. Accurate assessment of motion in this area is directly dependent upon proper positioning. The largest degree of sagittal motion occurs between C-4 to C-5 and C-5 to C-6 vertebral motion segments.[69]

According to Henderson and Dorman,[73] the sagittal excursion distance measured between the posterior superior vertebral body in flexion and extension indicates articular fixation if less than 25% of the sagittal diameter of the vertebral body is at the particular level. Radiographic instability should be considered if the excursion exceeds 75% of the sagittal vertebral body diameter.

These values should be used only as a general guideline for analysis and not as an absolute measure. It is important to visualize the overall shape or contour of the cervical spine in the flexed and extended positions. Normal flexion should demonstrate a smooth kyphosis of the cervical curve with uniform widening of the interspinous spaces between C-3 and C-7. A localized angular kyphosis with excessive widening of the interspinous space is an indication of ligamentous injury[74] even if the sagittal excursion values fall between 25% and 75% of the sagittal vertebral body diameter. Localized anterolisthesis upon flexion or retrolisthesis upon extension is often an indication of abnormal intersegmental translation due to decreased ligamentous integrity. This

form of instability may often present with a reduced sagittal excursion distance upon templating as the pivotal tilt motion is replaced by excessive translatory glide motion. These data could be mistakenly interpreted as fixation rather than instability. Manipulative therapy may thus be inappropriately delivered to an unstable segment.

Increased translatory motion is defined as 3.5 mm or more of horizontal movement measured from the posterior inferior corner of the vertebral body between the flexion and extension views. Some investigators use a more conservative figure of 2 mm.[78] When multiple levels of 1 mm or 2 mm of anterolisthesis and retrolisthesis occur in flexion and extension, respectfully, this is often indicative of slight ligamentous laxity rather than an acute injury.[74]

It is of little value to perform flexion and extension studies when generalized muscle spasm is present following acute trauma. Ligamentous injury with instability may be masked and appear to represent hypomobility or even normal motion. These segments often will demonstrate hypermobility or aberrant translation when the protective acute spasm subsides. Therefore, it may be more useful to order these studies as follow-up examinations when the patient can flex and extend maximally without hindrance from generalized spasm.

REFERENCES

1. Davis SJ, Teresi LM, Bradley WG, et al. Cervical spine hyperextension injuries: MR findings. *Radiology*. 1991;180:245–251.
2. Goldberg AL, Rothfus WE, Deeb ZL, et al. The impact of magnetic resonance imaging on the diagnostic evaluation of acute cervicothoracic spinal trauma. *Skeletal Radiol*. 1988;17:89–95.
3. Herkowitz HN, Rothman RH. Subacute instability of the cervical spine. *Spine*. 1984;9:348–357.
4. Hirsch SA, Hirsch PJ, Hiramoto H, et al. Whiplash syndrome, fact or fiction? *Orthop Clin North Am*. 1988;19:791–795.
5. Maimaris C, Barnes MR, Allen MJ. Whiplash injuries of the neck: a retrospective study. *Injury*. 1988;19:393–396.
6. Miles KA, Maimaris C, Finlay D, et al. The incidence and prognostic significance of radiological abnormalities in soft tissue injuries of the cervical spine. *Skeletal Radiol*. 1988;17:493–496.
7. Norris SH, Watt I. The prognosis of neck injuries resulting from rear-end vehicle collisions. *J Bone Joint Surg [Br]*. 1983;65:608–611.
8. Patijn J. Complications in manual medicine: a review of the literature. *J Manual Med*. 1991;6:89–92.
9. Rogers LF. *Radiology of Skeletal Trauma*. vol. 1. New York: Churchill Livingstone; 1982.

10. Schmitt HP. Anatomical structure of the cervical spine with reference to the pathology of manipulation complications. *J Manual Med.* 1991;6:93–101.

11. Wyatt L. *Handbook of Clinical Chiropractic.* Gaithersburg, Md: Aspen Publishers, Inc; 1991.

12. Yochum TR, Rowe LJ. *Essentials of Skeletal Radiology.* vol 1. Baltimore: Williams & Wilkins; 1987.

13. Clark CR, Igram CM, El-Khoury GY, et al. Radiographic evaluation of cervical spine injuries. *Spine.* 1988;13:742–747.

14. Dvorak J. Inappropriate indications and contraindications for manual therapy. *J Manual Med.* 1991;6:85–88.

15. Elster AD. Quadriplegia after minor trauma in the Klippel-Feil syndrome. *J Bone Joint Surg [Am].* 1984;66:1473–1474.

16. Edeiken-Monroe B, Wagner LK, Harris JH. Hyperextension dislocation of the spine. *AJR.* 1986; 146:803–808.

17. Hildingsson C, Hietala SO, Toolanen G. Scinitigraphic findings in acute whiplash injury of the cervical spine. *Injury.* 1989;20:265–266.

18. Regenbogen VS, Rogers LF, Atlas SW, et al. Cervical spine cord injuries in patients with cervical spondylosis. *AJR.* 1986;146:277–284.

19. Masters SJ, McClean PM, Argarese JS, et al. Skull x-ray examinations after head trauma. *N Engl J Med.* 1987;316:84–91.

20. Ballinger PW. *Merrill's Atlas of Radiographic Positions and Radiologic Procedures.* 7th ed. vol 1. St. Louis: Mosby-Year Book, Inc; 1991.

21. Aebi M, Nazarian S. Klassifikation der Halswirbelsaulenverletzungen. *Orthopade.* 1987;16:27–36.

22. Allen BL, Ferguson RL, Lehman TR, et al. A mechanistic classification of closed, indirect fractures and dislocations of the lower cervical spine. *Spine.* 1982;7:1–27.

23. Batnitzky S. Radiology of cervical spine trauma. *Radiol Soc North Am.* 1989;301.

24. White AA, Southwick WO, Panjabi MM. Clinical instability in the lower cervical spine. *Spine.* 1976;1:15–27.

25. Wilberger JE, Maroon JC. Occult posttraumatic cervical ligamentous instability. *J Spinal Disord.* 1990;3:156–161.

26. Holdsworth FW. Fractures, dislocations and fracture-dislocations of the spine. *J Bone Joint Surg [Br].* 1963;45:6–20.

27. Kettner NW, Guebert GM. The radiology of cervical spine injury. *J Manipulative Physiol Ther.* 1991;14:518–526.

28. Bohlman HH. Acute fractures and dislocations of the cervical spine. *J Bone Joint Surg [Am].* 1979; 61:1119–1140.

29. Marar BC. The pattern of neurological damage as an aid to the diagnosis of the mechanism in cervical spine injuries. *J Bone Joint Surg [Am].* 1974; 56:1648–1654.

30. White AA, Johnson RM, Panjabi MM, et al. Biomechanical analysis of clinical stability in the cervical spine. *Clin Orthop.* 1975;109:85–96.

31. Dall DM. Injuries of the cervical spine: does anatomical reduction of the bony injuries improve the prognosis for spinal cord recovery? *S Afr Med J.* 1972;46:1083–1090.

32. Norton WL. Fractures and dislocations of the cervical spine. *J Bone Joint Surg [Am].* 1962;44:115–138.

33. Felson BA, ed. *Roentgenology of Fractures and Dislocations.* New York: Grune & Stratton; 1978.

34. Jonsson K, Niklasson J, Josefsson PO. Avulsion of the cervical spine ring apophyses: acute and chronic appearance. *Skeletal Radiol.* 1991;20:207–210.

35. Rechtman AM, Borden AG, Gershon-Cohen J. The lordotic curve of the cervical spine. *Clin Orthop.* 1961;20:208–215.

36. Fineman S, Borrelli FJ, Rubinstein BM, et al. The cervical spine: transformation of the normal lordotic pattern into a linear pattern in the neutral posture. *J Bone Joint Surg [Am].* 1963;45:1179–1183.

37. Hohl M. Soft tissue injuries of the neck in automobile accidents. *J Bone Joint Surg [Am].* 1974; 56A:1675–1682.

38. Weir DC. Roentgenographic signs of cervical injury. *Clin Orthop.* 1975;109:9–17.

39. Harris JH, Edeiken MB, eds. *The Radiology of Acute Cervical Spine Trauma.* 2nd ed. Baltimore: Williams & Wilkins; 1987.

40. Rowe L, Steiman I. Anterolisthesis of the cervical spine-spondylolysis. *J Manipulative Physiol Ther.* 1987;10:11–20.

41. Dihlmann W. *Joints and Vertebral Connections.* New York: Thieme Medical Publishers, Inc; 1985.

42. Shapiro R, Youngberg AS, Rothman SL. The differential diagnosis of traumatic lesions of the occipito-atlanto-axial segment. *Radiol Clin North Am.* 1973;11:505–526.

43. Jacobson G, Adler DC. An evaluation of lateral atlanto-axial displacement in injuries of the cervical spine. *Radiology.* 1953;61:355.

44. Young JW, Resnik CS, DeCandido P, et al. The laminar space in the diagnosis of rotational flexion injuries of the cervical spine. *AJR.* 1989;152:103–107.

45. Pearce JM. Whiplash injury: a reappraisal. *J Neurol Neurosurg Psychiatry*. 1989;52:1329–1331.

46. Peterson CK, Wei T. Vertical hyperplasia of the cervical articular pillars. *J Am Chirop Assoc.* 1987; 24:78–79.

47. White AA, Panjabi MM. *Clinical Biomechanics of the Spine*. 2nd ed. Philadelphia: JB Lippincott Co; 1990.

48. Ricciardi JE, Kaufer J, Louis DS. Acquired os odontoideum following acute ligament injury. *J Bone Joint Surg [Am]*. 1976;58:410–412.

49. Hawkins RJ, Fielding JW, Thompson WJ. Os odontoideum: congenital or acquired. *J Bone Joint Surg [Am]*. 1976;58:413–415.

50. Hensinger RN, Fielding JW, Hawkins RJ. Congenital anomalies of the odontoid process. *Orthop Clin North Am*. 1978;9:901–912.

51. Wilkinson RH, Strand RD. Congenital anomalies and normal variants. *Semin Roentgenol*. 1979;14: 7–18.

52. Hensinger RN, Lang JE, MacEwen GD. Klippel-Feil syndrome: a constellation of associated anomalies. *J Bone Joint Surg [Am]*. 1974;56:1246–1253.

53. Strax TE, Baran E. Traumatic quadriplegia associated with Klippel-Feil syndrome: discussion and case reports. *Arch Phys Med Rehabil*. 1975;56:363–364.

54. Pennie B, Agambar L. Patterns of injury and recovery in whiplash. *Injury*. 1991;22:57–59.

55. Penning L. Prevertebral hematoma in cervical spine injury: incidence and etiologic significance. *AJR*. 1981;136:553–561.

56. Templeton PA, Young JW, Mirvis SE, et al. The value of retropharyngeal soft tissue measurements in trauma of the adult cervical spine. *Skeletal Radiol*. 1987;16:98–104.

57. Reymond RD, Wheeler PS, Perovic M, et al. The lucent cleft, a new radiographic sign of cervical disc injury or disease. *Clin Radiol*. 1972;23:188.

58. Krämer J. *Intervertebral disk diseases*. 2nd ed. New York: Thieme Medical Publishers, Inc; 1990.

59. Greenman PE. Principles of manipulation of the cervical spine. *J Manual Med*. 1991;6:106–113.

60. Murphy F, Simmons JC, Brunson B. Ruptured cervical discs 1939–1972. *Clin Neurosurg*. 1973;20:9–17.

61. Dvorak J, Baumgartner H, Burn L, et al. Consensus and recommendations as to the side-effects and complications of manual therapy of the cervical spine. *J Manual Med*. 1991;6:117–118.

62. Eder M, Tilscher H. *Chiropractic Therapy, Diagnosis and Treatment*. Gaithersburg, Md: Aspen Publishers, Inc; 1990.

63. Poppel MH, et al. Basilar impression and platybasia in Paget's disease. *Radiology*. 1953; 61:639–642.

64. Monu J, Bohrer SP, Howard G. Some upper cervical norms. *Spine*. 1987;12:515–519.

65. Bohrer SP, Klein A, Martin W. "V" shaped predens space. *Skeletal Radiol*. 1985;14:111–116.

66. Resnick D, Niwayama G. *Diagnosis of Bone and Joint Disorders*. vol 3. Philadelphia: WB Saunders; 1981.

67. George AW. A method for more accurate study of injuries to the atlas and axis. *Boston Med Surg J*. 1919;181:13:395–398.

68. Litterer WE. A history of George's line. *J Am Chirop Assoc*. 1983;24:39–40.

69. Lind B, Sihlbom H, Nordwall A, et al. Normal range of motion of the cervical spine. *Arch Phys Med Rehabil*. 1989;70:692–695.

70. Fielding JW. Normal and selected abnormal motion of the cervical spine from second cervical vertebra to seventh cervical vertebra based on cineroentgenography. *J Bone Joint Surg [Am]*. 1964;46:1779–1781.

71. Dimnet J, Pasquet A, Krag MH, et al. Cervical spine motion in the sagittal plane: kinematic and geometric parameters. *J Biomech*. 1982;15:959–969.

72. Anderson AL. Lecture notes, Western States Chiropractic College, 1975.

73. Henderson DJ, Dorman TM. Functional roentgenometric evaluation of the cervical spine in the sagittal plane. *J Manipulative Physiol Ther*. 1985;8:219–226.

74. Bohrer SP, Chen YM, Sayer DG. Cervical spine flexion patterns. *Skeletal Radiol*. 1990;19:521–525.

75. Conley RW. Stress evaluation of cervical mechanics. *J Clin Chirop*. 1974;3:46–62.

76. Grice AS. Preliminary evaluation of fifty sagittal cervical motion radiographic examinations. *J Can Chiro Assn*. 1977;21:33–34.

77. Hviid H. Functional radiography of the cervical spine. *Ann Swiss Chirop Assoc*. 1963;3:37–65.

78. Lewis LM, Docherty M, Ruoff BE, et al. Flexion-extension views in the evaluation of cervical spine injuries. *Ann Emerg Med*. 1991;20:117–121.

Chapter 4

Imaging of Hyperextension Injuries of the Spine

Damon Sacco and Jay A. Kaiser

INTRODUCTION

Plain film radiography remains the initial imaging study of choice in the acute evaluation of cervical spine trauma. Properly performed radiographs allow for the accurate determination of overall structural integrity, as well as spinal alignment, and give an estimation of soft tissue thickening anterior to the spine. However, it has been shown that the two-dimensional representation given by plain X-rays can, in a significant number of cases, fail to diagnose fractures, especially those involving the posterior elements. Furthermore, soft tissue anatomy within and adjacent to the spinal canal (i.e., intervertebral discs, spinal cord, and anterior and posterior longitudinal ligaments) is not seen on plain X-rays. In the past, linear tomography and myelography were used to attempt to see these structures. More recently, however, the noninvasive modalities of computed tomography (CT) and magnetic resonance imaging (MRI) have emerged as the procedures of choice in the definitive evaluation of clinically significant injuries. This is due in part to their ability to perform multiple imaging planes, as

well as providing improved soft tissue resolution. Both imaging modalities are noninvasive and generally require no intravenous or intrathecal infusion of contrast.

The purpose of this chapter is to define the appropriate utilization of MRI and CT in the evaluation of cervical spine trauma and to provide guidelines for determining the severity of injury based on scan findings. The strengths and weaknesses of each modality are discussed to provide a basis for determining the correct scan to order in individual cases. A complete discussion of the physics of the modalities is beyond the scope of this chapter. However, a brief discussion of how the images are generated is important to provide a basis for understanding the information obtained by the different scanning techniques.

TECHNICAL CONSIDERATIONS OF COMPUTED TOMOGRAPHY WITH MULTIPLANAR RE-FORMATION

CT images represent cross-sectional representations of the body produced by sending a thinly collimated beam of X-rays with directly opposed electronic detectors. The signal from the detectors is then sent to a computer, which turns the digital information received into a picture. The tissues within the course of the X-ray beam are differentiated by their varying electron densities and therefore their varying X-ray attenuation. Tissues with a high attenuation such as air appear black. Soft tissues will be seen as varying shades of gray. Spatial resolution and contrast resolution are dependent on the technical quality of the scanner, the size of the patient, the size of the area to be studied, and the scanning matrix. Larger patients and those with thick shoulders will result in more "noise" on the images. A high-resolution CT is obtained by the use of serial adjacent thin-section scans, not more than 2 mm thick, through the area of interest. Using the data from the axial images, computer-generated multiplanar re-formations (MPR) in the sagittal and coronal planes are an integral part of the examinations. The images are then filmed twice to delineate optimally either soft tissue or osseous anatomy.

MAGNETIC RESONANCE IMAGING

Magnetic resonance imaging, as opposed to CT, does not employ the use of ionizing radiation to generate the images. Instead, the patient is placed in a large magnetic field that leads to alignment of the free mobile protons in the body either with or against the field. The area to be imaged is then subjected to repeated short bursts of radio waves of a specific radio frequency (RF). This frequency, also called resonant frequency, is dictated by the strength of the applied external magnetic field. These short bursts of RF energy into the body excite the hydrogen nuclei or protons; with termination of the RF pulse, the excited protons relax and release the RF energy that they absorbed. This released RF energy by the protons is detected by sensitive receiver coils within the instrument. This signal is encoded with information as to its point of origin within the imaging plane. Since the detected signal is very weak, numerous measurements of RF pulses into the body are made, and an image is constructed. This characteristic absorption and release of energy is called nuclear magnetic resonance.

The process of returning from the excited state to the equilibrium state, with the release of RF energy, is called relaxation. The process of relaxation is characterized by two independent time constants, T1 and T2. The T1 relaxation time is also referred to as the longitudinal relaxation time and reflects the time required for realignment of the protons with the applied magnetic field. The T2 relaxation time is also referred to as the transverse relaxation time and reflects the time it takes the protons to lose coherence following excitation. The T1 and T2 relaxation times are intrinsic physical properties of tissue. The MR signal intensity that is displayed on the images is mainly dependent on the T1, T2, and proton density (i.e., number of mobile hydrogen ions) of the tissue being evaluated.

The repetition time (TR) represents the time between RF pulses; and the echo time (TE) represents the time between the application of the RF pulse and the time of recording the MR signal. These parameters, TR and TE, are set prior to acquiring the image. By varying the scanning parameters (TR and TE), the relative contributions of the T1, T2, and proton density of the tissue will determine image contrast. A T1-weighted image, which emphasizes the T1 properties of the tissue, is produced with a short TR (<1000 milliseconds) and a short TE (<30 milliseconds). T1-weighted images are ideal for evaluating structures containing fat, subacute or chronic hemorrhage, or proteinaceous fluid, since these materials have a short T1 and yield a high signal on T1-weighted sequences. The T1-weighted sequence yields images with high signal-to-noise ratios and provides excellent anatomic detail.

Images with a long TR (>1500 milliseconds) and a short TE (15 to 30 milliseconds) are referred to as proton-density or spin-density studies. With spin-density images the signal intensity reflects the absolute number of mobile hydrogen ions or protons in the tissue.

A T2-weighted sequence requires a long TR (>1500 milliseconds) and a long TE (>45 milliseconds). On T2-weighted studies the signal intensity is related to the state of hydration of the tissue. Any tissue rich in free or extracellular water (e.g., cerebrospinal fluid, cysts, necrotic tissue, edema, fluid collections, neoplasms, and the normal nucleus pulposus) will demonstrate increased signal intensity.

As opposed to CT/MPR, in which the only directly acquired plane is the axial plane and all other planes of imaging require computed re-formation from the axial images, with MRI any desired imaging plane can be directly acquired. This is a limitation of CT/MPR, as the resolution of the reformatted image is limited by the slice thickness of the axial images from which it was generated; with CT/MPR of the cervical spine this is generally on the order of 1.5 mm. Additionally, if motion occurs during the acquisition of the axial images, misregistration artifacts can degrade the reformatted images. Computer-generated sagittal and coronal images generally are not necessary with MRI data. Until recent advances, MRI was limited to a slice thickness of approximately 3.5 mm, whereas CT axial images could be obtained as thin as 1.5 mm. This gave CT greater axial resolution and an ability to perform more axial images through the disc space or nerve root canals. However, with the use of stronger magnetic fields and more powerful gradients, MRI can now obtain images with a slice thickness less than 1.0 mm. In addition to direct acquisition of an imaging plane, MRI has the capability of imaging an entire volume of tissue. This data set, or volume, can then be sectioned into any desired plane of interest.

Because MRI requires placing the patient in a large magnetic field, there are certain patients for whom the test is contraindicated. With the application of a powerful magnetic field, torque may be applied to a metallic object placed within the field. Patients with intracranial aneurysm clips cannot be imaged because of the possibility of torquing the clip off the neck of the aneurysm. For the same reason, patients with metallic middle ear implants, intraocular metallic foreign bodies, some prosthetic cardiac valves, or strategically located small pieces of metal (i.e., intraspinal shrapnel) should not be imaged. Because the patient is also exposed to RF pulsations, voltage may be induced in pacemaker leads or metallic leads from other neuro-biostimulating devices, and examination of patients with such devices is contraindicated. Although at this time there is no evidence to indicate harmful effects to an embryo from exposure to magnetic or RF fields, most imaging centers are not studying women who are in their first trimester of pregnancy. Some patients cannot be imaged because of claustrophobic reactions. Since the scanner has a bore significantly smaller than that of a CT scanner, claustrophobia is a common problem, occurring in up to 8% to 10% of patients, depending on the scanner design. Many of these patients can be scanned with the use of mild sedatives. For a more detailed discussion of MR physics and imaging techniques the reader is referred to the text, *Magnetic Resonance Imaging*, by Stark and Bradley.[1]

NORMAL CT AND MRI CERVICAL ANATOMY

In the sagittal imaging plane, the normal cervical spine has a slightly lordotic curvature. The cervical vertebral bodies become broader and increase in size as the examiner extends caudally from C-3 to C-7. The cervical pedicles are short, cylindric, osseous structures that extend off the posterolateral aspects of the vertebral bodies to the articular pillars, and the paired osseous struts are referred to as the lamina. On an axial image at the level of the pedicles, the spinal canal is completely surrounded by an osseous ring composed of the vertebral body, the paired lateral pedicles, the articular pillars, and posteriorly the paired lamina. Extending posteriorly off the lamina is the spinous process. The intervertebral canals are enclosed by the pedicles, facets, and posterolateral margins of the cervical vertebral bodies. Since the intervertebral nerve root canals have a defined depth, width, and height, they should not be referred to as nerve root foramina. Because of their oblique course they are not ideally imaged by sagittal imaging but are best identified by oblique sagittal images, which are reformatted perpendicular to the length of the canal.[2]

The transverse foramina of the cervical spine usually extend from C-2 through C-6. These are identified as round or oval defects within the transverse processes of the cervical vertebral bodies on CT. The uncinate processes are best demonstrated on coronal and axial images. These consist of osseous ridges that extend off the lateral margins of the superior end-plates of the vertebral body; this articulation is referred to as the uncovertebral joint or joint of Luschka. Degenerative changes involving the uncovertebral joints, such as sclerosis, osteophytic ridging, and uncinate spurring, are best appreciated on axial or reformatted coronal images with CT/MPR (Figures 4–1 and 4–2).

The cervical vertebral bodies are interconnected by the anterior and posterior longitudinal ligaments. The anterior longitudinal ligament (ALL) extends from the anterior aspect of the foramen magnum caudally to the level of the sacrum. The ligamentous fibers blend with the outer annular fibers of the discs or annulus fibrosus. The posterior longitudinal ligament (PLL) extends from the posterior face of the clivus caudally along the posterior aspects of the vertebral bodies. The ligamentous fibers of the PLL also blend with the outer annular fibers of the disc. The PLL is not imaged as a separate structure on CT but is identified on MRI. The PLL is best seen on sagittal T2-weighted sequences, where it is identified as a linear structure of low signal intensity, which is black, be-

tween the posterior aspect of the cervical vertebral bodies and the high signal intensity of the CSF within the thecal sac. On T1-weighted sagittal images of the spine the PLL is not well seen, because the low signal intensity of the cerebrospinal fluid (CSF) on T1-weighted images becomes inseparable from the low signal intensity of the PLL. Tears of the PLL are best imaged on the T2-weighted sagittal sequence; however, calcification or ossification of the PLL is best imaged by CT/MPR.

Along the posterior aspect of the spine is the interspinous ligament, which extends between the spinous processes of the vertebral bodies. The transverse ligament is a fibrous band that extends across the atlas, along the posterior aspect of the odontoid process, to maintain close apposition of the odontoid process with the anterior arch of C-1. Tearing or rupture of the transverse ligament will be seen as widening of the predental space, the space directly anterior to the odontoid process and the anterior arch of C-1.

Axial images through the cervical cord reveal the cord to be round or elliptic. There is a normal, subtle enlargement of the cord from approximately the C-1 to the C-4 level. Eight pairs of spinal nerves arise from the lateral margins of the cord and exit through the intervertebral nerve root canals. Without intrathecal contrast the individual nerve roots cannot be imaged by CT/MPR but can be identified by MRI. The size and morphology of the cervical cord are probably best evaluated on sagittal T1-weighted images, where the cord is of higher signal intensity than the CSF. However, on a high-quality, high-resolution, multiplanar CT scan of the cervical spine, the cord can be identified within the thecal sac as a round or elliptic structure of slightly higher density than the adjacent CSF. Both CT and MRI will demonstrate the size of the central canal to determine whether central canal stenosis exists; however, MRI is superior to CT, as it can better demonstrate cord compression or the existence of cord edema secondary to the central stenosis.

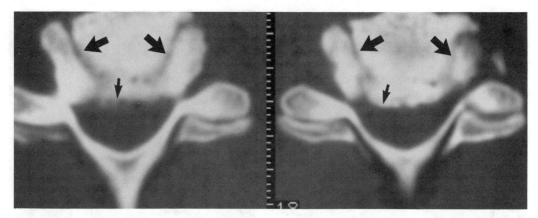

Figure 4–1 CT and MRI degenerative changes involving uncovertebral joints. Shown are 1.5-mm-thick axial CT images through the uncovertebral joints *(large arrows)*. Note the enlargement and hypertrophy of the uncinate processes with increased bone density. There is moderate osteophytic ridging also present along the posterior aspect of the adjacent end-plates *(small arrows)*. At this level, the central canal is the lower limit of normal in size. Note that the cervical cord cannot be identified within the central canal.

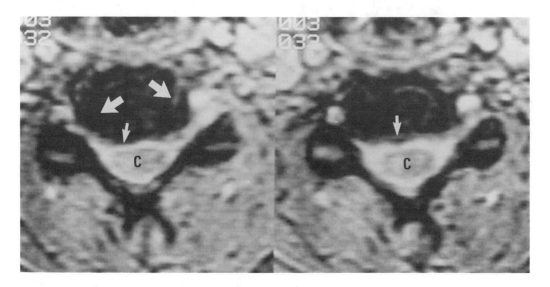

Figure 4–2 CT and MRI degenerative changes involving uncovertebral joints. The images correspond to 2-mm-axial T2-weighted images of the cervical spine. The uncovertebral joints are not as well demonstrated *(large arrows)*. Additionally, the posterior osteophytic ridging off the adjacent end-plates is not as well characterized *(small arrows)*. However, the cervical cord (C) can be identified within the thecal sac. The subarachnoid space is slightly effaced, but there is not evidence of cord compression.

Directly anterior to the ALL is the prevertebral space. This space contains fat and the longus colli and longus capitis muscles; it is contained anteriorly by the prevertebral fasciae. The prevertebral fasciae can be identified on sagittal T1- and T2-weighted MRI images as a linear black stripe that extends just anterior to the cervical vertebral bodies to approximately the level of C-6, where it curves anteriorly (Figures 4–3 and 4–4). Anterior bulging of

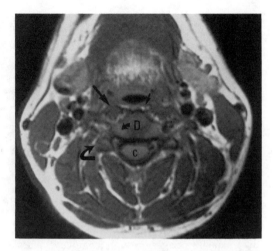

Figure 4–4 Axial T1-weighted MRI image of the cervical spine. Shown is a T1-weighted axial MRI image through the C-3 to C-4 intervertebral disc space. The disc *(D)* is of intermediate signal intensity. The uncinate processes of C-4 *(curved arrow)* are identified. The cervical cord is visualized in cross-section *(C)*. The small amount of fat within the prevertebral space and contained by the prevertebral fasciae *(small arrow)* is identified. The longus capitis muscles are also seen in cross-section *(large arrow)*. On this axial image, the C-3–C-4 facets (zygapophyseal joint) are partially visualized *(large curved arrow)*.

the prevertebral fasciae is a reliable sign of subjacent hematoma or edema within the prevertebral space.

ROLE OF CT AND MRI

MRI and CT have complementary roles in evaluating the cervical spine. MRI is the preferred modality to delineate soft tissue anatomy and to define chemical changes within the imaged region. On the other hand, CT is superior in evaluating osseous structures for subtle fractures, particularly those involving the posterior elements, and in evaluating osseous degenerative changes such as uncinate spurring, sclerosis, and subtle areas of osseous erosion. MRI, with its excellent soft tissue resolution, allows for better evaluation of the discs, spinal cord, ligaments, and paravertebral soft tissues such as muscles, tendons, and fat.[3] With fractures of the spine, accurate measurements

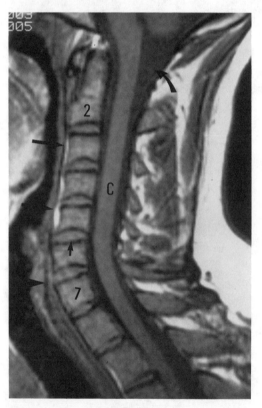

Figure 4–3 Sagittal T1-weighted MRI image of the cervical spine. The morphology of the cervical cord *(C)* is well delineated. The CSF on this sequence is dark *(curved arrow)*. This limits evaluation of the PLL as the low signal intensity of the ligament merges with that of the CSF. C-2 *(2)* and C-7 *(7)* vertebral bodies are marked. There is intermediate signal intensity of the intervertebral discs; however, the vertebral body end-plates, which were of cortical bone, are seen as linear areas of diminished signal intensity *(small arrow)*. The prevertebral fasciae are identified as a linear stripe of diminished signal intensity *(large arrow)*.

of bone displacement and subluxation can be better assessed by CT/MPR[4] (Figures 4–5 through 4–8).

However, MRI has the added value of being able to determine the presence of blood or blood products. It is therefore extremely useful in evaluating a patient for the presence of a cord contusion, epidural hematoma, or subarachnoid hemorrhage.[5] MRI can differentiate between an intramedullary hematoma or an area of cord edema, i.e., contusion (Figures 4–9 through 4–12). This differentiation is not trivial.[6] Patients with hyperextension injuries of the cervical spine can, if severe enough, present with central cord syndrome. This is a myelopathy that affects the upper extremities

to a greater degree than the lower extremities. MRI of the cervical cord in patients with central cord syndrome has been shown to be helpful in determining long-term prognosis.[7] Patients with a normal cord or mild cord edema, as demonstrated on MRI, have a better prognosis than those patients with intramedullary hemorrhage.[6]

Mild ligamentous injuries of the spine following hyperextension may present with a delayed onset of pain; neck pain may present up to 48 hours or more following the injury.[8] These mild ligamentous injuries, such as partial tears of the anterior longitudinal ligament, stretching of the disc annulus, or low-grade muscle strains, are not directly imaged by CT.

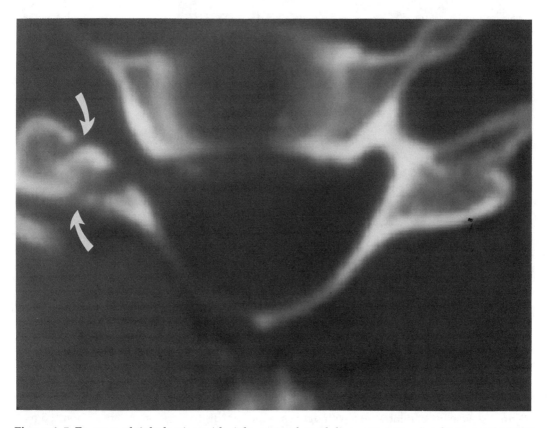

Figure 4–5 Fracture of right lamina with right posterolateral disc protrusion. Axial 1.5-mm-thick CT image, using bone window settings, demonstrates a slightly comminuted fracture involving the right lamina *(curved white arrows)*. The extent of the fracture is well demonstrated, and the fracture lines are well demarcated.

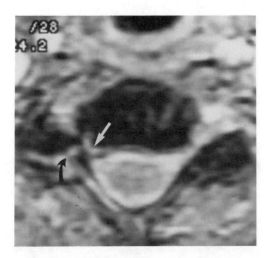

Figure 4–6 Fracture of right lamina with right posterolateral disc protrusion. Corresponding 2-mm-thick, axial T2-weighted MRI image of the cervical spine. The fracture through the right lamina *(curved black arrow)* can be appreciated but is better imaged by the axial CT image with bone window settings. A small right posterolateral disc protrusion is also identified *(white arrow)*.

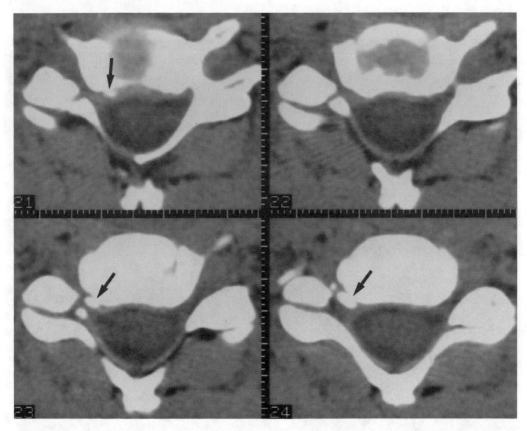

Figure 4–7 Fracture of right lamina with right posterolateral disc protrusion. A series of four 1.5-mm-thick axial images through the same level, using soft tissue window settings, also demonstrates small osseous fragments within the right lateral recess and entry zone of the right intervertebral nerve root canal. The posterolateral disc protrusion is more difficult to appreciate on these images.

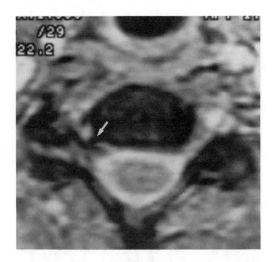

Figure 4–8 Fracture of right lamina with right posterolateral disc protrusion. Corresponding 2-mm-thick axial T2-weighted MRI image through a corresponding level also demonstrates low-signal-intensity defects within the right intervertebral nerve root canal *(white arrow);* these correspond with the above-described bone fragments. The bone fragments are better appreciated on the CT scan.

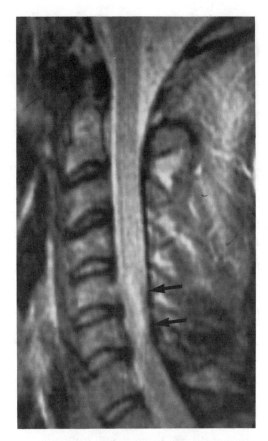

Figure 4–9 Nonhemorrhagic contusion. Sagittal T2-weighted image of the cervical cord reveals area of increased signal intensity within the cord at the C-5 to C-6 and C-6 to C-7 levels consistent with cord edema *(large arrows).*

Fortunately most of these injuries are mild and have a good prognosis. Rarely, more severe injuries, including unstable cervical fractures, can also present with a delayed onset of neck pain or only minimal complaints of neck pain.[9] Since chiropractic manipulation in an unstable spine could lead to further displacement, early evaluation with CT or MRI may be appropriate when significant trauma has occurred. Early recognition of injuries that would require surgical intervention is important not only to abate acute neurovascular compromise but also to prevent late disabling sequelae.

If the cervical spine is imaged with either CT or MRI shortly after a hyperextension injury, generally within 2 weeks, the prevertebral space should be evaluated carefully for the presence of soft tissue swelling. While normal plain film measurements of the width of the prevertebral soft tissues exist,[10] the advantage of MRI—and to some extent of CT—is the ability to image the edema and hemorrhage directly, making absolute measurements of tissue width unnecessary. The presence of soft tissue swelling can be an early and possibly the only sign of cervical instability.[10] Muscle spasm directly following the injury may give the false impression of a stable spine, making the finding of soft tissue swelling on imaging studies possibly the only clue that the patient may have an unstable injury (Figures 4–13 and 4–14).

Tears of the ALL, if imaged acutely or subacutely, are nearly always associated with

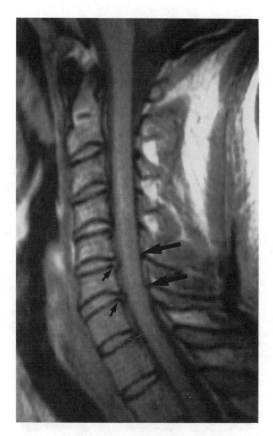

Figure 4–10 Nonhemorrhagic contusion. On this corresponding sagittal T1-weighted image of the cervical spine, note normal homogeneous signal intensity within the cord (*large arrows*). Also identified are small central disc protrusions at both the C-5 to C-6 and C-6 to C-7 levels (*small arrows*) and moderate central canal stenosis.

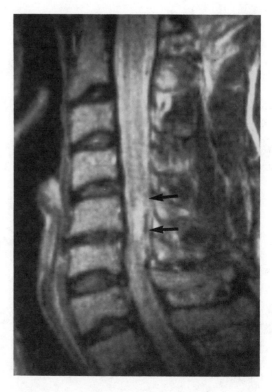

Figure 4–11 Region of hemorrhagic contusion. Sagittal T2-weighted image of the cervical spine reveals area of increased signal intensity identified within the cord at the C-5 level (*arrows*).

hemorrhage and edema of the prevertebral soft tissues.[11] The absence of edema or hemorrhage is a good sign that the ALL is intact. With MRI the ALL and PLL can be directly imaged, making identification of the location and extent of the tear possible. With CT the ALL is not directly imaged but injuries of the ALL can be inferred by the presence of prevertebral swelling or, in more severe cases, the presence of avulsion fractures off the anterior aspect of the vertebral body end-plates.[10]

Evaluation of the paravertebral muscle groups for possible injuries is best performed by MRI; however, severe muscle injuries may be appreciated on CT. Muscle injury may range from minor tears of the sternocleidomastoid muscle to partial avulsion of the longus colli muscle. Tears of the longus colli muscle are often associated with prevertebral hematomas and swelling. Muscle tears and strains on MRI are best imaged on the T2-weighted and STIR examinations. The STIR examination is a heavily T1-weighted sequence that suppresses the signal from fat. These injuries present as areas of high signal intensity within the injured muscle on both imaging sequences. Depending on when the patient is scanned, an associated hematoma may be better imaged on the T1-weighted study. This would be seen as an area of high

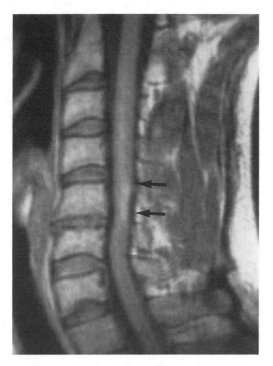

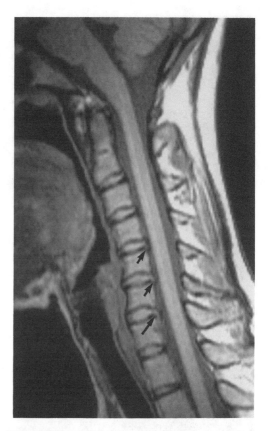

Figure 4–12 Region of hemorrhagic contusion. T1-weighted sagittal image of the cervical spine reveals a corresponding area of increased signal intensity within the cord posterior to the C-5 vertebral body *(arrows)*. This finding of increased signal intensity within the cord on both the T1- and T2-weighted images is indicative of intramedullary hemorrhage.

Figure 4–13 Mild reversal of normal cervical lordotic curvature. Sagittal T1-weighted image of the cervical spine demonstrates mild reversal of normal cervical lordosis. Note is also made of mild annular bulging at the C-4 to C-5 and C-5 to C-6 levels *(short arrows)*, with a small central protrusion at the C-6 to C-7 level *(long arrow)*. Note the excellent demonstration of the cord morphology on this image, as well as the size of the central canal.

signal intensity within or surrounding the injured muscle. Although the sympathetic nerves are not directly imaged by either CT or MRI, injuries to the sympathetic nerves have been associated with injuries to the longus muscles as well as with tears of the ALL. This has been postulated as a possible cause of the associated cranial complaints commonly seen following hyperextension injuries of the cervical spine.

While most soft tissue injuries will heal relatively quickly with conservative therapy, if there is a tear of the annulus fibrosus the recovery period may be prolonged and incomplete.[7,12] Tears of the annulus are not directly imaged by either plain film studies or CT;

however, MRI has the ability to image tears of the annulus noninvasively. With MRI an annular fissure may be seen as a linear, high-signal defect extending through the outer annular fibers on the T2-weighted examination. Annular disruption may be inferred on CT/MPR and plain films by anterior widening of the disc space; with the history of a hyperextension injury this may be the only sign of a potentially unstable cervical spine injury.[13] When performing CT if there is no contrast

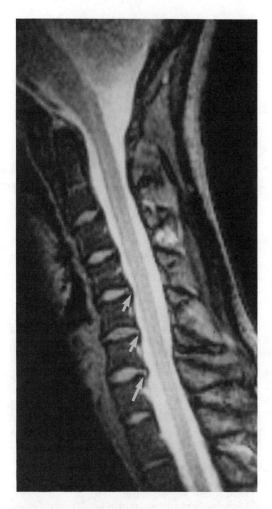

Figure 4–14 Mild reversal of normal cervical lordotic curvature. Corresponding sagittal T2-weighted image of the cervical spine also demonstrates the mild reversal of the normal cervical lordotic curvature. The small bulges at the C-4 to C-5 and C-5 to C-6 levels are also appreciated *(short arrows)*, with the protrusion also demonstrated at the C-6 to C-7 level *(long arrow)*. Note the high signal intensity of the CSF with respect to the cord, giving this sequence the "MR myelogram" effect.

herniations), and extrusions. The presence of such findings on CT would raise the suspicion of a disrupted annulus, possibly indicating further studies, such as discography, in the appropriate clinical setting.

The finding of radicular pain following injury does not necessarily imply disc herniation with compression of a nerve root. Radicular pain, or pain down an arm, following hyperextension injuries to the cervical spine has more commonly been associated with traumatic neuritis and spasm of the scalenus muscle.[12] Both of these causes of radicular pain would not be appreciated on either MRI or CT imaging. While disc protrusions and extrusions with demonstrable nerve root impingement rarely occur with true direct hyperextension injuries of the cervical spine, if there is rotation or torsion of the neck during the injury, as there often is during a motor vehicle accident, disc herniation may occur[12] (Figure 4–15).

Imaging of acute disc herniation using MRI following cervical spine trauma has been reported as high as 23% even with an intact neurologic exam.[14] Additionally, if there is a history of significant head or facial trauma the incidence of associated soft tissue injuries to the cervical spine increases greatly and has been shown to be present in up to 100% of cases.[15] Another cause of neck pain and radiculopathy is the presence of perineural or epidural hematoma.[15] Both CT and MRI are very sensitive and specific in determining the presence of disc herniation; however, MRI has a greater sensitivity and specificity in detecting hemorrhage that may be associated with the injury.

As noted, both modalities are excellent in evaluating the morphology of the annulus and distinguishing annular bulges, protrusion, and extrusion. Mild disc bulging and lateral protrusions may result in nerve root irritation and impairment of root conduction[12] (Figures 4–16 and 4–17). This has been postulated not only as a cause of radicular pain but also as a possible etiology of cranial symptoms, which are often complained of following hyperextension in-

within the disc space, CT will not directly image annular disruption or annular fissuring, but it is sensitive to changes in the morphology of the annulus and can detect the presence of annular bulges, protrusions (i.e., contained

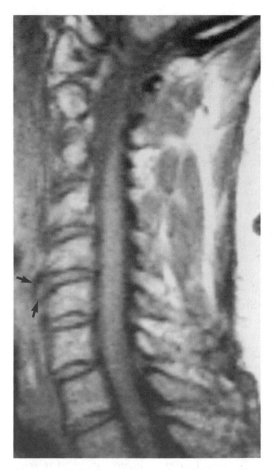

Figure 4–15 Patient with previous history of hyperextension injury of cervical spine. Sagittal T1-weighted MRI image demonstrates prominent anterior protrusion at the C-5 to C-6 level *(arrows)*.

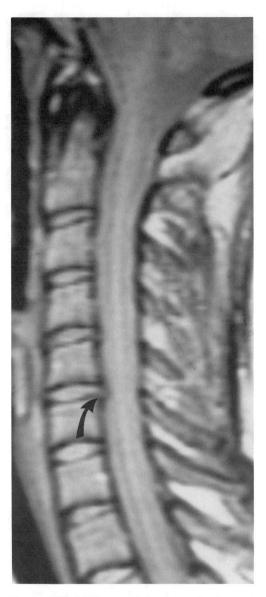

Figure 4–16 MRI scan of the cervical spine; patient has complaints of neck pain following hyperextension injury. Sagittal proton density MRI image of the cervical spine reveals posterior bulging of the annulus at the C-5 to C-6 level *(curved arrow)*. Apart from this finding, the cervical spine was unremarkable.

jury of the cervical spine.[16] Numerous communications between the cervical somatic nerve roots and the sympathetic chain have been described.[17] The C-4 nerve root communicates with the superior cervical ganglion of the sympathetic chain through a branch off the postganglionic fibers. Irritation of the C-4 nerve root may then lead to cranial complaints such as headache, vertigo, tinnitus, and facial pain, also known as the Barré-Lieou syndrome. Tamura[16] has demonstrated the existence of posterolateral protrusions at the C-4 level with myelo-

graphy in those patients with cranial complaints. Although myelography is now commonly not employed in the evaluation of the

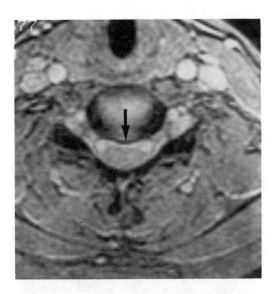

Figure 4–17 MRI scan of the cervical spine; patient has complaints of neck pain following hyperextension injury. Corresponding axial T2-weighted image. This demonstrates mild, symmetric, outward bulging of the annulus (*straight arrow*). There is slight effacement of the anterior subarachnoid space; however, the cord is not compressed. Also note the normal appearance of the intervertebral nerve root canals.

cervical spine, the presence of posterolateral protrusions can also be determined with MRI and, with slightly less accuracy, CT.

Innervation of the cervical intervertebral disc has been described by Bogduk as being primarily via the vertebral nerve.[18] Although the vertebral nerve is predominantly derived from the sympathetic nervous system, it does have connections with the cervical ventral rami. Hence, the vertebral nerve may not be exclusively autonomic in nature and also may convey somatic afferents. This interplay between the autonomic and somatic nervous systems may contribute to the cranial complaints following hyperextension injuries to the spine. Although the vertebral nerve itself cannot be imaged directly by either MRI or CT, demonstration of a disrupted annulus by either imaging modality or discography may indicate the etiology of the patient's neck or

radicular pain. However, it should be stressed that demonstration of an annular tear or herniation by itself does not always imply pain-generating pathology. Many annular tears are asymptomatic during discography and are often detected as incidental findings on imaging studies (Figure 4–18).

Additionally, degenerative disc disease in cervical spondylolysis can be seen on both MRI and CT in asymptomatic individuals. This finding of asymptomatic degenerative disc disease in cervical spondylolysis tends to increase in frequency with increasing age (Table 4–1). Asymptomatic disc herniations with resultant central canal stenosis and mild cord compression have been demonstrated with MRI.

Particularly in the elderly patient, the radiologist and the referring clinician must be careful about attributing clinical symptoms to structural abnormalities that may be regarded as age-related changes.[19,20]

It can be seen from the above discussion that MRI and CT are not mutually exclusive in the evaluation of the cervical spine. CT with its excellent osseous detail and MRI with its superior soft tissue resolution together are currently the most powerful noninvasive means of evaluating the spine.

Because of the invasive nature of myelography it has now been relegated to a very limited role in the evaluation of the cervical spine. If multiplanar CT and MRI are available, myelography generally is not necessary and would add little to the diagnostic work-up. Some imaging centers with access to both CT and MRI have supplemented the standard multiplanar CT scan of the cervical spine with a fast sagittal T2-weighted sequence that provides the "MRI myelogram" effect. This combination of CT and limited MRI provides the bone detail of CT and also adds the ability to evaluate cord morphology and the effects of thecal sac compression with MRI. Because one of the major advantages of CT/MPR over MRI is its ability to distinguish bone from soft tissue, the combination of CT/MPR and MRI has limited the use of myelography and CT myelography.

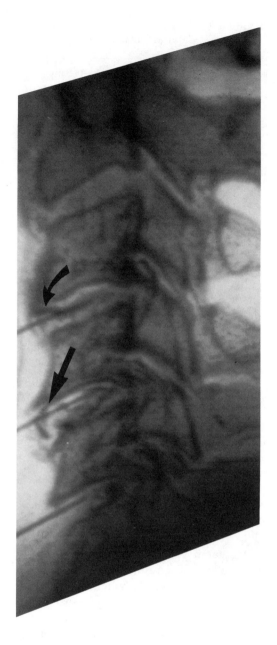

Figure 4–18 Cervical discography demonstrating annular tears at both the C-3 to C-4 and C-4 to C-5 levels. Upon opacification of the anterior fissure at the C-3 to C-4 level *(curved arrow)*, the patient's pain was reproduced. However, upon opacification of the anterior fissure at the C-4 to C-5 level *(straight arrow)*, no pain was evoked.

Table 4–1 Asymptomatic Degenerative Disc Disease and Spondylosis of the Cervical Spine: MRI

	% of Age	
Finding	*45–54*	*>64*
Disc space narrowed	24	67
Disc protrusion	20	57
Osteophytosis	20	37
Spinal cord impingement	18	26
Cord compression	5	9

Source: Reprinted from Teresi, L.M., et al., Asymptomatic Degenerative Disk Disease and Spondylolysis of the Cervical Spine: MR Imaging, *Radiology* Vol. 164, pp. 83–88, with permission of the Radiological Society of North America, Inc., © 1987.

FACTORS AFFECTING THE SEVERITY OF INJURY

In patients who have experienced a hyperextension injury of the spine, it is important to evaluate the spine for coexisting conditions that may predispose the patient to a more severe injury than might normally be expected by the stated mechanism of injury. Such predisposing conditions include cervical spondylolysis, central stenosis, congenital segmentation anomalies, and previous surgical fusion of the cervical spine. Patients with pre-existing spondylolysis or central spinal canal stenosis may be rendered quadriperitic even without a fracture or dislocation injury.[21,22] In such patients there is diminished overall mobility of the spine, particularly at the involved levels. This may predispose the first adjacent mobile segment to an injury to the cord or disc. Developmental or acquired cervical spinal stenosis with its associated diminished volume of the central canal has been shown to be a predisposing condition to neural dysfunction following spine trauma.[23–25]

SPINAL STENOSIS

Spinal stenosis is defined as local, segmental, or generalized narrowing of the central canal by osseous or soft tissue elements. Stenosis may be congenital, developmental, or acquired. Congenital stenosis is related to disturbed fetal development, and developmental stenosis is secondary to a growth disturbance of the posterior element. Acquired stenosis is narrowing of the spinal canal secondary to degenerative changes.[26] Both CT and MRI are able to provide extremely accurate measurements of the size of the central canal and assess for the presence of congenital, developmental, or acquired central stenosis.[27] Additionally, both modalities can assess and evaluate the extent of cervical spondylolysis, the presence of which can adversely affect the patient's prognosis.

By obtaining direct axial or sagittal images or reformatted images of the spine from either axial MR or CT images, the size of both the central and intervertebral nerve root canals can be determined accurately. MRI is able to evaluate the true sagittal dimension and cross-sectional area of the thecal sac, thus obviating the need for CT myelography. A true osseous diameter can be obtained orthogonal to the long axis of the cervical central canal off the sagittal images. Plain films and CT measurement of normal central canal diameters have been well established (Exhibit 4–1).

Osseous ridging or spurring off the uncinate processes and end-plates is appreciated on both MRI and multiplanar CT; arguably the osseous changes are probably better appreciated by CT. Thickening or redundancy of the ligamentum flavum is also well seen by both CT and MRI. Calcifications of the PLL, which may contribute to central stenosis, are best evaluated by multiplanar CT. Both the cranial to caudal and posterior extension of the PLL calcification are well defined by multiplanar CT.

In patients who present with cervical myelopathy or radiculopathy, thin-section high-resolution CT has been an excellent screening examination.[28] Because of its reduced soft tissue resolution, CT does not directly image neural impingement or compres-

Exhibit 4–1   Normal Sagittal Diameter of Cervical Canal by CT

C-3 to C-6	=	14–14.5 mm
Standard deviation	=	1.3–2.1 mm
Relative central stenosis	<	12.5 mm
Absolute central stenosis	<	10.5 mm

sion. However, CT is excellent in differentiating between disc herniation and spondylotic spurs (Figure 4–19).

The importance of MRI is in its ability to delineate the effect of spondylotic changes on the neural elements in either the central or intervertebral nerve root canals. Osseous stenosis itself may not result in cervical myelopathy, and MRI is extremely helpful in demonstrating the effects of the osseous or soft tissue encroachment on the neural structures (Figure 4–20). Recent studies have shown that the best predictors of the clinical course in myelopathic patients, the effect of surgical intervention, and the pathologic changes of the spinal cord are the degree of cord compression and measurement of cord volume.[29,30] Patients with high-signal-intensity areas within the cord on MR images responded less favorably to surgical or medical treatment.[31]

FACET ARTHROSIS

Degenerative changes involving the posterior facets can also result in reduced mobility of the cervical spine. Although the posterior articulating facets (i.e., zygapophyseal joints) are imaged by both MRI and CT, multiplanar CT surpasses MRI in assessing the severity or presence of degenerative changes involving the facets.[32] The extent of joint space narrowing is easily evaluated by multiplanar CT. Degenerative erosive and sclerotic changes involving the facets are also well characterized by multiplanar CT. The precise location and size of facet spurs can be determined, as well as evaluated for the presence of calcifications

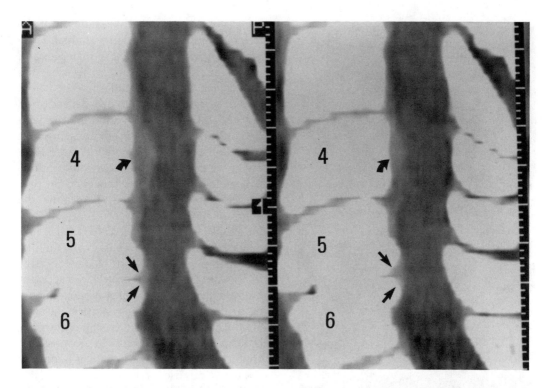

Figure 4–19 Combination study CT/MPR and sagittal T2-weighted MRI scan. Sagittal reformatted CT images of the cervical spine at soft tissue window settings reveal soft tissue density posterior to the C-4 vertebral body *(curved arrow)*. There is appreciable compression of the thecal sac at this level. At the C-5 to C-6 level, there is evidence of disc degeneration with narrowing of the intervertebral disc space and vacuum phenomena. Posterior osteophytic ridging off the adjacent end-plates is also noted *(small arrows)*.

involving the joint capsule. Although rare, the presence of a congenital spondylytic defect involving the facets can also be determined. Trauma to the facets, particularly when there are pre-existing degenerative changes, may be the etiology of many of the symptoms following hyperextension injury to the spine. Neck pain and possibly radiculopathy may be the result of referred facet pain via articular branches off the cervical dorsal rami that innervate the periarticular fibrous tissue.[18] Additionally, this may also contribute to the complaints of vertigo following hyperextension injuries by affecting the primitive "righting reflex" by causing inaccurate afferent input to the vestibular nuclei.[33]

ASSESSING TIME OF INJURY

If no examination of the spine prior to the injury is available, assessing the time of injury can be difficult with imaging studies alone. In the acute phase, findings such as a prevertebral hematoma, cord contusion/edema, and fractures obviously can be associated with the acute traumatic event. Difficulty may arise when the patient presents several months or even years following injury for an imaging study and there is the need to determine the temporal relationship of the findings to the injury. Assessing the "age" of a disc herniation can be difficult and is fraught with problems. Both the nucleus pulposus

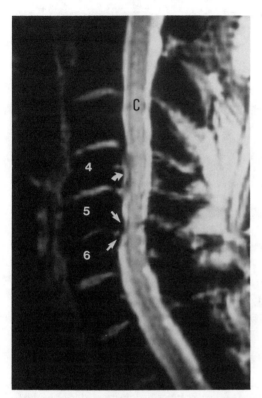

Figure 4–20 Combination study CT-MPR and sagittal T2-weighted MRI scan. Sagittal MRI study reveals a mass of high signal intensity posterior to the C-4 vertebral body *(curved arrow)*. Appearance is consistent with an extruded disc fragment from the C-4 to C-5 intervertebral disc space. Note complete effacement of the anterior subarachnoid space. However, the cord (C) is not compressed. The disc space at the C-5 to C-6 level is noted to be narrowed and of slightly diminished signal intensity. Posterior osseous ridging can be appreciated at the C-5 to C-6 level as well *(arrows)*.

and annulus fibrosus consist mainly of water, collagen, and proteoglycans, with the major differences being the relative concentration of the components, level of hydration, and the particular type of collagen that predominates.[34] On T2-weighted MRI studies the high signal intensity in the central portion of the disc is related to the well-hydrated nucleus pulposus and the inner annular fibers.[22] With

aging, there is a gradual breakdown of the proteoglycans in the nucleus, gradual desiccation of the mucoid nuclear material, and loss of anatomic delineation between the nucleus and the inner annular fibers.[35] Radial tears or fissure then lead to disc degeneration and desiccation, as these communicate with the central nuclear material, allowing disc herniation and loss of proteoglycans.[36] Following disc herniation the disc will continue to degenerate/desiccate; however, no prospective studies exist that determine the length of time necessary for a normally hydrated disc to become desiccated after it herniates. Hence, given the scenario of a middle-aged patient with coexisting degenerative disc disease and annular protrusions at one or multiple levels who presents months following an injury for imaging, accurate assessment of the temporal relationship of the findings to the injury may be impossible. Additionally, assessing the state of hydration of the cervical discs is more difficult than it is for the lumbar intervertebral discs. One reason for this is the relatively smaller size of the cervical disc, compared with that of the lumbar spine. With the small cervical discs it may be difficult to detect subtle decreases in the signal intensity of the nucleus pulposus, a sign of early disc degeneration/desiccation. Other factors such as operating field strength, type of surface coil used, and size of the patient may all contribute to relative signal intensity of the disc, making accurate assessment of the degree of disc hydration difficult.

It should also be stressed that it is quite possible to herniate a previously degenerated/desiccated disc; in this case, even in the acute phase it may be difficult to determine the time of injury by MRI alone unless the herniation is associated with a hematoma or edema of adjacent soft tissue structures. As always, the findings on imaging studies must be correlated with the patient's symptoms. The clinical findings, in combination with the findings on the imaging studies, may give the best estimate as to when the injury occurred.

INDICATIONS FOR OBTAINING IMAGING STUDIES

Because of the relatively high cost of imaging studies, as well as the exposure to ionizing with CT, an imaging study should not be a routine test in the evaluation of any patient who presents following a neck injury. Indications that would necessitate obtaining a study would include progressive neurologic deficit, significant head injury, incomplete neurologic lesions such as anterior or central cord syndrome, and Brown-Séquard syndrome; it is also indicated for any patient who presents with a complete neurologic lesion and for whom treatment or decompression is planned to promote nerve root recovery. Other predisposing indications include pain greater than expected by the mechanism of injury, failure of conservative management or poor outcome, inability to tolerate conservative therapy or a stabilization program, and unusual features of presentation such as nocturnal pain or atypical pain distribution.

Often it may be necessary to obtain imaging studies if the patient has a long history of neck pain and other somatic complaints, including cranial symptoms, following injury but has not been previously studied and carries no diagnosis. It may also be necessary to obtain a study to define or document a diagnosis, as in personal injury and disability cases.

As imaging technologies advance and continue to develop it will become increasingly important for the clinician also to gain a greater understanding of the technology so that it can be used to its greatest advantage. Both MRI and CT are extremely complex technologies, but used properly and interpreted accurately they are also extremely powerful tools in the evaluation of cervical spine injury.

REFERENCES

1. Stark DD, Bradley WJJ. *Magnetic Resonance Imaging*. St Louis: CV Mosby Co; 1988.
2. Modic M, Masaryk T, Ross J, et al. Cervical radiculopathy: value of oblique MR imaging. *Radiology*. 1987;163:231–277.
3. Emery S, Pathria M, Wilber R, et al. Magnetic resonance imaging of post traumatic spinal ligament injury. *J Spinal Disord*. 1987;2:229–233.
4. Bergstrom K, Nyberg G, Pech P, et al. Multiplanar spinal anatomy: comparison of CT and cryomicrotomy in postmortem specimens. *Am J Neuroradiol*. 1983;4:590–592.
5. Beers G, Raque GH, Wagner G, et al. MR imaging in acute cervical spine trauma. *J Comput Assist Tomogr*. 1988;12:755–761.
6. Schaefer D, Flanders A, Northrup B, et al. Magnetic resonance imaging of acute cervical spine trauma: correlation with severity of neurologic injury. *Spine*. 1989;14:1090–1095.
7. Davis S, Teresi L, Bradley W, et al. Cervical spine hyperextension injuries: MR findings. *Radiology*. 1991;180:245–251.
8. Selecki B. Whiplash. *Aust Fam Physician*. 1984;13:243–247.
9. Cox G, Barish R. Delayed presentation of unstable cervical spine injury with minimal symptoms. *J Emerg Med*. 1991;9:123–127.
10. Penning L. Prevertebral hematoma in cervical spine injury: incidence and etiologic significance. *AJNR*. 1981;136:553–561.
11. Goldberg A, Rothfus W, Deeb Z, et al. Hyperextension injuries of the cervical spine: magnetic resonance findings. *Skeletal Radiol*. 1989;18:282–288.
12. MacNab I. Acceleration injuries of the cervical spine. *J Bone Joint Surg [Am]*. 1964;46:1797–1799.
13. Clinton E, Gillula L, Murphy W, et al. The widened disk space, a sign of cervical hyperextension injury. *Radiology*. 1981;141:639–644.
14. Rizzolo S, Piazza M, Cotler J, et al. Intervertebral disc injury complicating cervical spine trauma. *Spine*. 1991;16:187–189.
15. Jonsson H, Bring G, Rausching W, et al. Hidden cervical spine injuries in traffic accident victims with skull fractures. *J Spinal Disord*. 1991;4:251–263.
16. Tamura T. Cranial symptoms after cervical injury: aetiology and treatment of the Barré-Lieou syndrome. *J Bone Joint Surg [Br]*. 1989;71:283–287.

17. Bogduk N. The innervation of the cervical intervertebral disc. *Spine.* 1988;13:2–6.

18. Bogduk N. The clinical anatomy of the cervical dorsal rami. *Spine.* 1982;4:319–329.

19. Boden SD, McCowin PR, Davis DO, et al. Abnormal magnetic-resonance scans of the cervical spine in asymptomatic subjects. *J Bone Joint Surg [Am].* 1990;72:1178–1184.

20. Teresi LM, Lufkin RB, Reicher MA, et al. Asymptomatic degenerative disk disease and spondylolysis of the cervical spine: MR imaging. *Radiology.* 1987;164:83–88.

21. Taylor A. The mechanism of injury to the spinal cord in the neck without damage to the vertebral column. *J Bone Joint Surg [Br].* 1951;33:543–547.

22. Yu S, Haughton V, Ho P, et al. Progressive and regressive changes in the nucleus pulposus, part 2: the adult. *Radiology.* 1988;169:93–97.

23. Eismont F, Clifford S, Goldberg M, et al. Cervical sagittal spinal canal size in spine injury. *Spine.* 1984;9:663–666.

24. Epstein J, Carras R, Hyman R, et al. Cervical myelopathy caused by developmental stenosis of the spinal canal. *J Neurosurg.* 1979;51:363–367.

25. Murone I. The importance of the sagittal diameters of the cervical spinal canal in reaction to spondylosis and myelopathy. *J Bone Joint Surg [Am].* 1974;56:30–36.

26. Roberson G, Llewellyn H, Taveras J. The narrow lumbar spinal canal syndrome. *Radiology.* 1973;107:89–97.

27. Schnebel B, Kingston S, Watkins R, et al. Comparison of MRI to contrast CT in the diagnosis of spinal stenosis. *Spine.* 1989;14:332–337.

28. Miysaka K, Isu T, Iwasaki Y, et al. High resolution computed tomography in the diagnosis of cervical disc disease. *Neuroradiology.* 1983;24:253–257.

29. Fujiwara K, Yonenobu K, Ebsara S, et al. The prognosis of surgery for cervical compression myelopathy: an analysis of the factors involved. *J Bone Joint Surg [Br].* 1989;71:393–398.

30. Fujiwara K, Yonenobu K, Hiroshima K, et al. Morphometry of the cervical spinal cord and its relation to pathology in cases with compress myelopathy. *Spine.* 1988;4:1212–1216.

31. Takahashi M, Yamashita Y, Sakamoto Y, et al. Chronic cervical cord compression: clinical significance of increased signal intensity on MR images. *Radiology.* 1989;173:214–219.

32. Carrera G, Haughton V, Syverrsen A, et al. Computed tomography of the lumbar facet joints. *Radiology.* 1980;134:145–148.

33. LaBan M. Whiplash: its evaluation and treatment. In: *Physical Medicine and Rehabilitation: State of the Art Reviews.* Philadelphia: Hanley & Belfus, Inc; 1990:293–307.

34. Ghosh P. *The Biology of the Intervertebral Disc.* vol 2. Boca Raton, Fla: CRC Press; 1988.

35. Miller J, Schmatz C, Schultz A. Computed tomography in degenerative spinal stenosis. *Clin Orthop.* 1981;161:221–234.

36. Lipson S, Muir H. Proteoglycans in experimental intervertebral disc degeneration. *Spine.* 1981; 6:194–210.

Chapter 5

Neurodiagnosis for Neck Injuries

Kulveen Sachdeva

INTRODUCTION

Electrodiagnostic studies play a significant role in the evaluation of a patient with cervical trauma. They provide the means to test the physiologic integrity of the nerves and their function. The following studies are indicated in cases of complicated cervical trauma in which there could be different disease processes, such as disc disease, resulting in cervical root compression, or traction injuries to either the roots or the brachial plexus (see Figure 5–1):

- nerve conduction studies
- electromyography
- somatosensory evoked potentials

Each of these studies has different sensitivities, depending on the site of the lesion. For example, nerve conduction studies are more sensitive in a peripheral neuropathy as opposed to electromyography, which is more sensitive in cases of radiculopathy. Therefore, a combination of different studies is performed, based on the patient's history. Electrodiagnostic studies are an extension of the physical examination and should be correlated to the radiologic investigations.

NERVE CONDUCTION STUDIES

Stimulation of a nerve generates an action potential that can be recorded from the muscle innervated by the nerve or along the nerve at a different site. In this fashion, sensory and motor nerves can be tested. The readily available nerves that can be tested in the upper extremity include the median, ulnar, and radial nerves. Less commonly studied nerves include axillary, musculocutaneous suprascapular, and thoracic nerves.

Motor Nerve Conduction

Stimulating a nerve and recording over the muscle innervated by that nerve provide an action potential that is referred to as a compound muscle action potential (CMAP). In the case of the median nerve the abductor pollicis brevis is used as the recording site. The active recording electrode should sit over the muscle belly, whereas the reference electrode is placed over the tendon of the muscle, distal to the active electrode (Figure 5–2).

A 20% to 30% supramaximal intensity impulse is required to ensure the activation of all the axons innervating the muscle.[1] A biphasic

124   MOTOR VEHICLE COLLISION INJURIES

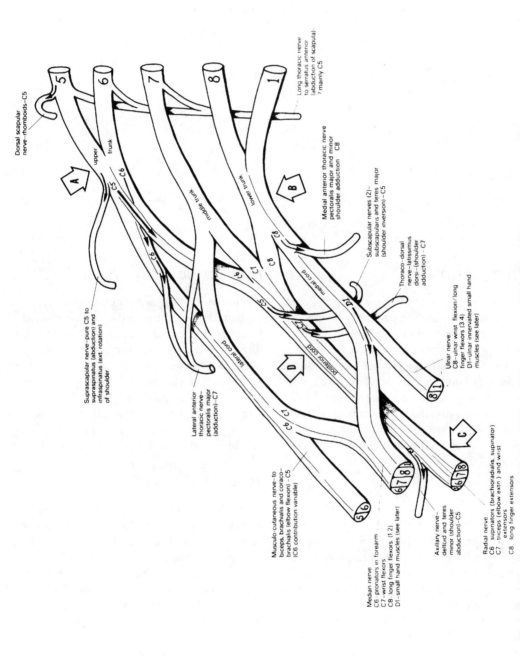

Figure 5–1 Scheme of the anatomy of the brachial plexus showing the eventual destination of all root components. *Source:* Reprinted from *Neurological Differential Diagnosis* by J. Patten, p. 204, with permission of Springer-Verlag, © 1987.

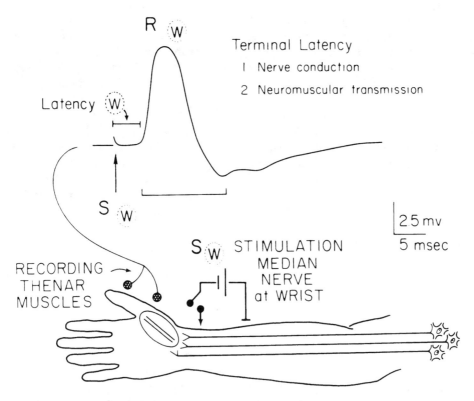

Figure 5–2 Compound muscle action potential recorded from the thenar eminence after stimulation of the median nerve at the wrist. The distal or terminal latency includes (1) nerve conduction from the stimulus point to the axon terminal and (2) neuromuscular transmission, including the time required for generation of the muscle action potential after depolarization of the end-plate. *Source:* Reprinted from *Electrodiagnosis in Diseases of Nerve and Muscle: Principles and Practice*, 2nd ed., by J. Kimura, with permission of F.A. Davis Co., © 1989.

wave is obtained and latency is calculated. Latency is the interval between the onset of the stimulus and the onset of the response, and indicates the integrity of the fastest conducting fibers. The amplitude is calculated from peak to peak, and reflects the axonal integrity of the nerve. Dropout of the axons results in decreased CMAP amplitude. Finally, the conduction velocity is calculated. This is achieved by obtaining two CMAPs through stimulation of two different sites on the nerve and recording at the same muscle. Accurate measurement of the distance between the two points ensures true motor nerve conduction velocity. Velocity is dependent on the myelin content of the nerves. Consequently, any demyelinating process will present as decreased nerve conduction velocity.

Sensory Nerve Conduction

Unlike motor nerves, sensory nerve recording and stimulation are performed over the course of the nerve. There are two methods of stimulation used for testing:

1. orthodromic
2. antidromic

Orthodromic stimulation is performed on a distal nerve and recording is done proximally over the course of the same nerve. For example, palmar stimulation is used on the median nerve distally while recording proximally over the wrist. Antidromic stimulation is achieved when recording is distal to the stimulated site.

For sensory nerve responses the amplitude is calculated from peak to peak, and latency is determined at the first peak because the takeoff is usually not a precise point. The sensory fibers degenerate only with a lesion distal to the sensory ganglion.[1] Therefore, the presence of a normal sensory potential may indicate a lesion proximal to the sensory ganglion, such as root avulsion in which clinical sensory symptoms are present. In the case of plexopathy or neuropathy, however, sensory symptoms coincide with sensory conduction abnormalities.

Commonly Tested Nerves in the Upper Extremity

The median nerve carries a fairly superficial course in the arm, allowing easy access to testing. The sensory component is tested distally at the wrist, using either orthodromic or antidromic stimulation. Palmar stimulation with recording at the wrist is particularly helpful in identifying compression or entrapment of the median nerve at the carpal tunnel. Motor testing is accomplished by recording at the abductor pollicis brevis and stimulating at the wrist, elbow, axilla, and Erb's point. Double-crush injuries indicate involvement of the roots and carpal tunnel after cervical trauma. Median nerve testing in that respect is a very important part of the evaluation. Responses recorded from the third digit evaluate the C-7 root, middle trunk, and lateral cord. First digit testing assesses C-6 to C-7 roots, upper or middle trunk, and lateral cord.[1]

The ulnar nerve also carries a superficial course in the upper extremity. Recording is performed at the abductor digiti minimi and stimulation is provided at various points, i.e., wrist, elbow, above the elbow, axilla, and Erb's point. Alternatively, the forearm muscles, like the flexor carpi ulnaris or flexor digitorum profundus, may be used to record ulnar motor conduction.[2] This nerve carries great relevance when evaluating posttraumatic thoracic outlet syndrome. The ulnar nerve studies are used to differentiate between C-8 and T1- root lesions from the lower trunk, medial cord of the plexus, and the nerve itself.[1] The radial nerve, on the other hand, reflects the integrity of the C-6 and C-7 root, upper and middle trunk, and posterior cord of the plexus.[1]

F Wave Studies

After obtaining the CMAP by using supramaximal stimulation with an antidromic technique, F waves are obtained. This is a form of late response and has a much smaller amplitude than the M wave. The wave helps to evaluate the proximal segments of the nerves and can be tested for most of the nerves of the upper extremity.

Abnormalities in the F wave can be seen in various neurogenic processes, including neuropathies and radiculopathies. Several studies suggest the use of F wave studies in root injuries.[3-5] In milder cases of root involvement, and especially if there is predominant sensory involvement, F wave studies may not reveal any abnormalities. In the case of thoracic outlet syndrome with a neuronal component,[6] latencies of the F waves may be delayed. Although comparison of left to right may be helpful in unilateral lesions of the root and plexus, F wave studies in and by themselves may not be reliable.

ELECTROMYOGRAPHY

Clinical electromyography (EMG) refers to a diagnostic procedure in which electrical activity of the muscle is tested. Action potential from depolarization of the muscle fibers or muscle groups can be detected by the use of needle electrodes introduced into the muscles.

Responses are amplified and projected on an oscilloscope, where they can be evaluated both aurally and visually.

Motor unit potentials are generated secondary to depolarization. This potential refers to the summation of electrical activity of the muscle fibers belonging to the same voluntarily activated motor unit. There is an initial positive triphasic waveform as the impulse approaches, arrives, and departs from the active electrode.[1] The amplitude of the action potential depends on the spatial relationship between the cell and the needle tip. Muscle fibers of a motor unit under normal situations fire in a synchronized fashion. In a typical denervated muscle, the fibers tend to fire independently, generating spontaneous activity (Figure 5–3). This is perhaps the most important component of electromyography.

Procedure

The proficiency of an EMG to detect nerve injury lies in its ability to find abnormalities in the electrical activation of the muscle as a result of injury to the nerve innervating that muscle. Each muscle must be tested separately at multiple sites. Normal findings in one area do not exclude the possibility of pathologic changes in another area of the same muscle. There are four steps to this evaluation:

1. insertional activity
2. spontaneous activity
3. motor unit potentials
4. interference pattern

The needle electrode used may be either a monopolar needle electrode or a concentric needle electrode. Activity generated is displayed on an oscilloscope. Exploration must be performed in all four directions of the muscle at two to three levels of insertion, depending on the size of the muscle. It is useful to select key muscles for detailed analysis and to obtain the maximal amount of information; for example, select the deltoid muscle to

evaluate the C-5 root, the triceps muscle to evaluate the C-7 root.

Insertional Activity

This burst of activity is generated in the muscle from the insertion of a needle[7] and lasts only a few milliseconds. The insertional activity is produced by the trauma of placing the needle electrode into the muscle. This activity is described as being normal, increased, or decreased. The most common cause of decreased activity is fibrosis of the muscle. Increased activity is seen during denervation or inflammation of the muscle, for example, as occurs in polymyositis.

Spontaneous Activity

In the resting muscle there should be no persisting spontaneous activity in the muscle after insertion of the needle electrode. The only circumstance in which spontaneous activity is noted is when the needle lies in close proximity to the end-plate. This is known as "end-plate noise."[1] End-plate noise and end-plate spikes are activities generated at this point and represent extracellular miniature end-plate potentials.[8]

Any other activity seen in a resting muscle is considered pathologic. This pathologic activity in descending order of frequency may consist of fibrillation potentials, positive sharp waves, fasciculation potentials, myokymic discharges, and complex repetitive discharges. Spontaneous activity must be reproducible in at least two different sites within a single muscle before it can be considered a definite abnormality. There is a lag period of about 2 to 3 weeks after injury before denervation patterns can be detected upon electromyographic testing.

Both fibrillation potentials and positive sharp waves represent single-fiber activation.[9] Fasciculation potentials are spontaneous discharges of an entire motor unit. Myokymia indicates repetitive firing of a motor unit. Complex repetitive discharges result from rapid firing of many muscle fibers in sequence. Most

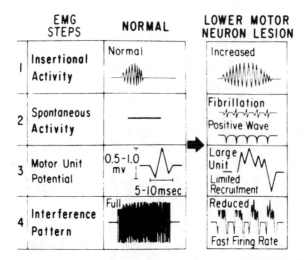

Figure 5–3 Typical EMG findings in lower motor lesions. They include prolonged insertional activity, fibrillation, limited recruitment, and reduction of firing rates. *Source:* Reprinted from *Electrodiagnosis in Diseases of Nerve and Muscle: Principles and Practice*, 2nd ed., by J. Kimura, with permission of F.A. Davis Co., © 1989.

denervation activity is graded 1 to 4, depending on the severity, with 4 being the worst.

Fibrillation potentials are usually biphasic or triphasic spikes with initial positive deflections. Their duration is 1 to 5 milliseconds and their amplitude ranges between 50 and 300 μV. They fire at a rate of 5 to 15 Hz but vary from 2 to 30 Hz. Fibrillation potentials are one of the most frequently noted abnormalities in patients with diseases or lesions affecting the peripheral nervous system. Positive sharp waves often are seen in association with fibrillation potentials due to denervation. These waves have an initial sharp positive deflection followed by a long-duration negative phase.

Motor Unit Potentials

Motor unit potentials are summated electrical activity of the same voluntarily activated motor unit. The various aspects of the study include shape, size, and duration of the motor unit. Initially the patient is asked to activate the muscle minimally by contraction, during which the configuration of the motor unit is accessed. Classically, loss of neurons secondary to neurogenic processes results in de-

crease in the number of motor unit potentials. However, because of reinnervation, the configuration changes to being polyphasic. The normal motor unit potential has an amplitude of 0.5 to 2 mV and a duration of 3 to 15 milliseconds.

Interference Pattern

Interference pattern, also known as the recruitment pattern, is the test of the number of functioning motor units in a muscle. In situations in which there is an axonal dropout, decreased interference pattern is noted despite good effort of contraction of the muscle.

Nerve Root Stimulation

In this situation the nerve root is accessed by introducing a monopolar needle electrode into the paraspinal muscles while recording is done from selective muscles representing various myotomes in the limb.[10] Preliminary claims are that this procedure is the most sensitive for the detection of compressive radiculopathies.

SOMATOSENSORY EVOKED POTENTIALS

Somatosensory evoked potentials (SSEP) are elicited by electrical stimulation of an accessible sensory or mixed peripheral nerve and recorded by electrodes placed at selected locations over the spine and the scalp. The entire afferent pathways can be evaluated by this technique. The international 10–20 system for scalp electrodes is used.

In the upper extremity the nerves commonly tested include the median and the ulnar.

Following upper limb stimulation, potentials are generated. They occur at the level of the cervical medullary junction and lower medulla, probably in the dorsal column nucleus and medial laminescus. There are various factors in play while generating these potentials, as indicated by the large variety of disease processes that can cause abnormalities in the SSEP. These include segmental demyelination and axonal and neuronal loss.[11] The clinical value is further enhanced because of the close relationship between the evoked potential waveforms and specific anatomic structures. The peripheral sensory conduction can also be studied in the absence of distal sensory nerve action potentials, such as in the case of coexisting peripheral neuropathies.[11] Comparison of peripheral and central conduction times is possible.[1]

Lesions Associated with SSEP Abnormalities

Commonly studied lesions include those of the root and plexus. In cervical spondylosis SSEP do not differentiate between it and other cervical lesions. It is believed that amplitude abnormalities as opposed to latency abnormalities of the response may indicate more accurately root lesions secondary to spondylosis. However, these abnormalities do not help in indicating either disease severity or long-term prognosis in patients with spondylotic cervical disease. In the case of cervical spinal cord injuries SSEP are not able to indicate severity of the lesion, although preserved responses or their return after injury indicate either an incomplete lesion or a good prognosis.[12] Selective stimulation of digital nerves is used to elicit SSEP, with the first, third, and fifth digits corresponding to the C-6, C-7, and C-8 nerve roots, in the differentiation of radicular lesions.[13]

CONCLUSION

Electrodiagnostic studies play a very significant role in the evaluation of a patient with cervical trauma. This is the only investigation that can test the physiologic integrity of the peripheral nervous system. Furthermore, it helps to localize the different pathologies at different levels within the peripheral nervous system. However, just as in any investigational procedure, these studies also have their limitations. The first limitation is the lag time between the onset of symptoms or injury and the appearance of electrical abnormalities on testing. Second, false-negative results can be seen even in the presence of clinical and radiologic abnormalities. Third, false-positive results may be seen in patients with a pre-existing condition. These limitations, however, do not negate the useful diagnostic and prognostic information that can be obtained in a relatively noninvasive manner.

REFERENCES

1. Kimura J. *Electrodiagnosis in Diseases of the Nerve and Muscle: Principles and Practice.* 2nd ed. Philadelphia: FA Davis; 1989.
2. Felsenthal G, Brockman P, Mondell D, et al. Proximal forearm ulnar nerve conduction techniques. *Arch Phys Med Rehabil.* 1986;67:440–444.
3. Eisen A, Schomer D, Melmed C. The application of F-wave measurements in the differentiation of

proximal and distal upper limb entrapments. *Neurology*. 1977;27:662–668.

4. Fisher MA, Kaur D, Houchins J. Electrodiagnostic examination, back pain and entrapment of posterior rami. *Electromyogr Clin Neurophysiol*. 1985; 25:183–189.

5. Fisher MA, Shuvde AJ, Teixera C, et al. Clinical and electrophysiological appraisal of the significance of radicular injury in back pain. *J Neurol Neurosurg Psychiatry*. 1978;41:303–306.

6. Dorfam LJ. F wave latency in cervical rib and band syndrome. *Muscle Nerve*. 1979;2:158–159.

7. Weddell G, Feintein B, Pattle RE. The electrical activity of voluntary muscle in man under normal and pathologic conditions. *Brain*. 1944;67:178–257.

8. Wiederholt WC. "End plate noise" in electromyography. *Neurology*. 1970;20:214–224.

9. Daube JR. Needle examination in electromyography. American Association of Electromyography and Electrodiagnosis. Minimonograph #11. Rochester, Minn; 1979.

10. Wilboourn AJ, Aminoff MJ. The electrophysiological examination in patients with radiculopathies. American Association of Electromyography and Electrodiagnosis. Minimonograph #32. 1988.

11. Rossini PM, Cracco JB. Somatosensory and brainstem auditory evoked potentials in neurodegenerative system disorders. *Eur Neurol*. 1987;26:176–188.

12. Rowed DW, McLean JAG, Tator CH. Somatosensory evoked potentials in acute spinal cord injury: prognostic value. *Surg Neurol*. 1978;9:203–210.

13. Synek VM. Somatosensory evoked potentials after stimulation of digital nerves in the upper limbs: normative data. *Electroencephalog Clin Neurophysiol*. 1986;65:460–463.

Chapter 6

Basic Concepts of Soft Tissue Healing and Clinical Methods To Document Recovery

PART 1: SOFT TISSUE INJURY REPAIR

Richard A. Nolan and Lawrence S. Nordhoff, Jr.

INTRODUCTION

It is generally accepted that automotive collisions produce frequent chronic neck pain, with prognostic studies showing significant percentages of long-term symptoms. (See Chapter 11 for specific prognosis studies.) The persistence of neck pain and referred pain beyond the active repair process indicates that there is continued physical, chemical, and/or mechanical alteration or irritation of pain-sensitive tissues. Resultant scar tissue formation, in either fibrotic tissue or adhesions within or around joints or myofascial tissues, accounts for most of the chronic symptoms that the physician encounters in practice. Although all occupants who have been involved in a motor vehicle collision injury (MVCI) will undergo the same stages of repair, the doctor can have a dramatic influence in the healing outcome if early education and active management are initiated. The physician can inform the patient about the stages of repair and how they can enhance the healing process. Encouragement should be given to the patient for a self-role in the management process. The patient should be informed of the adverse effects of smoking, poor diet, poor posture, and excessive stress as well.

To understand the healing process in soft tissue injuries of the cervical spine, it is essential to discuss the basic physiologic response to such injury. The scar itself has been considered the result of the repair of a tissue injury and as such is a pathologic process. Glynn states, "Tissue injury, especially of a traumatic kind involving skin and superficial tissues, is so common and its repair by the formation of scar tissue so regular a consequence, that it may be regarded as almost a physiological, rather than a pathological response."[1] Hunt says, "Wound healing is a continuous sequence of signals and responses in which epithelial, endothelial, and inflammatory cells, platelets, and fibroblasts briefly come together outside of their usual domains, interact, restore a semblance of their usual discipline, and having done so resume their normal functions."[2] Figure 6–1 illustrates the complex nature of wound repair.

SOFT TISSUE INJURY AND SUBSEQUENT STAGES OF REPAIR

Most neck injuries involve overstretching forces that exceed the force applied, the distance stretched, or the rate of acceleration. Fig-

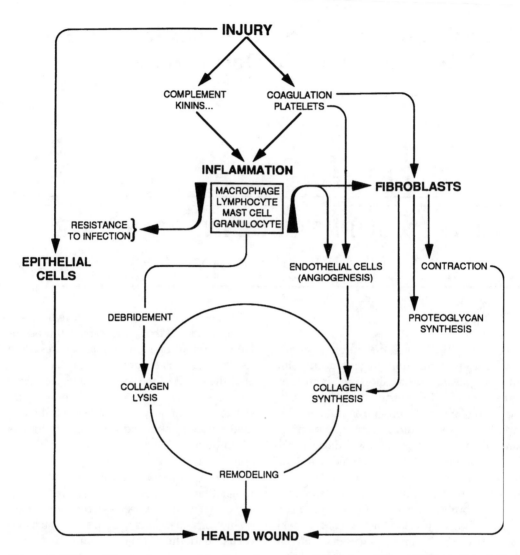

Figure 6–1 Flow diagram for wound healing. *Source:* Reprinted from Hunt TK, Basic Principles of Wound Healing, *Journal of Trauma*, Vol. 30, No. 12, pp. 122–128, with permission of Williams & Wilkins, © 1990.

ure 6–2 illustrates a stress-strain relationship between pathophysiologic failure and loading. The soft tissues that are traumatized will go through four stages of healing. Although several authors have referred to three or four stages of repair, there is in fact only one stage of repair. There are two prerepair stages that set the stage for repair to begin. The first stage involves simply the immediate effects of in-

jury, including bleeding, coagulation, and cell necrosis. The inflammatory response is primarily the means for the body to respond to the bleeding and necrosis and establish feedback so that an appropriate level of repair response can occur. In the repair stage the damaged cells are replaced with either the same type of tissue or scar tissue, depending on the degree of injury. The last stage occurs after all

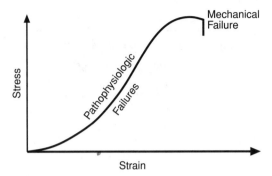

Figure 6–2 The stress-strain relationship for a one-dimensional tissue. Also shown is the zone of onset of pathophysiologic failure due to mechanical loading. *Source:* Reprinted with permission from Aldman B, An Analytical Approach to the Impact Biomechanics of Head and Neck Injuries, in 30th Proceedings, Association for the Advancement of Automotive Medicine, Montreal, 1986.

the damaged cells are replaced (repaired). It involves realignment of fibers according to the stresses put on them, usually called remodeling. Figure 6–3 illustrates the normal overlapping healing stages of the body. The body's intensity and quality of healing response and time frame depend on the extent of the injury, amount of motion stresses on the healing tissues, nutritional status, and genetic factors. Some patients just heal faster and better than others do. Further delineation of the processes follows.

Hemorrhage/Coagulation/Necrosis State

Rapid, high-force flexion/extension, lateral flexion, or rotational injuries of the cervical spine can result in overstretching that disrupts blood vessels and capillaries, muscle, fasciae, and ligamentous and neurologic tissues. The result is hemorrhage, coagulation, and possibly necrosis. The ruptured vessels in the confines and periphery of these injured tissues pour out blood, which is a protein-rich fluid containing the clotting factors that allow for a

fibrin clot to form in the surrounding injured tissues. Immediately after injury is sustained, the complex process of tissue necrosis, inflammatory reaction, and repair begins. Necrosis, literally "death" of the cell or tissues in the area of injury, is the ultimate injury. Lesser degrees of injury result simply in cell damage. The physiologic response to injury is an inflammatory one, whereby the body attempts to surround the area of injury and begin the repair process. This repair process may result in the need to remove the injured tissue and let regeneration (replacement of original tissue with scar tissue [connective tissue]) begin.

Trauma from motor vehicle crashes usually results in the death (necrosis) of many soft tissue cells. Up to the level of death the changes may be reversible. The hallmark of cell death is the occurrence of changes within the nucleus, which may include condensation, fragmentation, or lysis. A second hallmark of cellular death is disruption of the cell membrane, from which recovery is not possible. The reversible changes are permanently demonstrated in the cytoplasm with preservation of the cellular membrane and the nucleus. Once death has occurred the cell's own lysosomes digest the cell; this is the major physiologic change that takes place, along with a multitude of other events. Necrosis is usually the product of sudden, acute injury, whereas reversible changes are generally seen in the more chronic injuries, such as overuse-type syndromes.[3]

The source of trauma to the cell is usually direct physical force, the effect of which varies according to the injury site and the degree of force. The end result is either reversible or irreversible changes in the cell, and this can be determined in a very short time following injury by observing the degree of swelling and vascular disruption that reduces the oxygen supply to the tissues (hypoxia) or interrupts it (anoxia). The degree of cell injury is directly related to the amount of disruption as it relates to the oxygen demand for the various types of cells (e.g., skeletal muscle versus

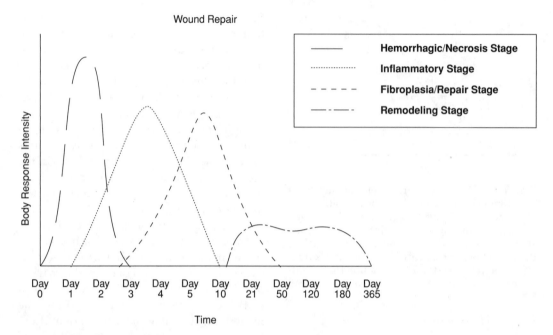

Figure 6–3 Stages of healing for soft tissue injuries over time. Healing includes two prerepair stages, repair, and remodeling stages.

myocardial muscle). Reversible changes are usually accompanied by swelling (edema), which results in enlargement of the tissues; whereas necrosis is not associated with swelling, but, in fact, is associated with contracture of the tissues.[3]

Shortly thereafter, the area is invaded by fibrocytes that when activated become fibroblasts. The fibrin is progressively replaced by collagen; this process takes several days to several weeks, depending on the extent of the area injured. At the same time, capillary ingrowth occurs by proliferation from the lining of the epithelial cells from the adjacent vessels through a budding process.[1] How this process takes place is not clear; however, it is believed that the increased metabolic demand created by the injured cells' presence, particularly the fibroblast, creates an environment stimulus level through which this process takes place. These capillaries begin the process of anastomosis and form loops that invade the fibrin. These loops in turn create a granular appear-

ance to the surface; that is, they turn into granulation tissue. The ensuing process is a complex one, involving enzymes to control the removal of the injured tissues, while at the same time, the collagen fibrils are formed. This is an intricate process involving anabolic, as well as catabolic, steps to provide for the synthesis of the collagen and complex proteoglycans to form the ground substance.[4]

Inflammatory Stage

The entire purpose of the inflammatory response stage is to surround the area of injury in an attempt to protect the surrounding uninvolved tissues and remove the debris from the cellular necrosis in order to pave the way for the upcoming repair process. The extent of this response is usually proportional to the amount of injury sustained. This may express itself as a mild reaction with a vascular and cellular response that is quite limited, versus a more intense reaction in which there is significant necrosis requiring phagocytosis, a process in which the neutrophils and macrophages remove the cellular debris and toxins from the area. The neutrophils are rapid-response cells that, upon arrival, release their digestive enzymes or begin the phagocytosis process. Shortly thereafter they themselves die. The macrophages are a slower-response cellular line that is responsible for the removal of the debris, including the necrosed neutrophils. The type of response will depend on the causative agents involved; for example, a bacterial agent will result in neutrophils, as opposed to a nonbacterial agent, which will result in macrophage invasion. In the event of foreign material, the macrophages will form giant cells, which are multinucleated cells capable of phagocytosing foreign material that may have penetrated as a result of the injury.[3]

The inflammatory response is of quick onset and once initiated is amplified by several chemicals, including bradykinin. This phase lasts up to 3 days.[5] The acute inflammatory response is characterized by a vascular component in which there is an increase in the blood flow and permeability of the vessel walls. The result is increased temperature in the affected tissues, with erythema and edema. The increased vessel response results in increased flow of blood. Concomitant with this is permeability of the vessel walls, which permits the flow of the blood components, including electrolytes, proteins, and cells, the cells being leukocytes and predominantly monocytes and neutrophils. Swelling results in pressure on the nerves, causing pain. Secondarily, there is limitation of motion and function based on the pain induced from the nerve pressure and limited function/use based on the cellular injury with its edema and pain.

Along with vascular dilatation comes an increased vascular supply with permeability that allows for increased fluid penetration. This serves to help carry away the debris, as well as to dilute toxins. In the more severe cases of permeability, fibrinogen and protein leaking into the tissue can form a network that will surround the area of injury and form a barrier for the egress, as well as the ingress, of further toxins and/or bacteria. In addition to the vascular events, there is a chemotactic event that takes place by the release of histamine from the mast cells. The local effects of trauma will cause dilatation of the vessels. Histamine furthers this event by causing dilatation and increased permeability of the small venules, which leak the plasma protein—particularly albumin—into the area, secondarily causing swelling through osmosis.

Repair Stage

The repair process following the injury is dictated by the severity of the injury. The injury will heal by full regeneration, having quality equal to that of tissue before trauma, or by fibrosis and/or scarring. In a case where there is cell trauma without necrosis, the process is one of regeneration. When cell necrosis takes place, the replacement is accomplished by the production of fibrous tissue, resulting in scarring or adhesions. The repair phase of fibroplasia lasts from 2 days to 6 weeks, at which time fibers have been repaired but the collagen fibers are not fully oriented in the direction of tensile strength.[6] Angiogenesis peaks at about 4 days.[7]

Regeneration is essentially replacement of the surrounding tissues by less similar cells and is the preferred process, since it reassures the restoration of function. This can occur in the case of cellular death; however, it is dependent on the ability of the surrounding cells to multiply. The regenerative process is limited to certain cells, such as liver mucosa, bone marrow, and epidermis. The most tenacious of these is the bone marrow, which can fully regenerate when only a few cells survive.

The fibrous form of repair is replacement of the necrotic tissue with collagen in an effort to bridge the gap formed by the tissue death. This is an expression of the body's attempt to strengthen the area to allow for function of the surrounding tissues. The fibrous tissue itself is a dense, minimally elastic tissue. The process begins with the invasion of capillaries and fibroblasts that provide the necessary components for the repair process, such as that of acute inflammation. Proliferation of the fibroblasts then sets the foundation for scar formation by reproduction of collagen that is progressively formed. A recent report concludes that scar tissue heals in a "haphazard manner."[8] Initially, the balance is in favor of the capillaries and fibroblasts. As the repair process continues, the balance moves in favor of the collagen tissue. The latter stage of this process is contracture of the fibrous scar, resulting in a very mild deformity depending on the size of the area that requires repair. Figure 6–3 illustrates a typical time chart for wound healing.

Remodeling Stage

The remodeling stage is of concern for the health care provider and the insurance company. After a person sustains an injury in an automobile crash, questions arise as to how long it takes for healing and what forms of therapy and rehabilitation are most appropriate. Soft tissue remodeling is the body's response to stress. For example, the heart remodels to high blood pressure by hypertrophy, muscles atrophy in space or after immobilization, and soft tissues remodel with activity. Remodeling occurs when the residual fibrous repaired soft tissues undergo reorganization and reorientation along the lines of stress. Carlstedt's review of the literature concludes that this process peaks at about 3 to 4 weeks and continues up to about 1 year.[9] This is the stage in which two activities take place, the first being realignment of the collagen source to increase the functional capacity of the collagen as it is stressed in normal usage. The tensile strength of collagen is dependent on the force imposed on it during the remodeling stage. The second event is that of replacement of the type III collagen with the preinjury type I collagen. The repair-type mature collagen, type III, is deficient in the number of cross-linkages within the tropocollagen subunits. It was determined by Frank et al.[10] that the normal ligament substance appearance has not been reproduced by the remodeling process even after 40 weeks, that this process appears to plateau at approximately 70% of the normal level. Remodeling beyond 6 months probably involves hypovascular tissues and injuries having extensive damage.

CHRONIC INFLAMMATION

Typically, chronic inflammation is a less intense response, with limited edema, hyperemia, and neutrophilic infiltration. The cellular component is generally that of lymphocytes, plasma cells, and—to a lesser extent—macrophages. The plasma cells produce antibodies that attach to the foreign material and allow the neutrophils and macrophages to phagocytose the material. The lymphocytes have a multifaceted role that appears to be involved with the recognition of foreign material at the level of host cells to isolate the foreign substances, transform into plasma cells to produce antibody, and direct traffic other than inflammatory cells, particularly macrophages. The macrophages continue to perform their phagocytosis, and they also supply the cytotoxic role.

The prominent feature of chronic inflammation, as opposed to acute inflammation, is proliferation of fibrous tissue in an attempt to confine the injured area and provide it with increasing strength. The formation of the fibrous tissue results in contracture distortion of the tissues, as well as the loss of normal function. Otherwise the inflammation responses essentially are identical, with the exception of the intensity of the response. There are many causes of chronic inflammation; however, in this chapter we are confining ourselves to the traumatic origin. Patients with fibrositis commonly have history of trauma, and the model shown in Figure 6–4 illustrates variations in cross-links, rubber-bandlike structures, small interlinking fibers between two muscles, and a healed wound with abnormal fiber orientation.

TYPES OF SOFT TISSUE INJURY

Peripheral nerve injuries can occur when tractional forces stretch the nerve beyond its tolerance level. This may be seen as a result of side collisions in which the occupant's head is laterally flexed, hitting the shoulder, and the brachial nerve plexus is put under tension. Actual nerve compression can occur in a patient with bony spurs in the cervical spine if tension forces are strong enough to pull the nerve over the bony encroachment. In peripheral nerve injuries the veins within can be injured, hemorrhage, and go through the repair process. The peripheral nervous system has the ability to repair or regenerate fully if the damage is not too extensive. It is also possible that physiologic disturbances, e.g., in nerve fibers, may occur at a lower strain than that needed for mechanical failure."[11]

Central nervous system tissue, such as the spinal cord and nerve rootlets, may also be injured in whiplash injuries of the neck. The damaged disc may put compression onto the cord if it is centrally bulging, or onto the nerve rootlet before it goes through the gutter of the intervertebral foramen below the level of the disc. Central nervous system tissue does not regenerate or repair; it either becomes fibrotic or scars over time. Damaged veins may leak blood via the effects of gravity and pressure down into the sheath and into the gutter of the intervertebral foramen. A study by Hoyland et al.[12] concluded that edema of nerve roots, compression, congestion, and resultant dilatation of intervertebral foraminal veins may be the mechanism in the development of perineural and intraneural fibrosis. Muscle tears (with capillary bleeding) of varying degrees always accompany post–MVCI neck pain. Muscles have a better circulatory supply than the other types of soft tissues in the neck, and as a result they usually will heal faster and

with fewer residual problems than ligament and tendon tissues. If fasciae surrounding the muscles are overstretched and injury is involved, seeping blood may move down the fascial planes and may cause adhesions from the repair process. Figure 6–4 illustrates possible soft tissue abnormalities that may develop in posttraumatic scarring. There may be cross-linking fibers, as seen in part A of Figure 6–4, interconnecting scar tissue fibers, rubber-bandlike structures, or irregularily shaped scar tissue formation.

Ligament and tendon repairs tend to be slower and are accompanied by more scarring than muscle tissue repair. There is a tendency for these tissues to overheal. This is largely due to a poorer vascular supply.[13] Tendons must have great tensile strength and must be able to glide great distances. Tendon strength requires an abundance of collagen, which may, as a part of normal repair, result in adhesions to the surrounding tissues, thus reducing its gliding capability. The presence of oxygen may very well parallel the repair process. Ligaments and tendons take about 6 weeks to heal, unless additional harmful stresses occur during the earlier stages of repair, such as micro- or macrotrauma. The ending scar tissue has less elasticity and strength than the original tissue. As Green states, "Sprains classically heal well with only some mild to moderate degree of permanent scarring and mild resultant permanent loss of elasticity of these tissues. Sometimes fibrous scarring in or near the joint capsule can occur as well, limiting the range of motion of that particular joint. This can permanently interfere with the injured areas' daily musculoskeletal functions."[14]

The intervertebral discs for adults have no regenerative ability. The disc receives fluid exchange from blood vessels in the periphery and by diffusion through the avascular portion of the disc. It tends to go through the usual inflammatory response and repair by scarring. Neovascularization will occur around the edges of the fragments of torn fibrocartilage.

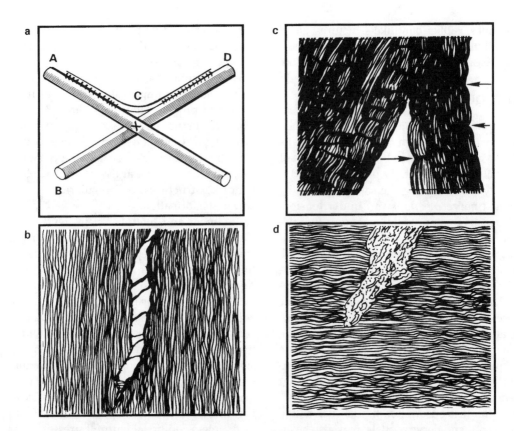

Figure 6–4 Illustration of four types of soft tissue abnormalities that may be seen after MVCI. a, An idealized model demonstrating the collagen cross-link interactions at the molecular level. *A* and *B* represent the pre-existing fibers, *C* represents the newly synthesized fibril, *D* represents the cross-links created as the fibril becomes incorporated into the fiber, and *X* represents the nodal point at which adjacent fibers are normally freely movable past one another. b, Interconnecting network of thin threads between fibers of fibrositis muscle. c, Fiber bundle from a glycerinated quadriceps muscle from a patient with fibrositis, showing rubber-bandlike structures along the fibers (*arrows*). d, Healed ligament with residual scar tissue area that has fibers that lie in an irregular manner.

Figure 6–4a: *Source:* Reprinted from Akeson W.H., Amiel D., and Woo S.L-Y., Immobility Effects on Synovial Joints: The Pathomechanics of Joint Contracture, 3rd International Congress of Biorheology, Symposium on Soft Tissues Around a Diarthrodial Joint, *Biorheology*, Vol. 17, No. 1, pp. 95–110, with permission of Pergamon Press, Ltd., © 1980.

Figure 6–4b and c: *Source:* Adapted from Bartels E.M. and Danneskiold-Samsoe B., Histological Abnormalities in Muscle from Patients with Certain Types of Fibrositis, *The Lancet*, April 5, 1986, pp. 755–756, with permission of The Lancet, © 1986.

WHEN DOES REPAIR STOP?

The question "When does repair stop?" frequently is asked by the insurance carrier paying for the collision injury. The claims adjuster wants to know whether the treatment parallels the repair process, and if so, how much future expense and time will be involved. As any doctor who has been in practice for a few years and has seen a couple of hundred whiplash injuries knows, there is variability among patients. Although several surgical and laboratory studies have shown remodeling occurring up to 1 year after injury, most active repair is completed by 6 to 8 weeks. When all torn or damaged fibers have reneurovascularized, the inflammatory stage and fibroblastic stages have ended, and the preinjury balance of synthesis has normalized, then repair is concluded. Each type of tissue (i.e., ligament, muscle, and tendon) has its own unique repair time.

The time needed is dependent upon the type of tissue traumatized, the location of the tissue, stresses during repair, extent of damage, quality and type of replacing scar tissue, and the age of the person. If one is evaluating nerve rootlet injury (central nervous system tissue), then only scarring/fibrosis occurs with little to no regeneration, and a longer time is needed. Tissues that are avascular or hypovascular, such as discs and ligaments, will usually take longer to heal as well. Early management with cryotherapy, mobilization,[5] manipulation, early controlled activity and exercises, and compliance by the patient can also speed repair time and enhance recovery. Just because the active repair process is finished does not indicate that the patient's progress will stop. Clinical experience has shown that most patients will show substantial decrease in pain/stiffness after 6 to 8 weeks and further moderate improvement for another 2 to 4 months. Between 6 months and 1 year the patient will continue to show slight improvement in symptoms, usually noting change in 3- to 4-week increments, rather than on a daily basis.

FACTORS THAT MAY COMPLICATE HEALING RESPONSES

There are several factors that complicate the normal repair process after MVCI. These include smoking, nutritional disorders, aging, diabetes, collagen diseases, severe injuries, and some medications. Of all of the following factors, the doctor can be most beneficial by having the patient stop smoking for a few weeks.

Nutritional Effects on Healing Process

Several surgical, laboratory, and clinical studies have been conducted in the past two decades evaluating nutritional factors that influence or retard injury/trauma repair.[2,15–24] Malnutrition is not uncommon in our society, due to poor dietary habits, weight loss programs, drugs, and certain disease states.[22] There are many factors that can retard soft tissue repair of an injury, and the nutritional status of the person injured is one of them. For example, a chronic alcoholic who is malnourished will have poor healing.[25] Most current studies evaluating nutritional effects on trauma have involved surgical wound cases; and, indeed, the importance of maintaining proper nutritional support after surgical trauma has been a mainstay of hospital management for years. Yet little research evaluating the effect of nutrition on nonsurgical injuries, such as whiplash, has been done. We know that the healing process can take place in an orderly fashion in the well-nourished tissues of a properly nourished individual, so there is every reason to expect nutrition to be a factor in the healing of MVCIs.

People in a protein-deficient state have a decrease in wound healing and in the rate at which the tensile strength of the wound progresses. Of the metals, zinc is the only one that has demonstrated a clear-cut effect on wound healing. It appears to be necessary as a precursor for collagen formation. High levels of zinc are found in wounds during the early stages of healing, when collagen biosynthesis is progressing, and then it drops to normal levels later on.

Vitamin-Mineral Recommendations

During the first 2 weeks after injury it is critical to create an optimal healing environment for the various damaged nerves, ligaments, and muscles that need adequate minerals, vitamins, water, and amino acids if they are to heal properly. A balanced diet with abstinence from dehydrating substances such as alcohol, caffeine, hot dogs, and too much red meat can be beneficial. During the first day after trauma the body is in its injury-shock phase. Nutritional changes are not advised for the first day because of the potential for disturbing the body's preprogrammed metabolic balance system.[26,27]

One review of literature concluded that after trauma, vitamin C levels are shown to decrease.[28] Ascorbic acid deficiencies produce the most adverse effects on wound repair.[6,25] Vitamin C has been confirmed as being essential to muscle, skin, and nerve repair, as well as to strong scar tissue formation.[16] It is recommended that 1000 to 3000 mg of this vitamin be taken per day for the first 6 weeks, spread out in three to four doses every day. Taking vitamin C will speed up the repair process. The patient should be given at least 500 to 1500 mg/day, depending on the severity of the trauma.[16,29] Vitamin C is needed for histamine breakdown and promotes collagen and elastin formation.[15,24,25]

One of the most extensive articles summarizing nutrition and repair suggests that the most important nutrients for healing include vitamin C, vitamin A, zinc, sulfur, and amino acids.[16] Also, additional vitamins such as vitamin E, which stabilizes cell membranes and speeds up the repair process, are recommended. Vitamin E is an antioxidant that prevents peroxide accumulation, thus preventing the harmful effects of free radicals on tissues.[16] It has the same effects as corticoids and may reduce scar tissue formation.[16] Vitamin B_1 helps in collagen formation and neural repair. Bioflavinoids and proteolytic enzymes can augment and increase the body's healing ability.[27]

Megadoses of vitamins and minerals are not suggested. A well-balanced, digestible vitamin supplement such as those termed *high-stress complex vitamins*, will suffice, with minor adjustments such as added vitamin C or iron in severely deficient patients. Some vitamin companies pack the pills so that they do not

break down well in the digestive tract. The authors have noted hundreds of vitamin pills on lumbar X-rays over the years, indicating that some brands are indigestible. Advise the patient to switch brands if results are not satisfactory. Nutritional counseling outside the doctor's office is usually not necessary for most patients unless a severe malabsorption problem exists or the doctor has inadequate expertise in this area.

Conditions That May Delay Healing

Occasionally patients have nutritional disorders that may complicate or slow the repair process after trauma. These patients heal more slowly and have more residual medical problems, thus a poorer prognosis. The repair process is complex and is dependent on the physiology of the body, which can be affected by aging, nutrition, systemic disease processes and medications (steroids).[3] Additional time is necessary to educate these patients, since they may not have had any advice on injury and dietary nutritional deficiencies. The following include some of the more common conditions or drugs that may affect wound repair:

- Pernicious anemia
- Chronic malnourishment,[25] for example, from stapling or surgical stomach removal, with the resultant inability to absorb certain nutrients. In the case of a partial intestinal removal the doctor needs to find out what part was removed and to correlate any deficiencies, such as liver failure with jaundice.[30]
- Iron deficiency anemia. Look at the sclera, ask about easy bruising, and perform lab tests to verify this condition (in severe cases).
- Eating disorders, namely, bulemia and anorexia
- Vitamin C depletion
- Alcoholism[25] resulting in a vitamin B_1 deficiency due to liver malfunction

- Caffeine overuse. Caffeine may add to the existing neuronal hyperexcitability in the already damaged oversensitive tissues.

- Drugs such as methysergide (headache medication) and diphenylhydantoin, which cause excess scarring for some unknown reason. Penicillamine prevents collagen cross-linking, and some sex hormones may inhibit angiogenesis.[30]

- Diabetes[30]

- Thyroid disorders

- Nutritional deficiency resulting from prolonged immobilization[31]

Cigarette Smoking

Cigarette smoking has several potentially negative effects for the injured patient:

- increased risk of prolapsed cervical intervertebral disc[32]

- higher risk of spinal surgical nonunion[33]

- reduced blood flow into vertebral endplates, reducing disc nutrition[34,35]

- oxygen reduction to discs[35]

- block of prostaglandin E_1, an anti-inflammatory chemical[36]

- lower acidic intradiscal pH[37]

- reduced fibrinolytic activity[5]

- associated coughing, which may increase intradiscal pressure[38]

- accelerated intervertebral disc degeneration[35]

- higher risk for developing myofascial pain syndromes[36]

It has been shown by several authors that smoking increases the incidence of back pain.[38] Smokers have been reported to have twice as great a chance of developing spinal pain and nine times as great a chance of failing to respond to surgery.[35] Cigarette smoking, which results in oxygen deficiency to already traumatized ischemic tissues, is not recommended for 4 to 6 weeks after the occupant has been in a motor vehicle collision. This rule applies to head injuries, cord injury, joint injury, soft tissue strain/sprains, and fractures as well. A comparative study of smokers and nonsmokers undergoing lumbar surgery found that smokers had a significantly higher incidence of surgical nonunion, possibly due to low oxygen blood gas levels.[33] Mandell et al. reported that spinal disorders are related to smoking, and that smoking reduces fibrinolytic activity that may result in more fibrous repair.[39] Battié et al.[34] found that smokers have 18% higher disc degeneration scores on magnetic resonance imaging (MRI) than nonsmokers, concluding that smoking may have a systemic effect of disc degeneration through vasospasms or arteriosclerotic changes. Kelsey et al.[32] found that the risk for prolapsed cervical disc was increased about 30% for each additional 10 cigarettes per day smoked during the year before the onset of symptoms. Hambly and Mooney[37] concluded from their data that exposure to cigarette smoke (10 cigarettes) consistently produces a biochemically sick disc for 2 weeks.

The authors suggest that smokers having acute neck injury, back injury, and head injuries be advised as follows: "Smoking during the first few weeks following an injury may interfere with the normal healing process. If you smoke during this time you may slow your recovery down or end up with pain that you would not have otherwise. This may result in your requiring more treatment, having worse prognosis, or being referred to another doctor." This statement is best reinforced with a couple of articles on the subject. Some patients may feel that the doctor just has it in for the smoker and does not have any research to back it up. If the doctor spends 2 to 3 minutes discussing the subject with the patient, the vast majority of smokers will comply. The objective is not to get the smoker to quit on a long-term basis, although beneficial, but rather to facilitate the repair response.

PART 2: QUANTITATIVE AND OBJECTIVE DOCUMENTATION OF SOFT TISSUE ABNORMALITY: PRESSURE ALGOMETRY AND TISSUE COMPLIANCE RECORDING*

Andrew A. Fischer

PRESSURE ALGOMETRY FOR DIFFERENTIAL DIAGNOSIS OF TENDERNESS AND EVALUATION OF TREATMENT RESULTS IN FLEXION/EXTENSION INJURIES

The vast majority of cases of flexion/extension injuries affect the soft tissues of the neck and upper back. In instances of bony damage the soft tissue injury is frequently a major cause of pain and dysfunction. Increased pressure pain sensitivity (PPS), that is, abnormal tenderness, is the most consistent finding in soft tissue dysfunction; therefore, this finding is essential for diagnosis. Pressure algometry (PA) quantifies the PPS, which is a measure of sensitization of nociceptive nerve endings, which causes pain and tenderness.

Pressure algometers are instruments that measure the amount of force (pressure) that will induce pain or discomfort. While several different types of algometers have been described recently,[40] the pressure threshold meter (PTM) has been proven most suitable for clinical diagnosis.[41] The PTM (Figure 6–5) is a pocket-sized mechanical instrument and is relatively inexpensive.

Normal values have been established[42] and clinical application of the instrument has been described.[41,43] The PTM consists of a rubber disc measuring head with exactly a 1-cm^2 surface, which is attached to an analog force gauge featuring a range of 10 kg with 0.1-kg divisions. The size of the measuring surface is critical, since larger surface includes more normal tissue around the *trigger points* (TrPs), inducing falsely high results. Too small a surface area of the head results in superficial skin pain reading and fails to transmit the pressure to the deep layers. Therefore, the deeper TrPs are missed. The analog scale is also important, since digital displays do not allow continuous reading, which is critical for increasing the pressure at an even pace.

Pressure threshold expresses quantitatively the sensitization of nociceptive nerve endings by products of tissue injury, which also cause tissue inflammation, pain, and increased sensitivity to pressure.

The measurement of pressure threshold (PTH) is very simple and can be accomplished in a few minutes.[41] First the patient is asked to

---

*This section is adapted from Fischer A., Quantitative and Objective Documentation of Soft Tissue Abnormality: Pressure Algometry and Tissue Compliance Recording, *Spinal Manipulation* Vol. 10, No. 2, with permission of the Foundation for Chiropractic Education and Research, © 1994.

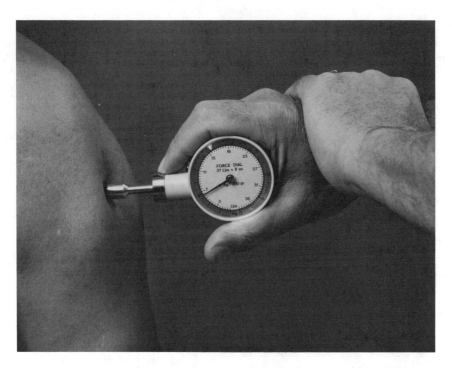

Figure 6–5 Pressure threshold meter (algometer) for quantification of pressure sensitivity. Distributed by Pain Diagnostics and Thermography Inc., 233 East Shore Road, Suite 108, Great Neck, NY 11023.

point with one finger to the area of the maximum pain. The area of maximum pain is usually over the TrP, but sometimes the patient indicates pain in the reference zone, which is specific for each TrP.[44] Therefore, it is important to compare the patient's pain patterns with the reference zones of the TrPs and if they coincide, the TrP causing the pain should be identified and measured. The PTM actually assists in this decision because the referred pain zone is always less tender, that is, has higher PTH than the TrP itself. The examiner palpates the area with his or her fingertip in order to pinpoint the maximum pain area, the most tender spot, and marks it. The meter is applied to the point of maximum tenderness, perpendicular to the muscle surface, and the pressure is increased continuously at the rate of exactly 1 kg/s until patient starts to feel pain. A bilateral comparison of pressure

threshold that exceeds 2 kg/cm^2 is considered abnormal.[43] If bilateral tenderness is present, then a nontender spot in the same or adjacent muscle is measured for reference, or normal values are used for comparison.[41] The reliability, validity, and reproducibility of the PTM[45] and other pressure algometers[46,47] have been proven independently.

Clinical Use of Pressure Algometry

In addition to quantitative diagnosis and differential diagnosis of tenderness, algometry also quantifies treatment results.[41] Both aspects are important for clinical practice. Algometry assists the health practitioner in the very crucial decision of how much pressure sensitivity is to be considered abnormal and diagnostic of trigger points, tender points, fibromyalgia, and muscle and joint dysfunction. PA provides unique information not obtainable by any other method. PA is the only quantitative clinical method for evaluating soft tissue disorders and injuries, including whiplash. Measurement of tenderness is very useful to convince the patient and insurance companies that myofascial pain, a treatable condition, is present. Quantitative data proving abnormal findings facilitate the approval for the treatment plan by insurance company.

Evaluation of Treatment Results

The evaluation of treatment results is also important. An increase of the PTH after the treatment session indicates the effectiveness of the employed procedure. A decrease in the readings indicates that the treatment was either too vigorous or too lengthy, or that an inappropriate procedure had been employed.[40] Long-term follow up of treatment results, usually at 2-week to 2-month intervals, is useful to demonstrate the degree of progress to the health practitioner, the patient, and the insurance company. Improved PA values confirm the need to continue treatment until complete healing is achieved.

The value of the PTM and its reliability in evaluation of treatment effects, such as spray and stretch therapy[48] as well as chiropractic manipulation,[49,50] have been documented.

TISSUE COMPLIANCE METER FOR QUANTITATIVE OBJECTIVE DOCUMENTATION OF MUSCLE SPASM AND TAUT BANDS OF MYOFASCIAL TRIGGER POINTS

The tissue compliance meter (TCM) is a clinical mechanical instrument[51] that consists of a force gauge ranging to 5 kg with a long shaft, which is fitted with a 1-cm^2 rubber disc (Figure 6–6).

When the rubber tip is pressed into the examined tissue at a known force, a disc-shaped collar fitted around the long shaft of a force gauge slides up, indicating the depth of penetration, on a scale attached to the shaft. The depth of penetration expresses the compliance or softness of the examined tissue in millimeters per kilogram of employed force. A harder consistency of the muscle indicates spasm or taut band of the myofascial trigger point. For clinical purposes, one or two measurements, usually 2 kg of force or 3 kg in larger muscles (glutei or large paraspinals), are sufficient and can be performed in a few minutes. For more precise documentation and for measurement of spasm in muscle layers at different depths, sequential measurement is preferred. This is performed at 1 to 5 kg of force in increments of 1 kg. The results are then plotted so that the force is represented on an X axis, and the depth of penetration in millimeters expresses the compliance on a Y axis.

Normal values of tissue compliance have been established, and the reliability and reproducibility of results have been proven.[52] Measurements are performed over the spasmodic muscle or taut band diagnosed by palpation; the contralateral normal tissue is used as reference.

A computerized tissue compliance recorder has been developed that automatically plots[48] compliance curves and in addition prints a table indicating compliance in 1-kg steps. See Figure 6–7 for sample graph.

Muscle spasm has been defined as a sustained, involuntary, usually painful contraction that cannot be alleviated completely by voluntary effort.[53] The primary method for diagnosis of muscle spasm is palpation. However, objective and quantitative documentation of the harder consistency in spasmodic muscles is useful not only for medicolegal purposes, but also to prove to the patient and to the insurance companies the presence of the abnormality. In addition, tissue compliance measurement can provide objective evidence of treatment effects after manipulation, physical therapy, injections, transcutaneous electrical nerve stimulation, and so forth. The TCM is the only clinical method that can document objectively the presence of soft tissue abnor-

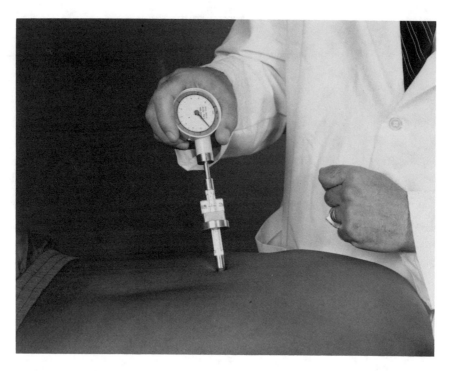

Figure 6–6 Tissue compliance meter for objective quantitative recording of muscle spasm and taut bands of myofascial trigger points. Distributed by Pain Diagnostics and Thermography Inc., 233 East Shore Road, Suite 108, Great Neck, NY 11023.

mality. The results are available immediately. Recent studies demonstrated that tissue compliance measurements are reliable; the results are reproducible within a 2-week follow-up.[54] Normal values for each segment of the spine were established for tissue compliance. Data are useful for evaluation of segmental abnormalities, as well as for documentation of treatment results.[54] An updated review of algometry, including the technique, has been published recently.[55]

CONCLUSION

Soft tissue and pain diagnostic instruments provide quantitative diagnosis of tenderness (trigger/tender) points. Tissue compliance makes possible quantitative, objective documentation of soft tissue abnormalities in clinical practice. Both instruments, the algometer and the TCM, provide unique information not obtainable by any other method. In addition to diagnosis, the instruments are useful to convince the patient as well as insurance companies that abnormality is present and requires appropriate treatment. The instruments also provide quantitative and objective evidence of treatment effects in clinical practice. The TCM and PTM are distributed by Pain Diagnostics and Thermography Inc., 233 East Shore Road, Suite 108, Great Neck, NY 11023.

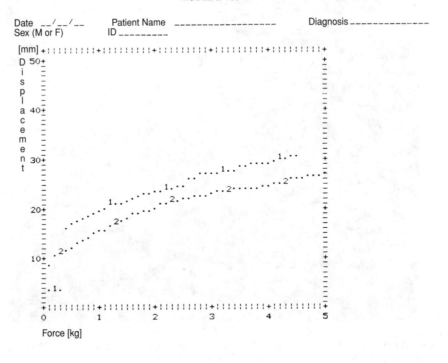

Figure 6–7 Recording by computerized tissue compliance meter (TCM-E100). When the tip of the meter is pressed into the examined tissue, the TCM prints out the displacement (i.e., the depth of penetration) on axis Y and the corresponding force on axis X. In addition, for each analog trace, the compliance is printed out numerically at the bottom.

REFERENCES

1. Glynn LE. The pathology of scar tissue formation. In: Glynn LE, ed. *Tissue Repair and Regeneration.* Amsterdam: Elsevier/North-Holland Biomedical Press; 1981.

2. Hunt TK. Basic principles of wound healing. *J Trauma.* 1990;30(suppl):122–128.

3. Kent TH, Hart MN. *Introduction to Human Disease.*

2nd ed. *Injury, Inflammation and Repair.* Norwalk, Conn: Appleton-Century-Crofts; 1987.

4. Gould JA III, Davies GJ. *Orthopaedic and Sports Physical Therapy.* vol 2. St Louis: CV Mosby Co; 1985.

5. Kellett J. Acute soft tissue injuries: a review of the literature. *Med Sci Sports Exerc.* 1986;18:489–500.

6. Jackson R. *The Cervical Syndrome.* ed 4. Springfield, Ill: Charles C Thomas; 1977.

7. Hunt TK. The physiology of wound healing. *Ann Emerg Med.* 1988;17:1265–1273.

8. Grodin A, Myerson GE, Malone TR. Soft tissue mobilization. *Sports Injury Management.* 1990;2.

9. Carlstedt CA. Mechanical and chemical factors in tendon healing. *Acta Orthop Scand Suppl.* 1987; 224:1–75.

10. Frank C, Amiel D, Woo SL-Y, et al. Normal ligament properties and ligament healing. *Clin Orthop.* 1985;196:15–25.

11. Aldman B. Living tissue properties. In: Aldman B, Chapon A, eds. *The Biomechanics of Impact Trauma.* Amsterdam: Elsevier Science Publishing Co; 1984.

12. Hoyland JA, Freemont AJ, Jayson MIV. Intervertebral foramen venous obstruction: a cause of periradicular fibrosis. *Spine.* 1989;14:558–568.

13. Maxwell C, Spiegel A. The rehabilitation of athletes following spinal injuries. *Spine State Art Rev.* 1990;4:481–489.

14. Green J. *Common Head, Neck, and Back Injuries.* Malabar, Fla: Robert E Krieger; 1988.

15. Boucek RJ. Factors affecting wound healing. *Otolaryngol Clin North Am.* 1984;17:243–264.

16. Bourne GH. Nutrition and wound healing. In: Glynn LE, ed. *Tissue Repair and Regeneration.* Amsterdam: Elsevier/North-Holland Biomedical Press; 1981.

17. Furst P, et al. *Nutritional Assessment in Severe Trauma, Nutritional Assessment Present Status, Future Directions and Prospects.* Columbus, Ohio: Ross Laboratories; 1981.

18. Gadisseux P, Ward JD, Young HF, et al. Nutrition and the neurosurgical patient. *J Neurosurg.* 1984;60:219–232.

19. Pollack SV. Three nutritional factors affecting wound healing. *Dermatol Surg Oncol.* 1979;5:8.

20. Rennie MJ, Harrison R. Effects of injury, disease, and malnutrition on protein metabolism in man: unanswered questions. *Lancet.* February 11, 1984:323–325.

21. Ruberg RL. Role of nutrition in wound healing. *Surg Clin North Am.* 1984;64:705–713.

22. Smith TK. Prevention of complications in orthopedic surgery secondary to nutritional depletion. *Clin Orthop.* 1987;222:91–97.

23. Tayer JA, Blackburn GL. Goals of nutritional support of acute infections. *Am J Med.* May 15, 1984.

24. Werbach MR. Wound healing. In: *Nutritional Influences on Illness, A Sourcebook of Clinical Research.* New Caanan, Conn: Keats Publishing; 1987.

25. Wright PH, Brashear HR. The local response to trauma. In: Wilson FC, ed. *The Musculoskeletal System, Basic Processes and Disorders.* Philadelphia: JB Lippincott; 1983.

26. Altemeyer KH, et al. Pathophysiology of post-traumatic metabolism and its clinical aspects. *Anaesthesist.* 1984;33:4–10.

27. Lawson GE, Walden T. Nutrition and the traumatized patient. *J Council Nutrition.* 1989;12:1–17.

28. Vitamin C, disease, and surgical trauma. *Br Med J.* February 17, 1979:437. Editorial.

29. Hirsch C, Zotterman Y, eds. *Cervical Pain.* vol 19. Proceedings of the International Symposium held in Wenner-Gren Center, Stockholm, January 25–27, 1971. Oxford: Pergamon Press; 1972.

30. Hunt TK. Disorders of wound healing. *World J Surg.* 1980;4:271–277.

31. Akeson WH, Amiel D, Woo SL-Y. Immobility effects on synovial joints, the pathomechanics of joint contracture. *Biorheology.* 1980;17:95–110.

32. Kelsey JL, Githens PB, Walter SD, et al. An epidemiological study of acute prolapsed cervical intervertebral disc. *J Bone Joint Surg [Am].* 1984;66:907–914.

33. Brown CW, Orme TJ, Richardson HD. The rate of pseudoarthrosis (surgical nonunion) in patients who are smokers and patients who are nonsmokers: a comparison study. *Spine.* 1986;11:943.

34. Battié MC, Videman T, Gill K, et al. Smoking and lumbar intervertebral disc degeneration: an MRI study of identical twins, 1991 Volvo award in clinical science. *Spine.* 1991;16:1015–1021.

35. Holm S, Nachemson A. Nutrition of the intervertebral disc: acute effects of cigarette smoking: an experimental animal study. *Uppsala J Med Sci.* 1988;93:91–99.

36. Shealy CN, Roger Cady R, Wilkie R, et al. Spinal and referred pain: nemesis of the harried physician. *J Neurol Orthop Med Surg.* 1988;9:305–306.

37. Hambly MF, Mooney V. Effect of smoking and pulsed electromagnetic fields on intradiscal pH in rabbits. *Spine.* 1992;17:S83–S85.

38. Deyo RA, Bass JE. Lifestyle and low-back pain: the influence of smoking and obesity. *Spine.* 1989;14:510–516.

39. Mandell P, Lipton MH, Bernstein J, et al. *Low Back Pain: An Historical and Contemporary Overview of the Occupational, Medical, and Psychosocial Issues of Chronic Back Pain*. Thorofare, NJ: Slack Inc; 1989.

40. Fischer AA. Diagnosis and management of chronic pain in physical medicine and rehabilitation. In: Ruskin AP, ed. *Current Therapy in Physiatry*. Philadelphia: WB Saunders Co; 1984:123–145.

41. Fischer AA. Pressure threshold measurement for diagnosis of myofascial pain and evaluation of treatment results. *Clin J Pain*. 1987;2:207–214.

42. Fischer AA. Pressure algometry over normal muscles: standard values, validity and reproducibility of pressure threshold. *Pain*. 1987;30:115–126.

43. Fischer AA. Application of pressure algometry in manual medicine. *J Manual Med*. 1990;5:145–150.

44. Simons DG. Myofascial pain syndrome due to trigger points. In: Goodgold J, ed. *Rehabilitative Medicine*. St Louis: CV Mosby Co; 1988:686–723.

45. Reevs JL, Jaeger B, Graff-Radford SB. Reliability of the pressure algometer as a measure of myofascial trigger point sensitivity. *Pain*. 1986;24:313–321.

46. Jensen K. Quantification of tenderness by palpation and use of pressure algometers. In: Friction JR, Awad E, eds. *Advances in Pain Research and Therapy*. vol 17. New York: Raven Press; 1990;165–181.

47. Ohrbach R, Gale EN. Pressure pain thresholds in normal muscles: reliability, measurement effects, and topographic differences. *Pain*. 1989;37:257–263.

48. Jaeger B, Reeves JL. Quantification of changes in myofascial trigger point sensitivity with pressure algometer following passive stretch. *Pain*. 1986; 27:203–210.

49. Vernon HT. Pressure pain threshold evaluation of the effect of spinal manipulation on chronic neck pain: a single case study. *CCA*. 1988;32:191–194.

50. Vernon HT, Aker P, Burns S, et al. Pressure pain threshold evaluation of the effect of spinal manipulation in the treatment of chronic neck pain: a pilot study. *J Manipulative Physiol Ther*. 1990;13:13–16.

51. Fischer AA. Clinical use of tissue compliance meter for documentation of soft tissue pathology. *Clin J Pain*. 1987;3:23–30.

52. Fischer AA. Muscle tone in normal persons measured by tissue compliance. *J Neurol Orthop Med Surg*. 1987;8:227–233.

53. Fischer AA, Change CH. Electromyographic evidence of paraspinal muscle spasm during sleep in patient with low back pain. *Clin J Pain*. 1985;1:147–154.

54. Waldorf T, Devlin L, Nansel DD. The comparative assessment of paraspinal tissue compliance in asymptomatic female and male subjects in both prone and standing positions. *J Manipulative Physiol Ther*. 1991;14:457–461.

55. Fischer AA. Pressure algometry (dolorimetry) in the differential diagnosis of muscle pain. In: Rachlin ES, ed. *Myofascial Pain and Fibromyalgia*. St. Louis: CV Mosby Co; 1994:121–141.

Chapter 7

Management of Minor Injuries

Lawrence S. Nordhoff, Jr., Daniel Murphy, and Michael L. Underhill

INTRODUCTION

Although research on motor vehicle collision injury (MVCI) is abundant, there is little standard for minor (no risk of fatality) auto injury management. This chapter focuses on various methods of managing the more common cases seen in the private practitioner's office. Our goals here are to provide a foundation for developing an effective treatment plan. We discuss various treatment and therapy methods, indications, and contraindications and make appropriate suggestions for their use. It is not the intent of this chapter to provide predetermined treatment plans but instead to provide a sound basis for the treating doctor in developing his or her own plan.

The protocol for basing clinical and other decisions is often inadequate today because of lack of attention in the educational institutions. Most federally and privately funded MVCI studies focus on serious to fatal accidents, with mild injury receiving only limited attention. The resulting lack of understanding concerning the nature of MVCI, its mechanisms, and its influencing factors may result in less than ideal management. Bland believes

that "whiplash patients probably are more often mistreated than optimally treated."[1] This chapter presents and discusses a model of treatment protocol to help fill the current void.

There are a number of areas of concern in the management of MVCIs. We have to ask ourselves, What is the logical sequence of treatment from initial patient contact to release? What initial steps should be taken in patient management? What are the means of determining a patient's progress, and are they adequate? What criteria can we use in determining when the patient has achieved maximal improvement, and at what point should treatment be concluded? In summary, can we develop a model that physicians can employ in the treatment and management of the MVCI? Figure 7–1 outlines an algorithm for the management of uncomplicated (nonsurgical) neck and back injuries. This algorithm was developed by the authors and is not a fixed system. It is intended as a general guide; the individual practitioner can modify it to the specific patient and the type of healing response.

When determining which therapeutic approach to use in the office and at home, the

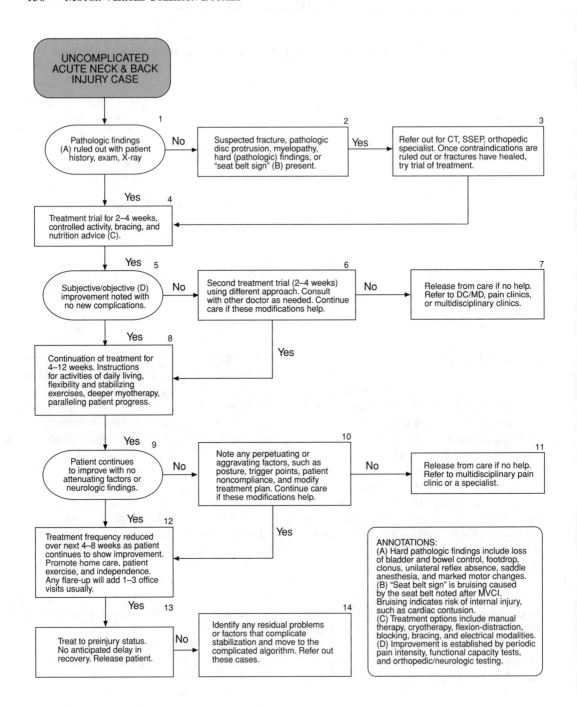

1 Pathologic findings (A) ruled out with patient history, exam, X-ray

No →

2 Suspected fracture, pathologic disc protrusion, myelopathy, hard (pathologic) findings, or "seat belt sign" (B) present.

Yes →

3 Refer out for CT, SSEP, orthopedic specialist. Once contraindications are ruled out or fractures have healed, try trial of treatment.

Yes

4 Treatment trial for 2–4 weeks, controlled activity, bracing, and nutrition advice (C).

Yes

5 Subjective/objective (D) improvement noted with no new complications.

No →

6 Second treatment trial (2–4 weeks) using different approach. Consult with other doctor as needed. Continue care if these modifications help.

No →

7 Release from care if no help. Refer to DC/MD, pain clinics, or multidisciplinary clinics.

Yes

8 Continuation of treatment for 4–12 weeks. Instructions for activities of daily living, flexibility and stabilizing exercises, deeper myotherapy, paralleling patient progress.

Yes

Yes

9 Patient continues to improve with no attenuating factors or neurologic findings.

No →

10 Note any perpetuating or aggravating factors, such as posture, trigger points, patient noncompliance, and modify treatment plan. Continue care if these modifications help.

No →

11 Release from care if no help. Refer to multidisciplinary pain clinic or a specialist.

Yes

Yes

12 Treatment frequency reduced over next 4–8 weeks as patient continues to show improvement. Promote home care, patient exercise, and independence. Any flare-up will add 1–3 office visits usually.

Yes

13 Treat to preinjury status. No anticipated delay in recovery. Release patient.

No →

14 Identify any residual problems or factors that complicate stabilization and move to the complicated algorithm. Refer out these cases.

ANNOTATIONS:
(A) Hard pathologic findings include loss of bladder and bowel control, footdrop, clonus, unilateral reflex absence, saddle anesthesia, and marked motor changes.
(B) "Seat belt sign" is bruising caused by the seat belt noted after MVCI. Bruising indicates risk of internal injury, such as cardiac contusion.
(C) Treatment options include manual therapy, cryotherapy, flexion-distraction, blocking, bracing, and electrical modalities.
(D) Improvement is established by periodic pain intensity, functional capacity tests, and orthopedic/neurologic testing.

CT = computed tomography.
SSEP = Somatosensory evoked potential.

Figure 7–1 Neck and back injury algorithm. Management of acute uncomplicated cases following motor vehicle collisions.

professional must make sure that it is appropriate for the stage of repair, type of tissue injured, and the unique healing characteristics of the patient. The treatment goal should focus on improving repair, reducing pain, limiting scar tissue formation, reducing the duration of pain, lessening the amount of related disability, and attempting to return the person to productive home and occupational life. The extent of the inflammatory and reparative processes may vary at different stages during the course of an injury. Therefore, to achieve optimal treatment results, the dominant healing process and symptomatic regions should be addressed primarily. As the repair process continues over time, the dominant condition and symptomatic regions may change and so must the treatment.[2] For care to be effective, Cyriax feels that the treatment must reach the site of the lesion and exert a beneficial influence there.[3]

As we discuss various posttraumatic conditions, it is advantageous to be familiar with the pathophysiologic processes of trauma. A thorough understanding of Chapter 6, from the initial injury to the chronic residuals of fibrosis of repair, is valuable. But first we shall examine the broader clinical context of the MVCI.

Historically, treatment for MVCI varies from doing nothing for the patient to a variety of modalities or treatment methods. They include prescribing medications, application of ice or heat packs, traction, rest, neck collars, chiropractic spinal adjustments, massage, exercises, electrical therapy, acupuncture, and lifestyle advice. More recently, deep tissue myotherapy and more aggressive forms of rehabilitation have been used.

POSTTRAUMATIC SPINAL MANIPULATION

We will discuss the benefits of spinal joint manipulation to restoring and maintaining normal joint motion during the repair process after an MVCI. In this chapter, the terms *ma-nipulation* and *adjustment* are used interchangeably. This text does not describe the various adjustive techniques available, since there are numerous literary sources readily available. Expanding current knowledge of the benefits of manipulation in the overall rehabilitation of patients with MVCI is critical, because many health, insurance, and legal professionals misunderstand or underestimate this aspect of rehabilitation.

Benefits and Goals of Spinal Manipulation

Chiropractors have been adjusting patients' spines for decades and have found that most nonsurgical neck and low back traumatic conditions respond very well to this method of management. Chapter 17 explores patients' satisfaction with this type of therapy. Reports have shown that spinal manipulation is effective in relieving cases involving neck pain, neck stiffness, headache, upper-extremity paresthesia, cervical radiculopathies, cervico-brachial neuralgia, and cervical disc bulging symptoms.[4–12] It also has been shown to be beneficial in early cervical arthrosis and spondylosis[13] and improves cervical hypo-lordosis.[14] White and Panjabi conclude that spinal manipulation is effective in 60% to 70% of patients.[15] Haldeman's review of literature concluded that clinical research on patients having manipulative therapy for relief of neck and back pain is favorable.[16] Fitzgerald's[17] and Greenman's[9] reviews are two excellent accounts of the benefits of spinal manipulation following cervical trauma.

The primary goals of manipulative therapy are to accomplish the following:

- Restore normal supportive tissue characteristics.[18]
- Restore normal biomechanical effects on other directly or indirectly attaching soft and bony tissues.
- Improve or restore joint articular function and mobility[19,20] by causing scar tissue cross-bindings and adhesions to rupture,

providing free motion to the tissue and breaking intra-articular fiber adhesions.[21] Significantly improve cervical range of motion (ROM),[22] causing myofascial tissues to interact more normally with other tissues as a result of improved spinal motion. Improve abnormal muscle tone and texture alterations.[23]

- Abort abnormal afferent/efferent reflexology.[24]
- Remodel periarticular paraphysiologic tissue after injury.[25]
- Increase joint motion proprioception, which will minimize pain[26] and improve joint function.
- Provide propriosensory retraining to improve efferent and afferent function.[27,28]
- Assist in aborting an adverse pattern of neurospinal learning.[29]
- Lessen coactivation of mechanically sensitive afferent structures.[30]
- Introduce mechanical energy in an effort to desensitize the denervation supersensitivity processes.
- Reduce vascular congestion or neurologic ischemia and resultant neural irritation in and near the intervertebral foramen that was initially caused by loss of joint motion.
- Provide pain blocking or relief[31,32] by improving pressure/pain thresholds.[33]
- Lessen sympathetic hyperactivity.[23]
- Increase joint sensory perception effects; i.e., improve function of proprioceptors, nociceptors, and mechanoreceptors. There is increased mechanical sensitivity of all types of receptors,[30] which may alter the physiology of small-caliber afferent axons to such a degree that they become hypersensitive to mechanical disturbances and in some instances develop impulse activity independent of stimulation.[30] In addition, manipulation may improve abnormal action potentials.[23]

Figure 7–2 shows that manipulation has the capability to work on joint adhesions, whereas active and passive ROM and massage do not work on these tissues.

Theory of Joint Manipulation

The following theories regarding spinal manipulation are widely held within the practicing chiropractic community. These ideas are primarily based on the clinical observations and experiences of the authors over the past 14 years, as well as on literature sources.

Joint manipulation provides the unique ability to mobilize periarticular tissues in a manner that is not possible through other means, such as joint or soft tissue mobilization.[17,26,34,35] This benefit to tissue healing is unique to joint manipulation, as only manipulation affects the periarticular tissue in the paraphysiologic ROM. Chiropractors carefully apply specific manipulative forces, utilizing the bones as levers and placing the desired motion into periarticular tissues. The resulting forces produce tension within the once-damaged and now healing fibrotically restricted joints. If in fact motion is essential for proper alignment of healing granulation tissue, then the periarticular paraphysiologic granulation tissues can be helped only through carefully applied joint manipulation. The chiropractor makes the determination as to what joints will be manipulated primarily through the quality of the joint play felt during passive motioning. He or she locates regions having abnormal resistive barriers to motion or joint play. A manipulative thrust is then carefully and gently delivered to the region having the resistive barrier to motion.

In summary, those who use manipulation use methodologies that improve the repair process through the various stages of healing. In each stage of repair, methods are used to lessen pain, reduce extent of injury, aid in remodeling of granulation tissue, break adhesions as they develop, and most important, at-

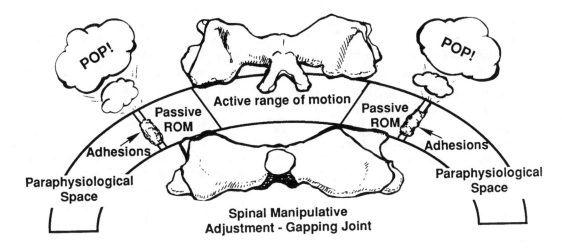

Figure 7–2 Spinal manipulation gaps the spinal joint.

tempt to prevent a potential chronic pain syndrome from developing.

The authors have found that spinal manipulation is most effective if used in combination with myotherapy, maintenance of good posture, exercises, stretching, and the use of proper ergonomics.

How Soon after Injury Should Adjustment Begin?

The beneficial role of spinal adjustment in all phases of injury has been commonly accepted in the chiropractic community. So the question is, How soon after injury should manipulation begin? In the acute stage, because of healing tissue fragility, it is certainly possible for excessive forces to aggravate or further damage the injured muscles or ligaments. If the injury history suggests a rapid-onset of severe disability, then the clinician must suspect that this is not typical for the normal inflammatory response to trauma. Unusually early intense disability starting before 12 hours *(red flag)* may suggest soft tissue hematoma or possible fracture.

Overall, the best rule is never to perform spinal adjustment on any patient whom the doctor is unable to bring to pre-tension positioning comfortably, what is known as the passive ROM. In general, it is probably best not to do any forceful adjustment for at least 2 or 3 days in any moderate to severe joint injury. Instead, gentle mobilization focused on regaining pain-free movement should be the goal in the acute stage.[36] When pain or spasm prevents the patient from achieving a comfortable position or does not allow the joint to move beyond the active ROM, focus your attention on reducing the inflammation first and educating the patient about home management. If pre-tension positioning is comfortably achieved, then gentle adjustments are easily tolerated by the acutely injured patient.

Delayed Joint Dysfunction after Trauma

Immediately after neck trauma, ROM examination often reveals mild to severe global motion losses due to pain and protective splinting muscle spasm. Usually within 5 to 7 days after trauma, patterns of cervical spine hypomobility or hypermobility start to appear as the pain and reactive muscle spasm begin to subside. Several mechanisms can cause joint dysfunction to appear early or as late as 6 to 8 weeks after injury.

Mechanisms for immediate local joint fixation include the following:

- inflammatory reactions that produce congestion and swelling in the joint spaces
- pain caused by tissue damage and chemical irritation
- reflex-induced muscle spasm that causes protective splinting
- joint misalignment

Mechanisms for delayed joint dysfunction include the following:

- shift in normal spinal joints' instantaneous axes of rotation, which are normally centered onto the disc, to the more pain-sensitive posterior facet structures (this is not a static malposition but rather a dynamic process)
- myofascial alterations that cause abnormal tension or tethering on joints or other myofascial structures
- instability caused by capsular ligament laxity
- edematous fluids and capillary bleeding that spread to uninjured tissues by effects of pressure build-up and gravity; spread of swelling to new pain-sensitive tissues, causing new or amplified symptoms

Contraindications for Cervical Spine Adjustment

Although there are few contraindications to adjusting the spine, the doctor must be aware of them. Contraindications for joint manipulation or adjustment include the following:

- fever indicative of serious disease, e.g., meningitis
- active infectious inflammation of spinal area

- spinal joints displaying hypermobility due to trauma, infection, rheumatoid arthritis, collagen disease, or surgery
- acute or healing fracture and advanced osteoporosis or bone loss
- pathology such as tumors or cancer near or adjacent to the joint area
- fused spine area, such as Klippel-Feil syndrome or surgical fusion (Do not adjust fused joints or compensating hypermobile segments directly above and below area of fusion. Restricted, nonfused joints above and below can be adjusted safely.)
- inability of the patient to relax prior to adjusting
- any vascular symptoms in the patient's medical history indicating possible vertebral artery compromise, e.g., blacking out when turning head; positive vertebral artery ischemia test
- any neurologic signs or symptoms, such as vertigo or blindness, that arise immediately after adjusting (*Under no circumstances should a second attempt be made in hopes of reversing symptoms!*)

APPLICATION OF CRYOTHERAPY AND HEAT AFTER INJURY

Doctors who either treat or give advice for neck injuries need sound rationale in determining which thermal therapy to recommend at the office and home for the stage of repair. Both heat and cold traditionally have been used to enhance healing, reduce pain, improve motion, and improve overall outcome of tissue repair and joint function. The predominant use of cryotherapy for early trauma management has recently gained more general acceptance in treating acute soft tissue injuries.[36–43] The authors of this text recommend cryotherapy for all acute and subacute MVCIs. In chronic injury, cryotherapy may be used in conjunction with heat for rehabilitation.

Several studies have been performed comparing the reparative outcome of injury with the use of ice or cold application. One study comparing ice and heat application to ankle sprains showed that recovery occurred an average of 15 days sooner with cryotherapy, which was especially effective when applied early. A study on ankle injuries concluded that cryotherapy combined with exercise was most successful in increasing blood flow on a long-term basis,[44] suggesting 10 to 15 minutes of ice before exercise. Heat packs[41] and other superficial heat, because of their inability to penetrate deep muscles, have limited therapeutic value in some cases.

Effects of Cryotherapy

The physiologic benefits of cryotherapy after trauma have been addressed by various authors. Following is a list of the more commonly accepted effects of cryotherapy:

- Reduces soft tissue cell metabolism[45,46] and oxygen consumption, allowing the uninjured tissues distal to the trauma to survive longer periods of ischemia, resulting in a decrease of secondary hypoxic injury.[47] This is one of the more important effects of using ice in acute injury.

- Reduces pain by breaking up the pain reflex cycle[48] and by acting as a counterirritant.[49] Cold has long-lasting effects on lowering nerve conduction velocity.[50,51] Cold has been shown to be more effective in reducing muscle electrical activity than heat.[52]

- Decreases overall inflammatory response,[36] although ice has been shown to increase swelling in the underlying superficial tissues.[53] This is due to ischemia in the normal surrounding tissues, which creates increased rebound perfusion. This swelling can be minimized with compression and elevation.

- Promotes vasoconstriction,[54] which reduces bleeding[49] and limits further exudation from the injured capillary beds into uninjured areas.[41]

- Speeds healing and reduces the time of disability.[25,46,53,55,56]

- Decreases muscle spasm.[37] Muscle spindles and Golgi afferents are temperature dependent.[57] Muscle spindles regulate muscle tension, and cold slows their rate of discharge, thus alleviating spasm.[56] Cold reduces spindle sensitivity.[58]

Effects of Heat

Heat has most benefits in the chronic injury patient and has limited use in management of acute or subacute stages of repair. Deep heat promotes blood flow and increases edema, both of which are already excessive after injury.[3] The length of time that heat will affect the body is much shorter than that for ice.[58] Heat is more useful in the chronic injury stage and should be used for treating stiffness and to increase blood flow in ischemic areas when indicated. All forms of heat should be avoided during the acute stage. This means avoiding prolonged warm showers or baths, hot tubs or saunas, and heat packs or electrical heating devices, including therapy equipment. Deep radiant heat is likely to perpetuate symptoms.[59] Generally speaking, heat does the following:

- Causes vasodilation, which increases blood flow.[60]

- Reduces pain[49] by raising the threshold to pain with long application.[41]

- Reduces muscle spasm.[61] By elevating muscle tissue temperature to around 42° C, it was found that type II afferent firing decreased and type 1b fibers increased from the Golgi tendon organs.[57] Reduction of spasticity is of short duration with heat.[58]

- Lessens joint stiffness and prepares stiff joints for exercise for a duration of 2 to 3 minutes. Increases connective tissue elasticity.
- May perpetuate or exaggerate pain and inflammatory responses.[46,58] Maxwell and Spiegel conclude that in disc nerve root compression, deep heat may cause increased edema and hyperemia, making symptoms worse.[62]
- Elevates tissue temperature down to 1 cm of depth but will have no effect beyond that. Deeper forms of heat (5 cm) can be accomplished by using ultrasound or short wave diathermy.[41]

How Soon after Injury Should Cryotherapy Be Used?

Early initiation of cryotherapy in the acute motor vehicle collision–related soft tissue injuries with continued intermittent use for an appropriate time frame has significant benefits in producing earlier and improved recovery. Cryotherapy should be applied as soon as possible, preferably within 2 hours after the injury. The authors' experience is that those patients who initiate cryotherapy early and continue to follow cryotherapy protocols as instructed have faster recovery and fewer residual chronic symptoms.

Frequency and Duration of Cryotherapy

Kellett recommends that patients apply ice every 2 to 3 hours after injury.[25] With frequent application, much of the swelling can be localized, thus reducing the likelihood of surrounding tissue and joint involvement. Compliance is usually easier to obtain from a person who is not working, but job schedules will still allow four or five applications a day if emphasized. The worker therefore should apply an ice pack first thing in the morning, before leaving for work; use it again during lunch and any available breaks; and use it

when first getting home, after dinner, and just before going to bed. Recommend that the patient use a timer to avoid overtreating or falling asleep with ice applied.

As a general rule, ice should be applied on the neck or back every 2 hours for 10 to 30 minutes at a time,[25] depending on the patient's underlying muscle mass (circulatory volume), insulating fat volume, and anatomy. For thin necks, Kottke et al. suggest 10 minutes; for medium to large, muscular necks, 20 minutes; and for those having an insulating fat layer, 30 minutes.[58] Extremity joints have less muscle tissue with resultant decreased circulatory capacity to dissipate cold. Therefore, extremities should be iced no longer than 10 minutes.

How Many Days Should Cryotherapy Be Used after Injury?

Microscopic capillary bleeding in deep anterior and posterior neck muscles has been shown on magnetic resonance imaging (MRI) to persist up to 2 to 5 days after MVCI.[63] Cryotherapy should be used for this time frame as a minimum. The authors suggest that, unless there is an intolerance or contraindication for cryotherapy, it should be used for 1 to 2 weeks. As long as there is functional joint loss due to inflammation, muscle spasm, or pain, ice will be beneficial.

Methods of Ice/Heat Application

The type of cryotherapy prescribed should take into account the size and architecture of the injured area and may include crushed ice, gel packs, chemical or blue ice, and other manufactured packs. The authors and manufacturers suggest using a thin towel or cloth over the ice pack to prevent burning or blistering. When using cryotherapy in acute injuries, it is important to inform the patient to use the ice on all areas that are injured. This does not mean that the patient has to use a dozen ice packs at the same time, but rather the routine should be varied so that all areas are iced. For example, consider a patient in a frontal crash with resulting pain and muscle spasms in all sides of the neck, anterior chest wall, and upper back. The patient would use two types of ice packs ideally, one that would wrap around the neck with Velcro straps and the other a flat sheet that could cover the back and chest wall at separate times.

In the clinic setting, heat typically is applied by moist packs containing silica gel. The packs are placed on the patient within thick covers to protect against burning. These packs are stored in hydrocollars filled with water kept at a constant temperature. For home use, a variety of electric heating pads is available. Some of the units may be used in conjunction with a wet towel for moist heat. Of course, caution should be used when using water and electricity together and only those pads that are specifically identified should be used wet. Other forms of heat therapy include heat lamps and diathermy.

Contraindications for Ice/Heat Application

There are a few contraindications to hot and cold therapy which should be reviewed. Therapy should not be used in the following cases:

- Recent history of heart attack or unstable cardiac conditions. Cryotherapy may cause sympathetic stimulation if used in the upper back region.
- Over tumors or when muscle diseases are present.[64]
- Conditions such as Raynaud's disease, Buerger's disease, multiple myeloma, leukemia, lupus erythematosus, and rheumatoid arthritis, as well as capillary fragility due to long-term steroid therapy.[48,65]
- Cold hypersensitivity or intolerance. Some people may exhibit histamine release reactions[37] when subjected to cold. Be aware of elderly patients with poor sensitivity to hot or cold.

DEEP MYOTHERAPY

As noted in Chapter 1, myofascial pain is one of the most common sources of chronic pain in the chronic MVCI case. Myofascial pain syndromes frequently develop after car crashes, even *minor* automobile collisions.[66] Myofascial pain can include tender muscles and trigger points. Deep myotherapy is a useful tool that addresses this specific condition. The soft tissues composing the musculoskeletal system include muscles, fasciae, tendons, tendon sheaths, ligaments, joint capsules, and bursae.[20]

In this section, our main focus is on the myofascial connective tissue structures of the neck, upper thoracic spine, and anterior chest. One primary reason to focus on the myofascial conditions in the cervical region is that a significantly greater proportion of cervical myofascial disorders exists than in lower back disorders.[67] Treatment of these soft tissues during the repair and remodeling stages of repair can lead the practitioner to gratifying results. Many physicians overlook or avoid this vital area of diagnosis and treatment.

A variety of management options are presented in the literature on myofascial pain. These include deep pressure massage, superficial to deep myofascial stretch and pressure, ice massage, exercise, and spinal manipulation. Other techniques for chronic conditions include use of vapocoolant spray and stretch techniques, acupuncture, ultrasound, galvanic stimulation, and medications. There is substantial literature available validating myotherapy. Myotherapy techniques have been the mainstay of posttraumatic soft tissue pain management for several decades and are not experimental in any fashion.

Myofascial pressure release techniques are generally quite safe, except for occasional bruising in some individuals.[68] The treating specialist must determine the proper time and force with which pressure should be applied. Pressure is typically applied for 15 seconds to a maximum of 2 minutes.[69] Skin rolling techniques and pinching are particularly valuable over areas with tight underlying structures such as the shoulders and trapezius areas. The area is lifted between two fingers and stretched, and the tissue is squeezed.[69] The skin is stretched in several directions, checking for adhesions. The sternocleidomastoid muscle can also be stretched in this manner while the patient is supine.

Vapocoolant "spray and stretch" techniques work in some cases, although caution must be employed when treating near the facial areas, as the sprays may be inhaled. Some patients will react with increased local tension.

Deep myofascial release techniques have been developed by Simons and Travell[68] and others.[69] The focus is to inactivate the trigger point by decompression of the focal ischemic area.[68] A number of specialized techniques can be useful. Small circular movements work well on deep lower cervical and suboccipital areas. The patient's head is rotated to the opposite side and the fibrotic areas are palpated and worked gradually deeper until they soften. Deep thumb or elbow techniques are useful to provide greater pressure in deeper myofascial areas. The scalenes, medial scapular, and trapezius myofascial areas are particularly well treated with this approach.

Transverse friction massage is useful to mobilize ligament, tendon, and muscle fibers. It has also been used to soften scar tissue[20] and mobilize painful adherent scarred areas.[40] As the name implies, the massage is accomplished by transverse friction, which is applied across the tissue fiber grain.[70] During the acute phase it can be used daily, but should be done lightly so as to move soft tissue structures without disrupting areas of tissue healing.[70] Treatment initially is performed for 1 to 2 minutes in a localized area. As healing progresses, treatment can be extended to 10 to 15 minutes. Deeper sweeps can be made into fibrotic areas at this point. After treatment with deeper measures, a lighter superficial massage should be given to promote relaxation. A soft tissue response should be felt.

Contact-relax and hold-relax methods[69] can be used to increase trigger-point area effectiveness. Spinal adjustments to release restrictions of joint mobility can improve and equalize joint range of motion. This will allow improved patterns for attachment of myofascial structures during the repair process. It will also minimize inordinate kinetic muscle stresses by improving any local alterations in the joint's motion quality.

In patients having chest wall pain 4 to 6 weeks after sustaining contusions from the shoulder harness or steering wheel, there are techniques available to lessen pain and improve biomechanical function of the intercostal muscles that develop myofascial adhesions. In one such technique, with the patient lying supine, the doctor uses the thenar aspect of his or her hand to locate the first palpable rib below the clavicle; while the doctor maintains a downward and inward push with the thenar area of the hand, the patient takes in a series of four or five slow deep breaths through the mouth. This technique works best when the doctor starts at the second or third intercostal junction, applies contact and push and breath, and then works down each intercostal junction with each breath. The patient will usually feel immediate relief of breathing pain. In patients having lateral chest wall pain, it is easier to have the gowned patient sit. As the patient bends laterally, the doctor pulls downward on the contralateral ribs with large sweeps of the hands; this technique is usually more comfortable for the patient if lotion is used. Myotherapy plays a very important role in managing microscopic and macroscopic repair of soft tissue injury. Unfortunately, these pain syndromes are frequently misdiagnosed and improperly treated. By adding myofascial therapy to treatment methods, doctors could certainly increase their overall effectiveness.

NECK AND BACK SUPPORTS

Several types of supports are available to the patient during the acute and subacute stages of injury. These supports provide partial or total immobilization, lessen pain, give support, and give proprioceptive awareness, thus lessening the risk of reinjury. It is important that the clinician be selective in whom is prescribed the support, if the support is to be used only during certain activities or continuously, and the length of time used. Discussions about the effect of immobilization on healing should help in making decisions.

Effects of Immobilization on Soft Tissues

When synovial joints are immobilized for prolonged periods, biomechanical, biochemical, functional, and morphologic changes occur in bone, muscle, cartilage, ligaments, and tendons.[71,72] These changes may include proliferation of fibrofatty connective tissue within the joint space, synovial fold adhesions, disorganization of cellular and fibrillar ligament alignment, collagen mass decline (5% in 9 weeks), and reduction of energy-load responses by one third.[71] Increased fatigability has been reported after immobilization,[73] probably due to decreased adenosine triphosphate concentrations and increased lactic acid in muscle tissues. Additionally, weakening of ligament insertion sites secondary to osteoclastic resorption of Sharpey's fibers and bone can occur.

Synovial joints need mechanical activity for homeostasis. Intermittent distraction and compression of joint surfaces must occur in order for proper exchange of waste products and nutrients to take place.[74] Hertling and Kessler feel that from a pathologic view, a joint that has lost motion, for example, from a tight joint capsule, fails to receive an exchange of nutrients in the areas where it is no longer moving.[74] Synovial joints having long periods of immobilization will exhibit reduction in concentrations of glycosaminoglycans (GAG) and water content. This alters tissue plasticity and lubrication efficiency, and reduces connective tissue matrix pliability.[75] GAG is reduced when force and motion do not occur.[75]

Water, along with proteoglycans, acts as a spacer and lubricant between fibers.[72] Loss of the water volume increases friction among the microfibrils and increases the potential for cross-linking or adhesion formation between collagen fibrils.[71]

An immobilized muscle will lose weight and will develop weakness throughout all ranges of motion, resulting in decreased muscle capacity. Periarticular tissues will cross-link without normal physical stretching forces.[59] Collagen fibers will be laid down in a haphazard manner because of the loss of the usual control on orientation imposed by mechanical forces of motion.[73] Joint immobilization is responsible for cartilage degeneration due to reduced joint lubrication, decreased metabolic activity, and reduced blood supply. Tissues will appear dry and less glistening, primarily in the interfacial planes.[60] Gross inspection of immobilized fibrous connective tissue showed a more "woody" texture.[71] An animal study concluded that after 3 weeks of immobilization, there were detrimental changes in axonal conduction velocities, muscle mass, and fatigability.[76]

Booth's study shows a decrease in the amount of protein synthesis in muscles within 6 hours of immobilization and decreased muscle strength. Muscle atrophy begins after skeletal muscle fixation in 1 to 3 days. This atrophy will occur in muscles fixed in resting or below-resting lengths.[77] A 20% decrease in muscle weight occurs in 7 days and 30% in 21 days.[78] Breaking strength of muscles immobilized 1 week was reduced by 20%.[78] By day 21 a 24% decrease in the ability of an immobilized muscle to elongate was seen and energy absorption was decreased by 45%. This caused a decrease of the so-called safety reserve of the immobilized muscles. Immobilization of muscle in a rest position causes rapid and significant loss of passive strength and tensile properties.[28]

Short periods of immobilization may result in profound alterations of the muscle and ligament properties, as well as joint wear and tear.

Animal studies on extremities show that short-term immobilization (as little as 4 days), as well as long-term immobilization (over 30 days), causes osteoarthroses.[79,80] Twelve weeks of immobilization may weaken ligaments and their insertion sites.[73] Note that the additional muscle weakness brought on by immobilization may complicate further an already injured person's healing outcome.[81] Prolonged cervical immobilization will cause muscle weakness, disuse atrophy, and muscle hyposensitivity[82] and can result in dependency on the part of the patient, making the condition more difficult to treat.[51]

We can see clearly that during rehabilitation, long-term rest and immobilization do not promote ideal healing of injured soft tissues and synovial joints. When indicated, immobilization devices must be used with caution. The authors recommend that patients use neck or back supports during any stressful activity such as riding in a car, housecleaning, or other tasks that require a lot of motion. The patient should take the support off every 3 to 4 hours for 30 to 60 minutes or remove the support if sitting still for a period of time in a controlled environment such as home. To promote maximum mobility and strength, controlled movement must be utilized. Joints and associated tissues need biomechanical motion in order to heal with minimal residual effects after injury. Current research indicates that generalized, non-traumatic, spinal joint motion may be significant in the maintenance of normal autonomic and neuromuscular tone.[72] Researchers suggest the use of selective, graded, and protected activity—not immobilization—for superior treatment outcome.[47] It has been demonstrated that management with controlled joint motion will preserve maximum mobility and strength without disturbing the new scar tissue formation. The amount of literature substantiating the need for early, controlled, soft tissue and joint motion and mobilization is overwhelming in management of these types of injuries. Similar early mobilization has been emphasized in recent years for patients undergoing surgery, as hospitals now ambulate such patients much earlier than they did a decade ago.

Cervical Collars

More selective and shorter-term use of cervical collars is now strongly advocated,[83] with strong recommendations for collar avoidance in the uncomplicated neck injury case during the course of treatment.[84] Several types of cervical collars or orthoses currently are available and include foam, leather, plastic, and combination materials. Cervical collars may even be custom-made, for example, the thermoplastic collar and the customized plaster of Paris collar. When selecting the type of orthosis, be sure to evaluate your treatment objectives. Decide whether you want to provide support, remind the patient to be cautious, provide a form of correction, limit certain types of neck motion, or obtain complete immobilization. Also consider whether the patient is likely to comply with instructions. A patient who is embarrassed to wear the collar in public may pose problems. If the doctor decides that a cervical collar is necessary, advise the patient what your goals are and what to expect with usage. Figure 7–3 outlines an appropriate cervical collar protocol.

Soft foam cervical collars provide little immobilization.[15] Although rigid collars do offer more limiting motion than soft collars, they do not adequately immobilize the neck in cases where complete immobility is needed. Rigid cervical collars restrict flexion-extension better than lateral flexion. Soft collars do not restrict flexion and act to restrict minimally extension and rotation.[85] Cervical-dorsal orthoses (e.g., Yale) and halo body jackets do offer adequate immobilization of the lower cervical spine.[41]

Cervical collars should be used in the following cases:

- Occult or suspected fractures. Philadelphia collar or rigid collar with head taped to board is best means to stabilize.

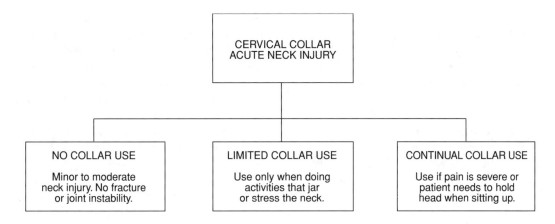

Figure 7–3 Cervical collar protocol for uncomplicated neck injuries.

- Severe ligamentous instability. Philadelphia collar or rigid collar is preferred.
- Severe neck pain, when patient has to lift or support the head when sitting up from the lying down position or when lying down. A soft collar of proper size is adequate.
- Severe muscle spasms.[51] The soft collar is usually adequate.
- Short-term use during activities that aggravate pain (this can include riding in a car or bending activities). Some states prohibit driving if the person is wearing a cervical collar.

Cervical collars should not be used in the following cases:

- Mild to moderate uncomplicated neck injury
- Mild to moderate pain levels when rest and ice application can reduce pain to a tolerable level
- Mild to moderate muscle spasm

How Long Should Collars Be Worn?

If cervical collars are indicated, the time of immobilization should be as short as clinically necessary because of adverse effects that may develop secondarily. Adverse effects include muscle atrophy, joint contracture, and a need for prolonged rehabilitation.[61] Only in the most severe cases is a cervical collar suggested, and then only for 7 to 10 days.[86,87] In a typical severe neck injury case that satisfies the collar use protocol, a soft collar would be worn frequently for 1 week, intermittently for the second week, and discontinued after 2 weeks.[87] More conservative authors recommend wearing collars for 2 to 6 weeks.[88] A number of studies have shown that, once provided with them, patients will wear cervical collars for many months.[27] Several authors feel that the use of prolonged cervical support is often useless, deplorable, and even dangerous.[82,89]

The collar should be removed at intervals to reduce the patient's dependency on the support.[59] The best times for removal are when sitting at home or in environments in which the patient will not have unexpected events occurring that require rapid head motion, such as when driving a car. The collar should always be worn during physically stressful situations, and such situations should be avoided during the first 10 days to allow for good tissue repair.

Application of Cervical Collars

The type and level of work, recreational, and home activity of the patient will have some determination in what type of collar best applies. As an example, a car salesperson needs to be able to turn the head while driving, but needs support also. The physician needs to look at his or her state's laws before recommending neck collars while driving, as some states may prohibit driving while using one. A construction worker who is lifting frequently will need a collar that is more durable. Some patients are just particular about the type of material and how the collar looks and feels. Remember, if the collar is uncomfortable, patient compliance is likely to be poor. Stressing the importance of proper use from the onset will avert most problems.

Proper cervical collar application should take into consideration the neck size of the patient. An adequate supply of cervical collars would include small, medium, large, and extra-large collars. The extent of injury and types of structures involved should be evaluated. For very severe sprain/strains or fractures, a completely rigid collar is indicated. For less severe injuries, softer, more comfortable collars can be used.

When providing a custom-made collar, such as thermoplastic or plaster of Paris, make sure that the collar is trimmed to allow movement of the clavicle and shoulder; in addition, make sure that the patient can swallow comfortably with no pressure on the throat.[90] The collar should be refitted and trimmed until fit and comfort are achieved.

Lumbar Supports/Cushions

Lumbar bracing can be a useful adjunct in patients having severe low back pain. Lumbar muscle spasms can increase the tendency to lose balance because of proprioceptive overstimulation of gamma fibers and sympathetic nerves in the erector muscles. Support in these areas can improve the balance system. One study of 200 MVCI patients found 33 patients having low back pain, and the severity of the lumbar pain was found to parallel the degree of vertigo during the course of treatment. The theory tested in this study, by having patients wear lumbar corsets and having equilib-

rium testing, was that the hypertonicity of the lumbar muscles led to vertigo and that bracing helped.[91] In MVCI patients having severe low back pain and/or sciatica a lumbar support can lessen the severity of the pain in many cases. There are numerous types and quality of supports available in the market.

A common complaint should alert the doctor that a lumbar belt might be useful: the patient comes in for treatment and relates that the treatment helps for only a few minutes. A belt can help stabilize the back after a spinal adjustment. As soon as the spine has been adjusted it is suggested that the brace be put on before the patient moves around. The belt will also increase the patients' proprioceptive awareness of the back, thus lessening the risk of reinjury.

The usual recommended time for intermittent or continuous use depends on the severity of the injury, the degree of symptom relief experienced by the patient, and home/work activity. Bracing is recommended during any painful activity.

Lumbar lordotic cushions can also be used for those patients having severe pain when sitting, especially if the office or vehicle seat support is poor and is aggravating their condition.

Cervical Pillows

Several authors believe that using cervical pillows can be helpful in the treatment of pain by offering support and should be considered an important adjunct in the treatment of acute or chronic cervical spine disorders.[2,92,93] There are biomechanical and pain-relieving benefits for patients using cervical pillows following a neck injury. This adjunctive support may relieve pain in many patients if properly used. With an ill-fitted pillow, however, pain and frustration usually result in low patient compliance. The patient should understand clearly the benefits and limitations of a cervical pillow before being sent home with one.

Biomechanically, the pillow or roll offers lordotic support to an inflamed, antalgic (forward) cervical spine that is reacting to the trauma by developing a straightened or kyphotic posture. This secondary, reflexive, forward antalgic posture of the neck is in response to the inflamed posterior spinal elements. The doctor should use caution in prescribing anything more than a small, rolled hand towel for an acutely injured patient. Sleep is very important to the repair process, and a poor pillow may account for disturbed sleep. In chronic injury, a larger supportive pillow under the injured neck can help alleviate pain and help prevent or reverse the neck straightening or kyphotic process. If initial X-rays show a marked cervical kyphosis, then a smaller roll will work better. The authors' experience is that too much early support can aggravate the patient's condition. If the pillow forces the neck into a hyperextended position, increased pressure on the facet joints may occur. Thus, in the acutely injured patient, pain-sensitive tissues may be inflamed further.

When using a cervical roll, it should be tucked under the mid- to lower-cervical region, allowing the head to lie on the mattress. The pillow support should be reinforced by neck extension exercises during the day and also by good postural habits.

Index Finger-Cervical Pillow Rule

The cervical roll should not be larger in diameter than the length of the patient's index finger. This will generally take into account the size and gender of the patient. It would not be appropriate to give a small person and a large person the same size pillow. Also, patients weighing under 150 lb should use softer pillows than patients weighing over 150 lb. Heavier patients will not get adequate support and will wear out the pillow more quickly if it is not firm.

Rib Cage Fracture Bracing

After chest wall injury some patients may have severe episodes of pain with slight torso motion, coughing, and sneezing. In particular, rib fracture cases may need the use of some type of elastic bandaging for several weeks. It is imperative that the doctor make the patient aware that there are risks of developing pneumonia if prolonged use occurs. In patients who are elderly or who have a history of respiratory disorders, the use of bracing must be limited. One practical suggestion is to have these patients keep a large, fluffy pillow nearby, if they need to sneeze or cough they should tuck the pillow tightly under their arms and bend their knees.

Wrist Bracing

Some type of support or bracing may be useful for patients having significant wrist pain or injury. Depending on the severity of the injury and/or pain and the type of work and sleep habits, the doctor may recommend intermittent (activity-based) or continuous use. For example, if the patient states that he or she is waking up with wrist pain after lying on the hand, the splint may be useful at night.

TRANSCUTANEOUS ELECTRICAL MODALITIES FOR SPINE INJURIES

Electrical modalities are used by some physicians and therapists for treating neck and back injury. Some use these modalities as the primary form of care while others use them in an adjunctive role. In addition, some use these modalities in one or all stages of repair. It also appears from the literature that some forms of therapy work better in one stage of injury than in others. Electrical modality usage has several management objectives, including enhanced healing by stimulating cell metabolism, micromassage, pumping exudates outside the injured area, or contracting muscles. Most electrical modalities work well for reducing severe spasm and pain, resulting in the patient's requiring less analgesic. Reduction of muscle spasm is an important part of the treatment because it decreases the ischemic effects of prolonged muscle contraction. Most electrical modalities have a window of time in which they are most effective, generally the first 4 to 6 weeks after injury. After 6 weeks, most of the repair process has taken place and remodeling is occurring. The clinical problems now involve primarily myofascial adhesions or joint-related problems.

When making the choice to use an electrical modality, as in any type of therapy, the doctors or therapists should ask themselves the following questions:

- What is the patient's stage of repair?
- What tissues do I want to help?
- What form of modality has the best affinity for that type of tissue?
- Will this form of therapy have short-term or long-term results?
- Can this patient do this therapy at home?
- What time parameters should I use for the therapy?

There are basically three types of transcutaneous electrical modality categories used by physicians and therapists to treat neck injuries: electrical nerve stimulation, electrical cellular stimulation, and electrical dense tissue mechanical-thermal devices.

Electrical Nerve Stimulation

Both transcutaneous electrical nerve stimulation (TENS) and galvanic current fall under the transcutaneous electrical nerve stimulator category, as both have an affinity for nerves. They include the traditional TENS unit and the galvanic current machine.

TENS

Several authors have encouraged the use of transcutaneous electrical neurostimulation in whiplash management.[61,94] One advantage of using TENS for management of posttraumatic pain is that there are no known adverse reactions to its use. Generally speaking, TENS provides short-term relief, but it can be valuable in some patients who continue to have severe

pain 8 to 10 weeks after trauma. Ease of patient application is an advantage, since the patient can take the equipment home and use it whenever pain arises.

The best results for TENS are experienced when the electrodes are placed on either side of the painful area or directly over the area. It is more effective if the pain is localized to a spinal lesion level. In the authors' experience TENS is effective in approximately 30% to 40% of patients who use the units as instructed.

It may be advantageous for the doctor to select a company that leases and/or sells TENS units. The company will send a qualified technician to the office or the patient's home to demonstrate use of the unit. Some companies will allow the patient a 30-day trial period to see whether the unit helps. They also will help the patient purchase the unit once effectiveness has been established. The technician should follow the patient closely, via phone, to make certain that the unit is being used properly or to suggest alternative frequencies if the patient is still having pain.

Caution is advised in use of these units around some pacemakers and the carotid sinus.[38]

Galvanic Current

Galvanic current is sometimes referred to as muscle stimulation current, as muscle contraction is the primary outcome of stimulating the nerves with galvanic current. Muscle stimulation can be used on the local, strained muscles to provide short-term edema reduction,[95] improve circulation, disperse exudates, and facilitate the normal modeling of repair. It can relax muscle spasms in innervated muscles and prevent muscle atrophy.[61] A recent article concluded that electrical stimulation can speed repair time and may improve resultant tensile strength.[96] Although the mechanism is unknown, electrotherapy may influence the migratory, proliferative, and functional capacity of fibroblasts.[96]

Electrical Cellular Stimulation

Microcurrent

Microcurrent is a relatively new development in the management of MVCI. It has an advantage over the other types of electrical therapies in that it does not have an affinity for any specific tissue. Instead, it creates a field at nearly the same electrical frequency as the natural human body's nervous system. It can be used for pain control and facilitating neck sprains/strains because of its general effect on stimulating cell metabolism.

Electrical Dense Tissue Mechanical-Thermal Devices

Ultrasound and Diathermy

Ultrasound and diathermy are included in this category and are known to have an affinity for very dense tissues such as bone and those dense tissues that attach directly to bone. Primary benefits includes deep heat, micromassage, and increasing metabolic activity. A recent study on ultrasound treatment of the human gastrocnemius muscle showed significant increases in blood flow up to 45 minutes after application.[97] These types of therapy, in the continuous setting, are best used in the subacute stage of repair. Pulsed ultrasound settings reduce the heating effect and can be used in acute injuries. Treatment should not exceed 3 to 10 minutes per field at any application.[61]

Some doctors feel that ultrasound will break up and destroy scar tissue once it has developed. However, there is no evidence in the literature that ultrasound has a direct affinity for myofascial tissues or scar tissue. This accounts for its inability to break down scar tissue within muscle. In essence, if the ultrasound head is placed over a joint, set at its highest level, and left on, the patient will eventually have severe pain as the result of bone and its surrounding periosteum being burned, not myofascial tissue. If the tissue cannot be burned at higher settings, how can it destroy scar tissue at the lower settings?

Since deep heat is the primary result of this type of therapy, there are some contraindications: (1) acute neck injury, (2) recent strokes, (3) recent transient ischemic attacks, and (4) any condition in which the blood-clotting factors are elevated, such as after recent child delivery. There are several potentially sensitive tissues in the neck region within range of these deep vibratory therapies. Therefore, care should be used to avoid these areas, which include the stellate ganglion, carotid sinus, brain, spinal cord, extensive peripheral neural structures (such as the brachial plexus), and the vertebral artery. Be particularly careful to avoid the stellate ganglion in patients with cardiac conditions.

CERVICAL TRACTION

Several authors have recommended the use of cervical traction for neck injuries sustained in automobile collisions, neck pain, herniated discs, cervical radiculopathy, and cervical arthritis.[61,88] Other authors have concluded that it has no additional benefit other than rest for neck injuries following MVCI. Pennie and Agambar,[98] who studied 135 MVCI adult patients, found that there was no benefit at 5 months postinjury for the cervical traction group, compared with the collar group. Cailliet believes that the value of traction for such conditions is still unproven, but it can be used to overcome periarticular contracture in some cases.[36] Although there is some debate as to the effectiveness of cervical traction, there is some evidence to support the claim that it may be an effective adjunctive therapy for subacute and chronic injuries.

Effects of Cervical Spine Traction

Some of the possible beneficial effects of traction follow:

- Temporary pain relief. Most evidence shows that the mechanical effects of traction are thought to be temporary.[15,50,99] Traction may result in modification of abnormal afferent impulse patterns from joint mechanoreceptors.[100] One study concludes that traction enhanced patient outcome in terms of greater mobility, less medication, and less pain.[101]

- Improved facet joint opening and gliding.[38,102] Traction improves joint mobilization[100] and temporarily alters spinal mechanics.[15]

- Release of dural, nerve root, and capsular adhesions.[15,103] Traction is also effective in reducing nerve root sleeve pull by preventing the formation of adhesions between the dural sleeves and the adjacent joint structures.[104] It has been shown to provide spinal ligament tension relief[102] and stretching of paravertebral muscles and intervertebral ligaments.[99,102]

- Widening of joint and articular surfaces and intervertebral foramina[38,42]

- Disc space separation, increased volume of disc, and/or bulge reduction[38,39]; relief of nerve root compression[103] and nerve root impingement[105,106]; release of entrapped synovial membrane

- Improved muscle and connective tissue fluid exchange[100]; improved circulatory status within the epidural spaces of the spinal and lateral nerve root canals[100,103]

- Relief from osteophyte impingement.[20] Particularly, traction is useful in the aging neck, where marked degenerative changes give rise to brachial symptoms.[107] The primary precaution in the aging spine is in use of traction with flexion. Patients with fibrosis and degenerative joint changes show little or no joint separation with traction because of ligament thickening.[54]

- Reduction of muscle spasm[15,100]

The authors' experience has been that if cervical traction is being used to stretch the upper cervical spine to relieve spasm and headaches, a pulling force of 15 to 20 lb works fairly well. On the other hand, if the objective is to stretch the lower cervical spine in patients with nerve root compression syndromes, additional weight (40 to 60 lb) is needed to transfer the distracting forces from the base of the skull. Note, however, that this may be counterproductive if high weights are used and possibly traumatic to areas already overstretched. It is possible to aggravate upper cervical pain and cause further injury if traction is used too early or if the patient's tolerance level is not established prior to usage. For patients whose lower cervical spine should be tractioned, it is preferable for the doctor to use his or her hands to focus the tractional forces directly on the appropriate segments.

Types of Cervical Traction

Intermittent Cervical Traction

One study compared static, intermittent, and manual neck traction, as well as no traction, for effects on neck pain. The study concluded that intermittent traction at 25 lb with a ratio of 10 seconds on and 10 seconds off had the best pain-relieving effects.[101] Intermittent cervical traction cycles at a ratio of 10 seconds on and 10 seconds off are employed to stimulate mechanoreceptors and increase circulation. This can be applied by motorized traction units or manually. These rhythmic traction forces produce twice as much joint separation as sustained traction[100] and yield results superior to those of other types.[101] The patient should be pretested before attempting this therapy, however.

Manual Traction

Intermittent manual traction is a technique in which the doctor or therapist grasps the cervical segments to be treated and manually applies a traction force. White and Panjabi conclude that a traction weight of 30 lb for 7 seconds will produce posterior separation of the cervical vertebrae.[15] This method is ideal when higher tractional forces are needed without using any jaw or chin pressure. It is possible to provide relief from radicular pain in the lower cervical region by interlocking the fingers, applying 35 to 40 lb of pressure, and obtaining a good tissue pull. Other forms of traction that focus forces at the base of the skull may offer less relief. One advantage is that the amount of traction can be lessened rapidly if the patient experiences increased pain.[40]

Sustained, Continuous Traction

Sustained, continuous traction for 10 to 60 minutes with a selected weight can be done with motorized machines, spring devices, over-the-door units, and in the supine or sitting position. Continuous traction with slight cervical flexion will open the posterior joints and may provide relief when inflamed. If a patient suffers loss or reversal of the normal cervical curvature in the subacute to chronic stages, traction using a wedge to cause cervical extension may help. A pillow under the neck while tractioning in an extension position will also work to increase lordotic cervical pressure. Cervical exercises in conjunction with this type of traction can help prevent worsening of the cervical lordosis and in some cases result in improvement or restoration.

Home Traction

A variety of traction units are available for home use. They include over-the-door units and spring systems that attach to a door or a wall, as well as units with weights. The weights may take any number of forms, including water bags, lead balls, and nylon sacks filled with lead shot.

When home traction has been recommended, the doctor should demonstrate in the office the proper setup and educate the patient as to its objectives. Keep in mind that some patients may not want to admit they are not following instructions properly. With overhead traction, the patient should face the door and have the neck in slight flexion. Instruct the patient to sit in a chair with armrests and try to relax. If the neck pull is too much, the patient should sit straight and then slump for traction. Home traction is generally used for 10 to 20 minutes,[38,92] depending on objectives and tolerance.

Traction Designed To Restore Cervical Curvature

There has been limited research into the effect of cervical-extension traction, where the goal is restoration of lordotic curvature in patients having lost or reversed their normal curves. Harrison et al.[108] report radiographic success after 10 to 14 weeks with this technique, combined with manipulative therapy. Other studies still need to be performed to evaluate the long-term effectiveness in maintaining spinal motion or more normal lordosis. This study did not look at whether this improvement made any difference in pain or functional capacity. Figure 7–4 illustrates a type of traction designed to improve cervical lordosis.

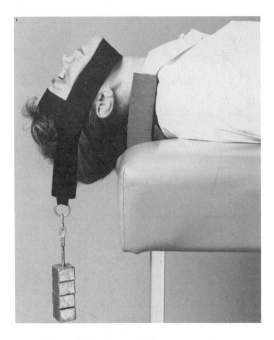

Figure 7–4 Wedge-weight traction. *Source:* Courtesy of Circular Traction Supply, Fountain Valley, California.

Traction Weight

Cervical traction weight needs to account for the pain level and stage of injury and accommodate for the amount of musculature in the neck. As a general rule, lower weights should be used until the level of patient comfort and any reactions can be established. Some authors feel that the weights should start at 15 to 20 lb and be increased gradually to 35 to 40 lb.[92] Other studies evaluating effects of neck traction with X-ray show that 15 to 20 lb of cervical traction weight is necessary to achieve any joint distraction. Radiographic studies show that with 20 to 25 lb, the intervertebral foramina and intervertebral spacing are increased.[92] When separation of vertebral bodies is desired, high tolerable traction forces for short periods work best.[100] Neck halters put most of the tractional forces into the upper cervical spine.

Angle of Traction Pull

The recommended angle of force for neck traction varies according to different authors and can range from 10° to 25° of flexion.[54,61] When deciding how much angle to use, the doctor should test the patient at varying angles until the most symptom-relieving benefits are manifested. Be sure to record the estimated angle. In more subacute or chronic conditions in which there is flattening or reversal of neck curvature, extension tractioning can be used, if tolerated well by the patient, in an attempt to restore or improve the curve.

Frequency and Duration of Traction

In cases of severe muscle spasm and radiculitis, cervical traction may help alleviate pain. If the patient is receiving intermittent traction at the office, use it two times a day at 10-second on-off intervals and taper off as the patient improves. Begin at 1 to 2 minutes in the initial stages and gradually increase to 5 to 15 minutes as tissue repair and patient toler-

ance improve. Home traction should be used two times a day if the desire is to reduce pain or improve neck function.

How Soon Should Traction Be Used?

Clinical experience has shown that moderate to heavy tractional force is contraindicated during the acute phase of cervical injury[59] or in patients with severe pain or torticollis. Mechanical traction is not suggested during the first 2 to 3 weeks after injury because sudden drops or increases in traction forces may cause increased pain. Before initiating traction as therapy, it is advisable to wait about 3 to 6 weeks, depending on injury severity. In the most severe cases, even further postponement is recommended.

Guidelines for Mechanical Cervical Traction

- First and foremost, know your equipment and make sure it is ready and safe before applying traction.
- Always adapt traction to the comfort of the patient.[20]
- Have the patient remove glasses and earrings and observe for hair pulling.
- Always test every patient with light traction first. Sometimes with ligamentous injuries, traction can cause pain. Traction weight is best when the patient says, "That feels good."
- Instruct patients as to what you are doing and what they should feel. Make sure they know that if they feel increased pain, numbness or pain in extremities, dizziness, or jaw pain they should say so immediately.[39] During traction, patients should be told to keep the teeth apart slightly[54] to minimize temporomandibular joint (TMJ) involvement. Bite blocks may be used when indicated. When using traction, the patient should not rotate or move the neck much, because neck ro-

tation while under traction can cause stretching of atlantoaxial ligaments, creating an inflammatory reaction.[54]

- Make sure that staff members applying traction in the office know exactly how it is to be set up and how the patient is to be positioned.

Contraindications for Cervical Traction

The following are contraindications for cervical traction:

- Heavier weights are contraindicated in patients with severe degenerative changes, particularly when causing significant stenosis.
- Patients with TMJ problems should not use a type of traction that puts excessive pressure over the jaw region. There are specially designed units for patients with TMJ conditions. Note prior history of TMJ problems and find out the vector of impact in any MVCIs. In the authors' experience, TMJ injuries occur usually in rear-end collisions in which the patient was not braced, resulting in rapid opening and closure of the jaw. TMJ injuries also result when there is direct jaw impact.
- Traction should be avoided in patients suffering severe pain. It should also be avoided in patients in whom the traction causes or worsens pain or results in paresthesia in the extremities.

ACUPUNCTURE

Acupuncture has been an effective tool for pain control for centuries. Little research is available on the effectiveness of acupuncture for whiplash injuries; however, two studies were noted in the literature.[109,110] A recent study of needle acupuncture for whiplash cases revealed that 71% to 91% had positive results.[111] A trial course of six acupuncture treatments has been recommended to determine whether a patient will benefit from this treatment.[61] Ultimately, some patients respond to acupuncture, just as some respond to other forms of therapy.

HOSPITALIZATION

It is not usually necessary to hospitalize patients with cervical injuries.[84,92] Hospitalization should be discouraged for the most part[54] unless there is moderate to severe head injury requiring frequent observation, unstable spinal fracture, skull fracture, spinal cord injury, vascular injuries having risk of complications, or injuries requiring surgical or extensive medical attention. National data show that 3% of MVCIs will require hospitalization,[112] requiring an average stay of 9 days.[113] Several studies have evaluated the effects of hospitalization versus home care for these injuries. McKinney et al.,[114] in a hospital study of 247 MVCI patients with neck sprains, showed that those patients who were hospitalized, as compared with those who had early mobilization, recovered on the average 1 month later.

DEVELOPING MANAGEMENT STRATEGIES

After completing an extensive review of the literature on spine injury management, it was found that most of the information available addresses the management of low back pain. This includes the recent Mercy Conference Proceedings.[115] Scientific study of the relative efficacy and mechanism of various procedures for the MVCI has begun only recently. Very little literature was found addressing management of the common injuries resulting from car crashes. Most of the recommendations found were based on clinical experience and were simply editorials. The variation among doctors in regard to treatment frequency and numbers of office visits is extreme.

An ideal management program for soft tissue injuries should take into account the nature and extent of the injury, stage of repair, and day-by-day changes in the patient's condition. The degree of severity and the specific types of symptoms should be evaluated with each individual's physical and psychologic uniqueness considered.[59] In other words, the treatment program should fit the patient as opposed to the patient's being fitted into the treatment program.[27] The motivation of the patient is also a critical factor to the pace of the recovery.[83] The treatment must be aggressive, but gentle.[36]

Some patients require daily treatment for up to 2 weeks, after which treatment frequency should decrease.[54] If the patient's functional capacity and pain levels are continuing to improve, then the treatment frequency should be decreased. As the patient continues to stabilize, the amount of pain should lessen and the amount of pain-relief time after an adjustment should continue to increase. The patient should be performing scheduled strengthening exercises as well as stretching at home to complement office therapy. If the patient has no flare-ups and seems to be holding his or her own, the lower frequency can be maintained until a stabilizing point is reached.

Fitzgerald[17] has recently suggested from his experience that these neck injuries should be treated with spinal manipulation for a 1- to 4-month period, starting with daily treatments for about 2 weeks and then three times a week for 4 to 6 weeks, followed with reducing frequencies.

INITIATION OF TREATMENT AFTER MVCI

Cailliet recommends that treatment be initiated early after injury, ideally within hours.[36] Dies and Strapp[116] found in their short-term MVCI study that patients with neck injury who had delays in treatment had lower levels of improvement. A recent hospital study was conducted on 158 patients with cervical syndrome treated by manipulative therapy; the study concluded that if the pain was present

for 6 months prior to initiation of treatment the patients' recovery rate was significantly less than it was for those having pain for less than 6 months.[12]

The main advantage the doctor has in early management is in being able to educate the patient on the injury repair process and on home care. With the proper instruction, the patient can take an active and beneficial role in his or her own care, including application of home therapies such as ice packs, performing specific rehabilitative exercises, and modifying activities of daily living. Once 4 to 6 weeks have passed, a significant portion of the reparative process has been completed, resulting in a disadvantage for the doctor who begins treatment later.

Factors Complicating or Delaying Recovery

There are several factors that may complicate or slow the recovery time for the MVCI case. (Read Chapter 11 on prognosis for more detailed information.) Complicating factors may include any of the following:

- Delay in starting treatment
- Disc protrusions of clinical and non-resolving significance
- Cervical fracture (excluding spinous process) or dislocation
- Head injury associated with the neck injury
- Presence of either headache or low back pain. These patients have been found to require more treatment than average.[116]
- Early upper and lower extremity radicular symptoms (usually associated with prolonged therapy)
- Long vacations or unusual work schedules that excessively interrupt the normal treatment schedule
- Reinjury or new injury of significant magnitude. New car crash injuries that occur within the first 2 to 3 weeks can create a challenge, especially if the first in-

jury resulted in any early radicular symptoms typical for disc or ligamentous injury.

- Complication by other nonrelated biomechanical factors, such as pregnancy, knee surgery, or use of crutches, which results in upper body and neck compensation and causes aggravation of symptoms
- Intractable pain that does not respond to any therapy. Multispecialty evaluation must be strongly considered.
- Earlier treatment involving rest as opposed to early mobilization. Patients so advised will require an additional month of treatment.[114] A sedentary lifestyle slows recovery.
- Nutritional and endocrine disorders, such as anemia, malnutrition, diabetes, hypothyroidism, nicotine addiction, and alcoholism
- Significant pre-existing degenerative joint disease processes, genetic fusion, recent major illnesses, or congenital spinal or soft tissue anomalies such as Klippel-Feil syndrome

When Should Active Curative Treatment Conclude?

In most mild, uncomplicated neck injuries, that is, those cases having no radicular pathology, disc damage, or severe myofascial pain syndromes, active curative treatment should no longer be required after 3 to 4 months. If the patient's daily activities, perpetuating factors, and physical weaknesses have been evaluated and managed, then only an occasional future pain-relieving treatment is indicated. At those times, the doctor should evaluate for any healing residuals and weaknesses that the patient might not be addressing adequately. The time when a patient's condition will stabilize is dependent on the injury severity, the type of tissue injured (muscles stabilize faster than ligaments), the patient's physi-

cal fitness, the patient's motivation to exercise and stretch, and postural and ergonomic stresses. Most authors believe that after about 1 year most patients will fail to make significant improvement. Farrell believes that soft tissue injury fibrosis in the neck will take approximately 1 year to reach its permanent status.[117] There are authors who believe that the time frame can be 6 months or 2 years also. (See Chapter 11 for more detailed information on prognosis.)

We believe that the doctor should close curative treatment based on two categories of recovery:

1. The patient reaches and has stabilized at the preinjury level for a reasonable time frame, typically 1 to 2 months. Any problems or complaints prior to the injury should be treated and billed outside the personal injury case.
2. The patient continues to have persistent symptoms after a reasonable treatment plan and has not shown any objective or subjective evidence of improvement over a 1- to 3-month period, depending on the individual's lifestyle, type of injury, and response to treatment. This is sometimes referred to as the point at which the patient has reached maximal medical improvement. All future supportive treatment should focus at keeping the injured person's pain and/or disability at the discharge level. In the more serious injuries where ligament remodeling is still ongoing, typically up to 1 year, and the patient has periods of pain, supportive care is focused on maintaining joint and soft tissue mobility and making sure the patient is continuing to exercise properly.

Are Flare-Ups Common during Course of Treatment?

It is fairly common for one symptomatic flare-up to occur during the time the patient is under care.[59] Typically, it occurs about 2 to 4 weeks after injury, when the patient's pain is starting to subside and he or she overdoes some activity at home or work. These flare-ups will usually require one to four additional office visits over 2 weeks or so. The patient should use ice during these flare-ups at home. The risk of exacerbations may be reduced if the doctor takes the time to discuss activities of daily living with the patient early in the treatment plan. The need to resume active treatment for more than one flare-up of pain indicates poorer prognosis potential.[118,119]

What Happens When a Second Injury Occurs?

The situation occasionally arises that the patient who is under active care for one MVCI now has a second crash injury. It is imperative that the physician document the new injury and any new symptoms or exacerbations of any old symptoms. If the new injury treatment goals and billing procedures are not clearly outlined to the insurance company and the patient, potential problems may arise. If either case goes to arbitration, deposition, or trial, the issues of liability will be a factor. It is recommended that in such cases the treating doctor should do the following:

- Obtain a complete history and perform a new examination. The history form must evaluate the patient's symptom intensity and frequency status just prior to the second injury. Each complaint must be ranked in severity, frequency, and effect on activity and performance.

- Evaluate the patient's status from the second injury closely. At the conclusion of the work-up of the second injury the doctor should have written notes on overall differences, including pain severity, frequency, and disability level. For example, just prior to the injury the patient had an overall pain intensity level of 3 in the neck region 10% of the time,

brought on only when bending the head forward at the computer station at work. Now the patient has a pain intensity level of 8 100% of the time.

- Address the medicolegal issues. The doctor should discuss the situation with the attorney, if the patient is represented, and the insurance carrier. One suggestion is that the doctor notify the first injury insurance company of the second injury and suspend all billing temporarily until the second injury is preinjury; that is, the first carrier will not be billed until the patient is just like he or she was just prior to the second injury. The doctor should let the company know that apportionment will be closely evaluated and that the patient's condition will be scrutinized thoroughly as to his or her status before and after the second injury.

Monitoring the Patient's Response to Therapy

In MVCI cases periodic reassessments are performed to determine whether improvement is occurring at an appropriate rate. The patient's response to treatment and the normal reparative responses over time need to be assessed at periodic intervals. These re-evaluations should be performed on a patient-by-patient basis depending on injury severity, pain levels, and degree of functional capacity loss. Typically the clinician will develop an initial problem list with treatment objectives being outlined, and at each office visit will make progress notations. When appropriate he or she will complete a more complex assessment of how the patient is progressing, sometimes in a subjective, objective, assessment, and plan (SOAP) format. SOAP notes are most appropriate in environments such as hospitals, which produce the constant hourly, potentially life-saving, incoming data from tests and other procedures requiring SOAP notes several times a day. However, in private practice, SOAP notes need to be done less often, as the clinician should be able to list conditions being treated on a travel card, noting the patient's response to therapy and other pertinent data. Periodic SOAP notes are done to indicate testing that needs to be performed; treatment is then given for a specified time, and the patient is re-evaluated to determine response to therapy. For example, if an antibiotic is given over a period of 10 days, the patient is instructed to take the medication four times a day for 10 days and then return to the office for reassessment. As the patient's improvement becomes more gradual over time, the process usually is performed less frequently. In chronic conditions, when the chiropractor is treating a patient beyond 6 months, assessment every 2 to 3 months is usually appropriate as long as there is no deterioration in the patient's status. The physician should be able to use any type of written format that he or she finds adequate to address the problems and progress of the patient.

Several outcome measurement systems currently are available to document and validate treatment results for MVCI cases. Some reliable measures available include the following:

- Multiple injury functional capacity test. The clinician can use parts of this system, which is covered in Chapter 10 in detail. The test is a 10-part, 2-page questionnaire that modifies the Oswestry low back disability system into a scale that incorporates the multitude of injuries and areas of disability common to MVCI cases.
- Periodic comparative pain intensity and/or pain frequency test forms. A sample form is given in Exhibit 7–1.
- Periodic comparative orthopedic and neurologic examinations. These examinations focus on regions where positive findings were found initially or previously. For example, tests are repeated that initially detected abnormalities such as range-of-motion limitations, reflex changes, positive pain provocation signs,

and soft tissue palpation changes.
- Pain drawings. Pain drawings have been found in one study to have a 0.85 retest reliability.[120] Although subjective, if they are plotted sequentially in a graph over time, they show objective proof of a patient's progress.

Three patterns of reassessment have been identified by the Mercy Conference[115]: interactive, periodic, and follow-up.

Interactive Reassessment

Since the practice of chiropractic inherently involves continual reassessment by virtue of the "hands-on" nature of the therapies, an interactive evaluation is achieved with each visit. This is done in order to arrive at an ongoing clinical impression and to determine the immediate need for chiropractic intervention.

Periodic Reassessment

Periodic reassessment is utilized when changes are likely to be seen over a more extended period of weeks or months. The dynamic nature of the recuperative process requires that periodic reassessment be performed to track the patient's progress and determine the need for continued care or the need to modify the management program.

Follow-Up Reassessment

Follow-up reassessment is performed at the end of the management program or when the patient has attained maximal clinical improvement. Such an assessment is often performed to ascertain the degree of residual deficit, such as disability ratings or the degree of recovery.

In all cases the patient should have an initial assessment with sufficient detail to determine the diagnosis and the course of treatment. The authors recommend that a pain intensity notation be made at each office visit and a more detailed assessment at periodic intervals, usually more frequently in the acute stage. At these periodic, more detailed reassessments, a

Exhibit 7–1 Patient Treatment Progress Form

Date: _____ Patient: _____

For Section 1, please relate your improvement in a percentage. For Section 2, describe on a scale of 1–10 how intense your pain level is currently. A 0 indicates that no symptoms exist. A 1-3 level is a mild level and indicates that your pain is an annoyance primarily. A 4–7 level is moderate pain that probably restricts or limits your activity to some degree. An 8–10 level is severe and means that the pain intensity is so great that some or complete disability exists. For Sections 3–5, please relate your improvement in a percentage. Please circle all shaded areas that best apply to your case.

SECTION 1: OVERALL ACTIVITY PROGRESS

I have made approximately ____% improvement in my overall ability to perform home, recreational, social, and work activities since the first date that I saw the doctor. (Circle the appropriate box.)

0%	10%	20%	30%	40%	50%	60%	70%	80%	90%	100%

SECTION 2: CURRENT PAIN INTENSITY LEVELS

Circle the box following the area of pain that best indicates your overall average-usual pain severity today.

Pain Intensity	None	Mild			Moderate				Severe		
Headache	0	1	2	3	4	5	6	7	8	9	10
Neck Pain	0	1	2	3	4	5	6	7	8	9	10
Mid-Back Pain	0	1	2	3	4	5	6	7	8	9	10
Low-Back Pain	0	1	2	3	4	5	6	7	8	9	10

SECTION 3: CURRENT PAIN FREQUENCY LEVELS

Circle the box following the area of pain that best indicates the average percentage of time you have pain today.

Pain Frequency	None	Occasional		Intermittent			Frequent			Constant	
Headache	0%	10%	20%	30%	40%	50%	60%	70%	80%	90%	100%
Neck Pain	0%	10%	20%	30%	40%	50%	60%	70%	80%	90%	100%
Mid-Back Pain	0%	10%	20%	30%	40%	50%	60%	70%	80%	90%	100%
Low-Back Pain	0%	10%	20%	30%	40%	50%	60%	70%	80%	90%	100%

SECTION 4: OVERALL SYMPTOM INTENSITY PROGRESS

I have made approximately ____% improvement in my overall symptom intensity since the first date that I saw the doctor. (Circle the appropriate box.)

0%	10%	20%	30%	40%	50%	60%	70%	80%	90%	100%

SECTION 5: OVERALL SYMPTOM FREQUENCY PROGRESS

I have made approximately ____% improvement in my overall symptom frequency since the first date that I saw the doctor. (Circle the appropriate box.)

0%	10%	20%	30%	40%	50%	60%	70%	80%	90%	100%

functional capacity evaluation can be performed using any of the disability systems available. The results can be noted in the doctor's progress notes or can be graphed on a functional capacity and pain intensity graph as shown in Chapter 11. Exhibit 7–1 illustrates a type of form that documents pain intensity and frequency responses to treatment.

MANAGEMENT OF SPECIFIC CONDITIONS

The proposed model for the physician treating MVCI is based on several fundamental concepts of patient recovery, cost containment, treatment effectiveness, and a general trend to shift passive care to more active, independent participation of the patient in managing some issues at home or at a gym. The proposed treatment model must consider the following objectives:

- has long-term clinical effectiveness
- eliminates treatment methods that can be performed by the patient at home
- promotes less dependence on the doctor
- encourages active participation and independence by the patient
- categorizes effectiveness of treatment options

Synovial Joint (Spine and Extremity) Injuries

Car crashes cause two general types of spine and extremity joint injuries: (1) to the facet joints and deep ligaments, synovial tissue, capsular ligaments, tendons, and disc structures within, immediately surrounding, and directly attaching to the joint; and (2) to the peripheral nerves, muscles and fasciae (soft tissues), and joints. The doctor takes into account the following concerns when determining the type and duration of management:

- Stage of injury and repair
- Degree of pain. Pain may limit the ability of the patient to relax before adjustment.

- Type of tissue injured. Some tissues have good vascularity and others have poor. Some tissues scar more.
- Accessibility of the specific tissue. For example, facet adhesions are not within reach of finger pressure, so other forms of therapy need to be considered.
- Unique dislikes and likes of the patient. Some patients hate ice application.
- Compliance likelihood when recommending exercises and stretching routines
- Ability of the patient to make appointments
- Eagerness of the patient to help with recovery
- Effects on patient of other people, i.e., attorneys, doctors, family, friends. Some patients may be motivated by an attorney to incur more costs to increase the likelihood of obtaining a larger settlement. Another crash victim may tell a patient that a certain therapy type helped him or her and advise the patient to use only that therapy.

In general, for all joint injuries the focus should be on early use of cryotherapy in acute injuries for 4 to 5 days, early controlled activity, gentle range-of-motion and isometrics, and progression to isotonics in an attempt to correct all abnormal joint biomechanical function. Once normal biomechanical function is restored, the clinician should attempt to maintain joint biomechanical function during the repair stages to optimize the nutritional and lubricant environment. Improved joint motion will facilitate any attaching muscle motion.

Temporary bracing (collars, lumbar supports, shoulder slings, tennis elbow braces, and wrist supports) should be used only when indicated and for a limited time. Long-term supports or orthotics may be indicated, such as cervical pillows in patients having loss of cervical curvature, heel lifts and foot orthotics, or a lumbar belt when heavy lifting will be done. Finally, the doctor needs to identify and eliminate or lessen the negative effects of any perpetuating factors, such as poor posture or ergonomic stressors.

Headaches/Migraines

In the acute-stage MVCI patient having headaches the objective initially is to reduce pain. In mild to moderate cases, ice applied to the base of the skull and neck, gentle manipulation (see contraindications), rest, and good posture may be enough. In the more intense headaches, medications may be needed to help the patient manage the pain. Neck ergonomic and postural modifications, such as avoiding forward or downward postures, avoiding holding the telephone between the neck and shoulders, and avoiding driving or vibration may be useful. As the headaches move from the acute stage to the subacute stage there is more focus on optimizing upper neck biomechanical function and providing some myotherapy to any injured muscles that have the potential for developing myofascial adhesions typical of MVCI headache sufferers. These include the sternocleidomastoid, massater, temporalis, trapezius, anterior scalene, levator scapular, and deep cervical muscles, primarily the suboccipital triangle. In chronic posttraumatic headaches the focus is on identification of latent or active trigger points, biomechanical alterations of spinal joints, drug-induced causes, and postural (slouch) and ergonomic causes. Deep myotherapy focused on neutralizing trigger points will help. Having the patient perform exercises that strengthen and stabilize cervicothoracic posture will more than likely reduce the frequency of the headaches.

Mild Head Injury and Chronic Postconcussion Syndromes

The chiropractor is in an ideal position to help the patient with mild head injury (MHI).

He or she can educate the patient, take time to give lifestyle advice, and treat the neck and back problems that can compound the patient's pain or disability. Often, MHI patients have associated cervical spine conditions, and management of these problems can lessen headaches and other cranial symptoms frequently associated with head injury. It is common to have head symptoms originating in the cervical soft tissue structures. Figure 7–5 illustrates an algorithm for acute uncomplicated MHIs. Far too often the MHI patient undergoes poor management resulting in long-term functional disabilities. The primary focus in MHI is to assess the patient initially for referral indicators (pathology); educate the patient, family, and employer on what to expect over the next 2 to 3 months and give them suggestions on how to cope; monitor progress, looking for deterioration or improvement; and perform a postconcussion evaluation at about 3 months to see whether a postconcussion syndrome has developed. If so, the patient is referred to a neuropsychologist. Management of the acute MHI patient by the physician involves several steps.

- Educate the patient about the typical course of symptoms.
- Educate the family about the support system.
- Educate the employer.
- Encourage the person to write down every task and appointment on a daily calendar.
- Obtain baseline symptoms for future reference if significant postconcussion syndrome develops.

Perform an initial evaluation of the patient with appropriate referral if indicated by pathologic findings. The alert patient having no neurologic findings can usually be sent home with monitoring by a responsible party. If the patient is sent home, an instruction form must be given to the patient and the responsible party. The doctor should always follow

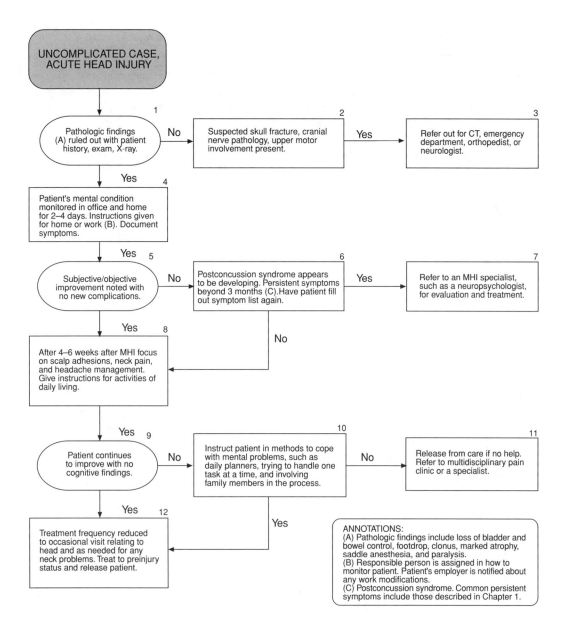

Figure 7–5 Head injury algorithm. Management of acute uncomplicated cases following motor vehicle collisions.

up the initial visit by calling the patient at home the same day to make sure that he or she is following instructions, to monitor neurologic status, and to answer any questions. The MHI patient and a responsible family member should be given an instruction sheet with the doctor's emergency telephone number (see Exhibit 7–2).

Early evaluation of symptoms classic to MHI will provide a baseline or reference point for any long-term problems that may occur. (See Chapter 1, which covers diagnosis of con-

Exhibit 7–2 Head Injury Home Instruction Form

GENERAL ADVICE

While checking the person with head injury, it is important for you the observer to pay very close attention to any mental or physical changes that might develop. When awakening the person with the head injury, be sure to fully awaken. If any of the following symptoms become worse or if there are any new symptoms that develop from the list below, call the doctor immediately.

Under no circumstances is this person to do any heavy lifting or other exertional activities (including sex) for the next _____ days. No alcohol, aspirin, or smoking is allowed for the next week.

> CHECK THIS PERSON EVERY _____ HOURS DAY AND NIGHT FOR _____ DAYS.

OBSERVE ANY MENTAL CHANGES

- ☑ Ease of arousability
- ☑ Abnormal behavior
- ☑ Worsening headache or persistent headache beyond 24 hours
- ☑ Decrease in awareness of home address (location), names (family), and time (date)
- ☑ Agitation or restlessness
- ☑ Memory loss
- ☑ Progressive drowsiness

OBSERVE ANY PHYSICAL CHANGES

- ☑ Weakness or numbness in the arms or legs
- ☑ Fever
- ☑ Unequal pupil size
- ☑ Convulsions or seizures
- ☑ Vomiting spells more than three times or continuous nausea
- ☑ Any vomiting without nausea before
- ☑ Inability to make a circle with thumb and index finger
- ☑ Balance problems
- ☑ Walking abnormality
- ☑ Speech difficulty
- ☑ Blurry or double vision
- ☑ Hearing loss

CHILDREN

Observe for excessive crying, headaches, temper tantrums, lack of initiative, acting immaturely, awkwardness in social activities, awkward athletic abilities, and disturbances in writing or artwork.

I, _____, have read the above instructions and understand them.

Date _____   Signature _____

---

cussion.) Obtaining a reference point on the patient can be very useful in cases involving future neuropsychologic evaluation. It is very difficult for a neuropsychologist to determine what was normal for the patient before the ac-

cident and what subsequent problems exist if initial records are not available or are limited in detail. When the doctor takes this portion of the history, it is a good time to educate the patient about possible problems.

Evaluate the MHI patient for cervical-thoracic problems. Many MHI patients suffer injuries to the neck and upper back regions as compressive forces are loaded directly from impact. Many of the headache problems, auditory and visual symptoms, and neck pain reflect indirect injuries. Early management of these problems can make the overall problems for the MHI patient more tolerable. If the head injury is causing headaches and is compounded by cervicogenic headaches, the combination can cause more disability.

Provide an informative letter to the employer about common symptoms and encourage working with the injured person. The employer needs to understand that it is common for the employee to have temporary memory problems and difficulty handling complex or multiple tasks. Keeping the patient employed during this process is critical. It can be devastating to a patient's recovery if he or she loses a job or an advancement opportunity because the doctor failed to inform the employer of possible symptoms (Exhibit 7–3).

"The most basic and effective intervention for minor head injury is early education and information of both the head injured person and the family. Such intervention does nothing to ameliorate the primary deficits, but it is the best course of action for reducing the severity of the secondary psychological reaction. Persons who know what may happen, how to understand it, and what to do, are simply less likely to become enmeshed in one of the dysfunctional syndromes."[121] Suggestions may include having the person use a system that lists activities that need to be done (i.e., a day calendar) for each day for 1 to 3 months or have the person perform one task at a time. Having a discussion with the immediate family or support members and educating the people close to the MHI patient about normal sequelae may make the difference in the continuity of the social environment. Teamwork and support are helpful in the recovery.

In the chronically injured MHI patient, management strategies focus on establishing the pre-existing status of the patient, what happened initially, what happened during the course of treatment, and present symptoms classic to the head injury. The physician must determine whether the current problems are creating an impairment/disability and if so, how severe. Typically, the doctor will have the patient complete periodic reassessments, looking for improvement, and then will perform a concluding comprehensive evaluation between 3 and 6 months, looking for any healed residual problems. Use the form in Exhibit 2–2 to evaluate any sequelae. If notable problems exist, the doctor will then need to assess disability levels, discuss options available to the patient, and determine appropriateness for referral to a specialist, usually a neuropsychologist with training and experience in MHI. The MHI patient and his or her family or support group may need counseling and further education about the problems that frequently follow MHI.

Thoracic Outlet Syndrome

The female occupant involved in a rear-end crash who has sternocleidomastoid and anterior scalene injuries and who later develops arm and/or hand numbness must be evaluated for thoracic outlet syndrome (TOS). This syndrome is usually seen in chronic cases and involves hypertrophy of the scalene muscles leading to neurovascular entrapment. Most MVCI cases involve neurologic compromise, and both postural and cervicothoracic instabilities need to be addressed. These patients almost always have a rounded, forward shoulder, stooped posture with the head positioned forward in relation to the shoulders. In addition many of these patients have atrophy in the muscles that maintain downward and inward scapular positioning. As a result, overhead pull-down and rowing-machine exercises will usually help to stabilize these patients. The clinician also must focus on reducing upward shoulder motion by modifying patient posture, doing deep muscle

Exhibit 7–3 Return to Work after Head Injury Form

Date

Dear Employer:

Your employee, _____, has recently been in an accident in which he/she sustained a mild head injury. Although your employee has had a concussion, he/she is capable of returning to work on a full-time basis. See below for any restrictions. As a direct result of this injury it is likely that this employee will have some difficulty in performing the following activities for the next 2 to 3 months. These symptoms should lessen gradually over time.

Common temporary problems may include:
- ☑ Difficulty handling multiple tasks at one time
- ☑ Memory difficulty, sometimes forgetting details
- ☑ Hard to keep mind on the job
- ☑ Irritability and fatigue

This employee needs your cooperation during the healing process. These symptoms may get worse at about 2 weeks after injury, but should start to subside afterward. Please try to understand these areas of difficulty. Your cooperation could improve the healing process. Suggestions include allowing the employee to keep a day calendar with all activities listed with times. Keeping the employee doing one task at a time and working together with the temporary memory difficulties will help the healing process as well. It is advised that the employer talk directly with the doctor to discuss this situation.

This employee has:
- ❑ No restrictions, return to work doing all normal regular work activities
- ❑ The following restrictions:
  - ❑ No lifting for ____ days
  - ❑ No bending head or stooping for ____ days
  - ❑ No driving any vehicle for ____ days
  - ❑ No operating dangerous mechanical/electrical equipment for ____ days
  - ❑ No job task that requires balancing at heights

---

stretches to lengthen the scalene and trapezius muscles, and stretching the pectoral muscles, which tend to be contracted, tender, and lead to rapid fatigue for many patients when they are tight. Myofascial adhesion and trigger point neutralization and elimination will help as well. Figure 7–6 illustrates an anterior scalene stretch as the patient rotates the head toward involved side and laterally flexes contralaterally as the clinician applies deep muscle stretching. Figure 7–7 illustrates a technique for the middle and posterior scalene muscles. The reader can review a recent book specifically written to address the posttraumatic thoracic outlet syndrome.[122]

Chest Wall and Hip Joint Injuries

Chest wall injuries resulting either directly from contusions incurred by the occupant's striking the steering wheel or dash or indirectly from anterior neck muscle bleeding seeping down between myofascial planes can create acute and chronic pain. Subscapular trauma can occur with torso rotational forces. Intercostal and subscapular myofascial adhesions can cause severe chest wall pain that may be intensified with torso motion or with inspiration. Myofascial techniques that the authors have found helpful include lifting the scapula off the rib cage, as shown in Figure 7–

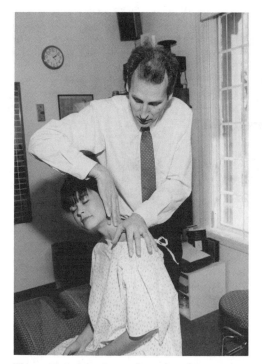

Figure 7–6 Anterior scalene stretch.

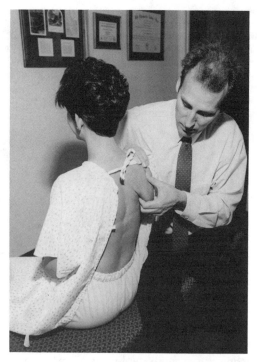

Figure 7–8 Subscapular lifting myofascial technique.

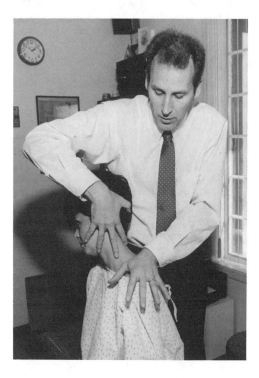

Figure 7–7 Posterior scalene stretch.

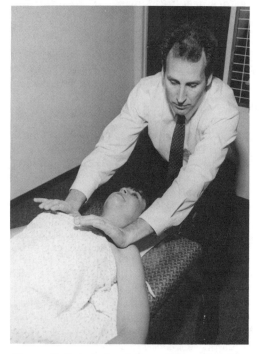

Figure 7–9 Anterior intercostal myofascial release technique.

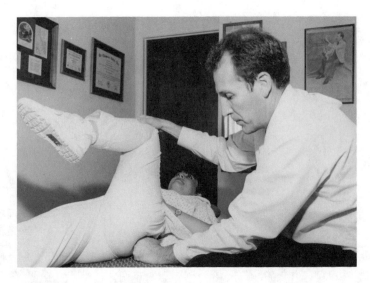

Figure 7–10 Posterior hip circumduction over a fulcrum point such as a fist.

8. Intercostal pain is helped with deep probing between tender ribs, with the clinician contacting the rib with the thenar eminence and pushing gently downward as the patient breathes deeply (Figure 7–9). Posterior hip pain is a common chronic complaint, with the clinician finding tenderness and myofascial adhesions in the deep gluteal and piriformis muscles and around the bursae. In frontal crashes these injuries occur by flexion over a lap belt; in rear-end crashes the injuries occur when the occupant rebounds forward in the second stage. The authors have found that a useful technique involves having the patient lie prone, and deep elbowing these regions, or having the patient lie supine and rotating the knee as the doctor's fist is held under the hip region, acting as a fulcrum (Figure 7–10).

REFERENCES

1. Bland JH. The cervical spine: from anatomy to clinical care. *Med Times.* 1989;117(9):15–33.

2. Smythe H. Referred pain and tender points. *Am J Med.* 1986;81(suppl 3A):90–92.

3. Cyriax J. *Textbooks of Orthopaedic Medicine: Treatment by Manipulation, Massage, and Injection.* vol 2. 11th ed. Philadelphia: Bailliére Tindall; 1984.

4. Ankermann VKJ, Ankermann A, Keil G, et al. Vertebragener kopfschmerz aus banaler ursache. *Z Physiother.* 1990;42:171–176.

5. Bogduk N. Headaches and cervical manipulation. *Med J Aust.* 1979;66:65–66.

6. Bourdillon JF. *Spinal Manipulations.* 3rd ed. London and New York: William Heinemann Medical Books Ltd and Appleton-Century-Crofts; 1982.

7. Carrick FR. Cervical radiculopathy: the diagnosis and treatment of pathomechanics in the cervical spine. *J Manipulative Physiol Ther.* 1983;6(3):129–137.

8. Droz JM, Crot F. Occipital headaches: statistical results in the treatment of vertebragenous headache. *Swiss Ann.* 1985;7:127–136.

9. Greenman PE. Manual and manipulative therapy in whiplash injuries. *Spine State Art Rev.* 1993; 7(3):517–530.

10. Jeffreys E, McSweeney T. *Disorders of the Cervical Spine.* London: Butterworth; 1980.

11. Triano JJ, Humphreys CR. Patient monitoring in the conservative management of cervical radiculopathy. *J Manipulative Physiol Ther.* 1987;10(3): 94–100.

12. Zhongda L. A study of the effect of manipulative treatment on 158 cases of cervical syndrome. *J Tradit Chin Med.* 1987;7:205–208.

13. Grieve GP. Manipulation therapy for neck pain. *Physiotherapy.* 1979;65(5):136–146.

14. Leach RA. An evaluation of the effect of chiropractic manipulative therapy on hypolordosis of the cervical spine. *J Manipulative Physiol Ther.* 1983;6(1):17–22.

15. White AA III, Panjabi MM. *Clinical Biomechanics of the Spine.* 2nd ed. Philadelphia: JB Lippincott Co; 1990.

16. Haldeman S. Manipulation and massage for the relief of pain. In: Wall PD, Melzack R, eds. *Textbook of Pain.* 2nd ed. Edinburgh: Churchill Livingstone; 1989: chap 69.

17. Fitzgerald PB. Manipulation and mobilization. In: Tollison CD, Satterthwaite JR, eds. *Painful Cervical Trauma: Diagnosis and Rehabilitative Treatment of Neuromusculoskeletal Injuries.* Baltimore: Williams & Wilkins; 1992.

18. Hoag JM, Cole WV, Bradford SG. *Osteopathic Medicine.* New York: Blakiston Div, McGraw-Hill Publishing Co; 1969.

19. Lewit K. Chain reactions in disturbed function of the motor system. *Manual Med.* 1987;3:37–39.

20. Zohn DA. *Musculoskeletal Pain, Diagnosis and Physical Treatment.* 2nd ed. Boston: Little, Brown & Co; 1988.

21. Paris SV. Spinal manipulative therapy. *Clin Orthop.* 1983;179:55–61.

22. Lewit K. Ligament pain and anteflexion headache. *Eur Neurol.* 1975;5:365–378.

23. Dishman R. Review of the literature supporting a scientific basis for the chiropractic subluxation complex. *J Manipulative Physiol Ther.* 1985;8(3): 163–174.

24. Wyke BD. The neurology of joints. *Ann R Coll Surg Engl.* 1967;41:25–50.

25. Kellett J. Acute soft tissue injuries: a review of the literature. *Med Sci Sports Exerc.* 1986;18(5):489–500.

26. Kirkalady-Willis WH. *Managing Low Back Pain.* New York: Churchill Livingstone; 1988.

27. Farbman AA. Neck sprain, associated factors. *JAMA.* 1973;223:1010–1015.

28. Janda V. Muscle spasm: a proposed procedure for differential diagnosis. *J Manual Med.* 1991;6:136–139.

29. Slosberg M. Spinal learning: central modulation of pain processing and long-term alteration of interneuronal excitability as a result of nociceptive peripheral input. *J Manipulative Physiol Ther.* 1990;13:326–336.

30. Gillette RG. A speculative argument for the coactivation of diverse somatic receptor populations by forceful chiropractic adjustments: a review of the neurophysiological literature. *Manual Med.* 1987;3:1–14.

31. Maitland GD. *Peripheral Manipulation.* 3rd ed. London: Butterworth-Heinemann; 1991.

32. Mennell JMCM. *The Musculoskeletal System: Differential Diagnosis from Symptoms and Physical Signs.* Gaithersburg, Md: Aspen Publishers, Inc; 1992.

33. Vernon H. Spinal manipulation and headaches of cervical origin: a review of literature and presentation of cases. *J Manual Med.* 1991;6:73–79.

34. Haldeman S. *Principles and Practice of Chiropractic.* 2nd ed. Norwalk, Conn: Appleton & Lange; 1992.

35. Jayson MIV. General aspects of back pain: an overview. In: Jayson MIV, Swezey RL, Knoplich J, et al. eds. *Back Pain, Painful Syndromes and Muscle Spasms: Current Concepts and Recent Advances.* London: Parthenon Publishing Group; 1990.

36. Cailliet R. *Neck and Arm Pain.* 3rd ed. Philadelphia: FA Davis Co; 1991.

37. Ciolek JJ. Cryotherapy: review of physiological effects and clinical application. *Cleve Clin Q.* 1985;52(2):193–201.

38. Cooper BC, Lucente FE. *Management of Facial, Head, and Neck Pain.* Philadelphia: WB Saunders Co; 1989.

39. Downer AH. *Physical Therapy Procedures.* 4th ed. Springfield, Ill: Charles C Thomas, Publisher; 1988.

40. Echternach JL, ed. *Pain.* New York: Churchill Livingstone; 1987.

41. Gould JA III, Davies GJ. *Orthopaedic and Sports Physical Therapy.* vol 2. St Louis: CV Mosby Co; 1985.

42. Loane SR. Cryotherapy, using cold to treat injuries. In: Appenzeller O, ed. 3rd ed. *Sports Medicine, Fitness, Training, Injuries.* Baltimore: Urban & Schwarzenberg; 1988.

43. McMaster WC, Liddle S, Waugh TR. Laboratory evaluation of various cold therapy modalities. *Am J Sports Med.* 1978;6(5):291–294.

44. Knight K, Aquino J, Urban C. A re-examination of Lewis's cold-induced vasodilation in the finger and ankle. *Athl Train.* 1980:15:248–250.

45. Barnes L. Cryotherapy—putting injury on ice. *Physician Sportsmed.* 1979;6:130–136.

46. Hocutt JE, Jaffe R, Rylander R, et al. Cryotherapy in ankle sprains. *Am J Sports Med.* 1982;10(5):316–319.

47. Knight KL. Cryotherapy in sports medicine. In: Schriber K, Burke EJ, eds. *Relevant Topics in Athletic Training.* Ithaca, NY: Monument Publications; 1978.

48. Michlovitz SL, Wolf SL. *Thermal Agents in Rehabilitation*. Philadelphia: FA Davis Co; 1988.

49. Claus-Walker J, Halstead LS, Carter RE, et al. Physiological responses to cold stress in health subjects with cervical cord injuries. *Arch Phys Med Rehabil*. 1974;55:485.

50. Kowal MA. Review of physiological effects of cryotherapy. *J Orthop Sports Phys Ther*. 1983;5:66–73.

51. Lenhart LJ. Post-traumatic cervical syndrome. *J Manipulative Physiol Ther*. 1988;11(5):409–414.

52. Prentice WE Jr. An electromyographic analysis of the effectiveness of heat or cold and stretching for inducing relaxation in injured muscle. *J Orthop Sports Phys Ther*. 1982;3(3):133–140.

53. Farry PJ, Prentice NG, Hunter AC, et al. Ice treatment of injured ligaments: an experimental model. *N Z Med J*. January 9, 1980;12–14.

54. Jackson R. *The Cervical Syndrome*. 4th ed. Springfield, Ill: Charles C Thomas, Publisher; 1977.

55. Basur RL, Shephard E, Mouzas GL. A cooling method in the treatment of ankle sprains. *Practitioner*. 1976;216:708–711.

56. Sawyer M, Zbieranek CK. The treatment of soft tissue after spinal injury. *Clin Sports Med*. 1986;5(2):387–405.

57. Mense S. Effects of temperature on the discharges of muscle spindles and tendon organs. *Pflugers Arch*. 1978;374:159–166.

58. Kottke FJ, Stillwell GK, Lehmann JF. *Krusens's Handbook of Physical Medicine and Rehabilitation*. 3rd ed. Philadelphia: WB Saunders Co; 1982.

59. Hohl M. Soft tissue injuries of the neck. *Clin Orthop*. 1975;109:42–49.

60. Grodin A, Myerson GE, Malone TR. Soft tissue mobilization. *Sports Injury Management*. Summer 1989, 1990.

61. Ruskin AP. *Current Therapy in Physiatry: Physical Medicine and Rehabilitation*. Philadelphia: WB Saunders Co; 1984.

62. Maxwell C, Spiegel A. The rehabilitation of athletes following spinal injuries. *Spine State Art Rev*. 1990;4(2):481–489.

63. Aldman B. Injury Biomechanics. Government/Industry Meeting and Exposition. Washington, DC: Society of Automotive Engineers; 1987; SP-731.

64. Gerhardt JJ, Reiner E, Schwaiger B, et al. *Interdisciplinary Rehabilitation in Trauma*. Baltimore: Williams & Wilkins; 1987.

65. Ritzmann SE, Levin WC. Cryopathies: a review. *Arch Intern Med*. 1961;107:186.

66. Moldofsky H. Sleep and musculoskeletal pain. *Am J Med*. 1986;81(suppl 3A):85–89.

67. Wolfe F. The clinical syndrome of fibrositis. *Am J Med*. 1986;81(suppl 3A):7–14.

68. Simons DG, Travell JG. Myofascial origins of low back pain, part 1: principles of diagnosis and treatment. *Postgrad Med*. 1983;73:66–77.

69. Chaitow L. *Soft-Tissue Manipulation, A Practitioner's Guide to the Diagnosis and Treatment of Soft Tissue Dysfunction and Reflex Activity*. Wellingborough, UK: Thorsons Publishing Group; 1987.

70. Chamberlain GJ. Cyriax's friction massage: a review. *J Orthop Sports Phys Ther*. 1982;4:16–22.

71. Akeson WH, Amiel D, Woo SL-Y. Immobility effects on synovial joints, the pathomechanics of joint contracture. *Biorheology*. 1980;17:95–110.

72. Lantz CA. Immobilization degeneration and the fixation hypothesis of chiropractic subluxations: a review of the literature related to the degeneration of connective tissue following joint immobilization. *Chiropractic Res J*. 1988;1(1):22–45.

73. Amiel D, Woo SL-Y, Harwood FL, et al. The effect of immobilization on collagen turnover in connective tissue: a biochemical-biomechanical correlation. *Acta Orthop Scand*. 1983;53:325–332.

74. Hertling D, Kessler RM. *Management of Common Musculoskeletal Disorders: Physical Therapy Principles and Methods*. 2nd ed. Philadelphia: JB Lippincott Co; 1990.

75. Akeson WH, Woo SL-Y, Amiel D, et al. The connective tissue response to immobility: biochemical changes in periarticular connective tissue of the immobilized rabbit knee. *Clin Orthop*. 1973;93:356–362.

76. Robinson GA, Enoka RM, Stuart DG. Immobilization-induced changes in motor unit force and fatigability in the cat. *Muscle Nerve*. 1991;14:563–573.

77. Booth FW. Effect of limb immobilization on skeletal muscle. *J Appl Physiol*. 1982;52(5):1113–1118.

78. Järvinen M. Immobilization effect on the tensile properties of striated muscle: an experimental study in the rat. *Arch Phys Med Rehabil*. 1977;58:123–127

79. Videman T. Connective tissue and immobilization: key factors in musculoskeletal degeneration? *Clin Orthop*. 1987;221:26–32.

80. Waddell G. A new clinical model for the treatment of low back pain. In: Roland MO, Jenner JR, eds. *Back Pain: New Approaches to Rehabilitation and Education*. Manchester, UK: Manchester University Press; 1989.

81. Gay JR, Abbott KH. Common whiplash injuries of the neck. *JAMA*. 1953;152:1698–1704.

82. Martin GM. Sprain, strain, and whiplash injury. *Phys Ther*. 1959;39:808–813.

83. Ameis A. Cervical whiplash: considerations in the rehabilitation of cervical myofascial injury. *Can Fam Physician*. 1986;32:1871–1876.

84. Greenfield J, Ilfeld FW. Acute cervical strain: evaluation and short term prognostic factors. *Clin Orthop*. 1977;122:196–200.

85. Podolsky S, Baraff LJ, Simon RR, et al. Efficacy of cervical spine immobilization methods. *J Trauma*. 1983;23:461–465.

86. Bennett RM, Smythe HA, Wolfe F. Recognizing fibromyalgia. *Patient Care*. July 15, 1989:60-83.

87. Carroll C, McAfee PG, Riley LH Jr. Objective findings for diagnosis of whiplash: comprehensive care can bring long-term relief. *J Musculoskel Med*. March 1986;57–76.

88. Lewis RC Jr. *Primary Care Orthopedics*. New York: Churchill Livingstone; 1988.

89. Gandee WS. Preferential use of ice vs heat. *Am Chiropractor*. February 1990: 36.

90. Lawton DS. Adult collars made with thermoplastic materials. *Physiotherapy*. 1984;70(9):355–359.

91. Hinoki M. Vertigo due to whiplash injury, a neurotological approach. *Acta Otolaryngol* Suppl (Stockh). 1985;419:9–29.

92. Hirsch C, Zotterman Y. *Cervical Pain*. vol. 19. Proceedings of the international symposium held in Wenner-Gren Center, Stockholm, January 25–27, 1971. Oxford: Pergamon Press; 1972.

93. Schafer RC. *Clinical Biomechanics, Musculoskeletal Actions and Reactions*. 2nd ed. Baltimore: Williams & Wilkins; 1987.

94. Richardson RR, Siqueira EB. Transcutaneous electrical neurostimulation: in acute cervical hyperextension-hyperflexion injuries. *Ill Med J*. 1981; 159(4):227–230.

95. Bettany JA, Fish DR, Mendel FC. Influence of high voltage pulsed direct current on edema formation following impact injury. *Phys Ther*. 1990; 70(4):219–224.

96. Weiss DS, Kirsner R. Eaglstein WH. Electrical stimulation and wound healing. *Arch Dermatol*. February 1990; 126:222–225.

97. Baker RJ, Bell GW. The effect of therapeutic modalities on blood flow in the human calf. *J Orthop Sports Phys Ther*. 1991;13:23–27.

98. Pennie BH, Agambar LJ. Whiplash injuries: a trial of early management. *J Bone Joint Surg. [Br]*. 1990;72:277–279.

99. Krämer J. *Intervertebral Disk Diseases: Causes, Diagnosis, Treatment, and Prophylaxis*. 2nd ed. New York: Thieme Medical Publishers, Inc; 1990.

100. Grieve GP. Neck traction. *Physiotherapy*. 1982; 68(8):260–264.

101. Zylbergold RS, Piper MC. Cervical spine disorders: a comparison of three types of traction. *Spine*. 1985;10:867–871.

102. Saunders HD. *Orthopaedic Physical Therapy: Evaluation and Treatment of Musculoskeletal Disorders*. Philadelphia: WB Saunders Co; 1982.

103. Rogoff J. *Manipulation, Traction, and Massage*. 2nd ed. Baltimore; Williams & Wilkins; 1980.

104. Jayson MW, Sims-Williams H, Young S, et al. Mobilization and manipulation for low back pain. *Spine*. 1981;6:409.

105. Cibulka MT. Evaluation and treatment of cervical spine injuries. *Clin Sports Med*. 1989;8(4):691–701.

106. Downie PA. *Cash's Textbook of Orthopaedics and Rheumatology for Physiotherapists*. Philadelphia: JB Lippincott Co; 1984.

107. Paterson JK, Burn L. *An Introduction to Medical Manipulation*. Lancaster, UK: MTP Press Ltd; 1985.

108. Harrison DD, Jackson BL, Troyanovich S, et al. The efficacy of cervical extension-compression traction combined with diversified manipulation and drop table adjustments in the rehabilitation of cervical lordosis: a pilot study. *J Manipulative Physiol Ther*. 1994;17:454–464.

109. Greenwold MT, Leong LA, Tan WC. Traditional acupuncture treatment for whiplash syndrome. *Am J Acupunct*. 1988;16(4):305–318.

110. Pearson EJ. Combined manual medicine and acupuncture in neck injury. *Manual Med*. 1990;5: 19–20.

111. Su HC, Su RK. Treatment of whiplash injuries with acupuncture. *Clin J Pain*. 1988;4:233–247.

112. Miller TR, Luchter S, Brinkman CP. Crash costs and safety investment. *Accid Anal Prev*. 1989; 21(4):303–315.

113. National Highway Traffic Safety Administration. *Report on Traffic Accidents for 1979–1980*. Washington, DC: US Department of Transportation, February 1982.

114. McKinney LA, Dornan JO, Ryan M. The role of physiotherapy in management of acute neck sprains following road-traffic accidents. *Arch Emerg Med*. 1989;6:27–33.

115. Haldeman S, Chapman-Smith D, Petersen DM Jr, eds. *Guidelines for Chiropractic Quality Assurance and Practice Parameters, Proceedings of the Mercy Center Consensus Conference*. Gaithersburg, Md: Aspen Publishers, Inc; 1993.

116. Dies S, Strapp JW. Chiropractic treatment of patients in motor vehicle accidents: a statistical analysis. *J Can Chiro Assn*. 1992;36(3):139–145.

117. Farrell M. Headaches and cervical manipulation. *Med J Aust*. 1980;1:34–35.

118. Hohl M. Soft-tissue neck injuries. In: *The Cervical Spine*. 2nd ed. Cervical Spine Research Society Editorial Committee. Philadelphia: 1989, JB Lippincott Co; 1989:436–441.

119. Kenna CJ. The whiplash syndrome: a general practitioner's viewpoint. *Aust Fam Physician*. 1984;13(4):256–258.

120. Margolis RB, Chibnall JT, Tait RC. Test-retest reliability of the pain drawing instrument. *Pain*. 1988;33:49–51.

121. Kay T. *Minor Head Injury: An Introduction for Professionals*. Southboro, Mass: National Head Injury Foundation; 1986.

122. Sanders RJ. *Thoracic Outlet Syndrome: A Common Sequela of Neck Injuries*. Philadelphia: JB Lippincott Co; 1991.

Chapter 8

The Rehabilitation Phase in Cervical-Thoracic Injuries

Gerald P. Keane

INTRODUCTION

One of the major changes in the approach to care of the whiplash (automobile crash) patient in recent years has been the increasing focus on the active approach in physical rehabilitation. The sports injury model of aggressive strengthening, flexibility training, and reconditioning has been more widely applied and accepted for the spinal injury patient, as well. The traditional method of treatment of symptoms of prolonged rest has been essentially abandoned. This approach tended to lead to a generalized deconditioning with associated and equally difficult to manage psychologic implications. The patient was, in many cases, made apprehensive and fearful, and was advised to exhibit extreme caution for fear of reinjury. The athletic model for rehabilitation and peripheral joint injuries, however, encourages early work on development of full range of motion, strengthening, and sports-specific training and reconditioning. This not only promotes the physical rehabilitation of the patient, but also is beneficial for psychologic well-being and in moving the patient more actively into return to his or her normal level of function.

One of the criticisms of chiropractic care, right or wrong, has been directed toward a perception of a somewhat passive interaction on the part of the patient. The chiropractic community, in my experience, has moved away from passive approaches only and moved into the more aggressive model of active rehabilitation. This is in concordance with the general approaches taken in the sports injury model, as mentioned earlier.

The whiplash syndrome lends itself particularly well to this kind of approach. The incorporation from an early stage of active aggressive intervention in conjunction with manual treatment and modalities is a very powerful tool in promoting as full a recovery as possible. There is the additional benefit of the sense of well-being that comes from the patients' feeling as though they are active participants in their own recovery program. Conversely, patients who want to be treated with only passive modalities and do not exhibit an interest in becoming actively involved in their own care can be identified as being at high risk for long-term failure. Patients who are reluctant to become active participants in the maintenance of their own health tend to do much more poorly on a long-term basis, in my experience.

In this chapter, I attempt to pick up the recovery process at a point where much of the early recovery phase has been accomplished or is already under way and look at some of the associated techniques that can be of great value in enhancing other aspects of medical treatment. These topics include independent stretching and exercise programs, the concept of cervicothoracic stabilization training, postural and ergonomic issues, and active long-term maintenance programs. It is assumed during the early phases of such treatment that the patient will continue to participate in more passive approaches, as well, in order to maintain pain control and allow as full and active a participation as possible. It is also assumed that many of the topics discussed here need to be incorporated from very early on to prevent secondary complications of disuse, atrophy, and deconditioning from setting in.

GENERAL GOALS

- Increase and restore the normal pre-injury range of pain-free motion, flexibility, strength, and endurance.

- Emphasize patient education that allows the patient to become self-managing and begins to incorporate the patient in his or her own recovery process as early as possible.

- Encourage an early emphasis on function and decrease the emphasis on individual pain complaints. This has the advantage of decreasing the potential for long-term development of chronic pain behavior.

- Undertake early intervention in postural education and development of proper spinal balance and alignment during activities of daily living.

- Gradually incorporate into treatment more progressive methods of strengthening and conditioning to allow the patient to increase physical capacity to preinjury levels. Early functional assessment and

setting of specific goals on a week-to-week basis can be of benefit. This gives patients a chance to gauge their progress and measures objectively those patients who are failing to move forward.

- Establish a level of independence that allows the patient to develop, as reasonably soon as possible, an independent exercise and conditioning program. This can usually be accomplished best in a home or local gym or health club.

- As the patient improves and recovers toward reasonable levels of functional capacity, encourage the patient toward early return to work and avocational activities.

ACUTE PHASE

During the earliest stages after the typical whiplash (automobile crash) injury, there is often a significant loss of range of motion in the affected areas due to both local spasm and pain inhibition. Early on, however, the patient should be brought through active-assist range of motion exercises both to maintain the range of motion that remains and to allow progression of soft tissue flexibility. During this phase, typically there is a great reliance on modalities and manual techniques to allow the patient to participate in such a program. The adjunctive use, when otherwise safe, of simple over-the-counter anti-inflammatory medication can also be of value for some patients. Short-term immobilization in a soft collar may have benefit, but usually not beyond the first few days postinjury. Prolonged use of restraints such as collars may only promote further loss of range of motion and therefore prolong the recovery process. The patient can be encouraged to use passive methods of heat to increase soft tissue extensibility, and these can also be provided by the chiropractor prior to initiation of exercise. Postexercise, I encourage the use of ice in the early phases to reduce swelling and edema.

Exercises for strengthening at this stage are generally only minimally tolerated. This is typical during the first 5 to 10 days postinjury. During this period of time, however, the patient can be instructed in isometric forms of pain-free muscle contraction. The patient is shown simply how to place the palm of the hand on the side of the head and gently push with resistance against the hand. Such contractions can actually be used to cause a contract/relax type of phenomenon, allowing gradual increase in range of motion as a result. The patient is usually started for 1 to 2 minutes three to five times a day. As the patient moves out of the acute phase of injury, more aggressive strengthening and subsequent stabilization training can be initiated.

Postural considerations at this point include teaching the patient proper methods of positioning the head and neck for sleep, in particular. It is very common for patients at this phase to find a great deal of difficulty in achieving a comfortable sleeping position. The use of appropriate placement of rolls, towels, pillows, and particular sleeping postures can all be of benefit. One relatively inexpensive method of achieving reasonable neck support is to instruct the patient in rolling a towel to a size that allows comfortable fitting into the cervical recess and using some surgical or masking tape to secure the roll in its position. Pillows can be used in a similar manner. Typically in this phase, patients are going to do best by lying on their side with a pillow underneath the space between the shoulder and neck to provide support or by lying in the supine position with similar support. A pillow placed between the knees in side-lying or behind the knees when lying supine can also be helpful in preventing rotation of the spine that will cause increased pressure and stress to the cervical and thoracic regions.

During this phase, the patient is also started on some gentle strengthening exercises, not only to work through the affected areas, but to maintain good mobility to the associated areas that tend to develop long-term secondary complications. It is very typical for the patient with a cervical spine/whiplash injury to develop secondary shoulder problems due to guarding and decrease in general use of the extremities. By starting the patient on an early stretching and active exercise program for the shoulder joints and upper back area, for example, these areas can often be exercised effectively early on. This may be started during a phase when cervical motion and stretching are tolerated to a much lesser degree.

Ergonomic considerations at this point typically revolve around trying to find some comfortable methods of posture and associated mechanical support to allow the patient to function when necessary. In the more severe injuries, patients typically are going to need a period of rest away from work activities to promote early healing and allow some recovery.

Progress at this point is measured primarily by symptomatic relief. It is essentially too soon at this stage to do much in the way of functional assessment, as typically the patient's level of pain tolerance will not allow such testing to be performed reliably. However, the chiropractic physician who is working with the patient should keep in mind that such a phase should be expected to move along fairly rapidly, that is, over a period of 2 to 4 weeks, at the most, before concern sets in about either the possibility of a more serious and unsuspected injury or the relative reliability of the patient's reporting of symptoms. This is not to suggest that all patients recover during this time. Unfortunately, there is a significant percentage of patients who do not have, even at long-term follow up, full recovery from whiplash types of injuries. It would be expected, however, that during this phase the average patient would be making progress; when such recovery is not occurring, careful assessment is indicated.

SUBACUTE PHASE

The subacute phase, by definition, is the period when patients are becoming less reliant on passive measures and can begin to participate more fully in their own active recovery. During this phase typically the patient continues to need the support of associated manual treatment, including mobilization as well as modalities. The mobilization techniques and modalities usually can be approached more aggressively during this phase, as range of motion begins to improve and soft tissue spasm and edema begin to decrease. This is the point where more active rehabilitation measures become particularly appropriate. This is also the phase when, oftentimes, the failure to move forward aggressively leads to a significant loss of potential for as full a recovery as possible.

Stretching exercises during this phase tend to become more aggressive. Both active and active-assist stretching can be begun; when necessary, passive stretching can also be undertaken. The patient at this phase is encouraged not only to work through the pain-free range of motion that is available, but to begin to work through mild stiffness and discomfort in order to improve flexibility and motion. The patient often needs careful supervision with such approaches, as some patients will tend to underdo and others will tend to move too aggressively and simply set themselves back in the recovery phase.

There is obviously some trial and error involved, but working to the point where there is some discomfort and gradually working gently against this type of restriction is the most reliable approach. Stretching should be continued again, not only in areas that are painful and where motion has been lost, but also in secondary associated areas, as discussed previously. All too often, a patient with a soft tissue/whiplash cervical injury presents at 3 to 4 months with a "frozen shoulder" due to lack of attention to such problems. Normal scapular mobility also needs to be maintained to allow full and symmetric rhythm of the scapular and glenohumeral joints.

Exercise at this point typically can begin to move past the gentle isometric phase. At this point, isotonic programs also can be initiated. Patients are taught to find their "neutral position." I define this as the position of greatest spinal comfort. They are then encouraged to exercise actively in this fashion to allow earlier and more aggressive intervention. They can then be encouraged to transfer this skill to gain improved tolerance for functional daily activities. Patients typically start with isometric exercises and move to a program of more active strengthening, using a variety of methods. These include Theraband, pulleys, and light, free weights. The STP neck exerciser is an inexpensive method to exercise the neck (Figure 8–1).

Some patients tend to focus on the amount of weight they are using early on, and this can be to their detriment. It is important to emphasize to the patient that proper technique and spinal positioning and alignment are paramount at this phase. All exercises should be carried out with good postural mechanisms. The chiropractor working with the patient should be carrying out the early phase of such a program in the office and under supervision to ensure that the techniques are properly applied. Failure to do so will often lead to injury from the exercises, again causing setbacks in the recovery process.

The patient should be encouraged to use weights and resistive methods that allow progression to the maximum amount that does not lead to a breakdown in proper technique. The patient should be discouraged from using substitute muscle groups that do not, in fact, exercise the area intended, but simply allow a false sense of improvement through improper muscle group substitution. At this phase, the patient typically is working with relatively light weights and increasing the number of repetitions to promote range of motion with exercise and muscle endurance. Once the patient can go through each particular exercise with 8 to 12 repetitions and a total of three

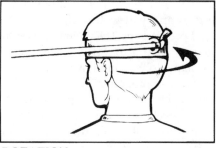

ROTATION

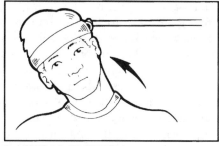

LATERAL FLEXION

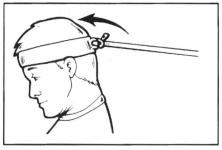

FORWARD FLEXION

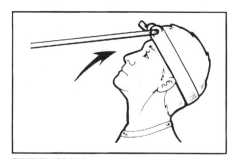

EXTENSION

Figure 8–1 STP neck exerciser, a simple, inexpensive, effective means to strengthen the neck in all planes of motion. *Source:* Reprinted from *For Your Neck Self Help Manual*, 1992 ed., by H.D. Saunders, with permission of Saunders Therapy Products, Bloomington, Minnesota.

sets, it is time to move forward in the amount of weight or resistance used.

At this stage, a variety of muscle groups need to be involved. These groups include the upper thoracic stabilizing musculature, including rhomboids, latissimus groups, trapezius, serratus group, and shoulder stabilizers including the rotator cuff muscles. General strengthening of the upper extremities, including both arm and forearm musculature, is also of benefit. See Figure 8–2 for some exercise examples using flexible bands and exercise balls. In female patients who have scapular winging and rhomboid atrophy, rowing machine and overhead bar pull-down exercises will be of great benefit in stabilizing persistent headaches and cervicothoracic pain. The patient at this point is also encouraged to

begin generalized cardiovascular reconditioning. This can include a walking program, exercise bicycle, or other forms of aerobic exercise. Careful cardiopulmonary assessment in this regard, of course, also must be undertaken.

Patients who are interested in swimming programs often will do poorly at this stage because of the rotational component involved with breathing during swimming exercises. Patients who enjoy this approach a great deal, however, may consider swimming with a snorkel and mask. Exercises that involve a fair amount of spinal compressive forces, such as running, tend to be poorly tolerated at this stage.

Postural mechanisms at this stage tend to focus on more long-term supportive approaches. For the patient who is not making as quick a recovery as possible or is having continued postural problems, use of some readily available market products such as cervical pillows and lumbar supports for driving may be of benefit. These are available through a wide variety of catalogs and supply stores in most areas. When the patient does make a decision to purchase such a supportive device, direct feedback from the treating chiropractor about proper choices in that regard can be helpful in keeping the patient from buying products that are useless and wasteful for a particular condition.

During this stage, monitoring of the patient's recovery on an objective basis becomes of value. This is important not only for the patient and the treating physician, as outlined above, but also for documenting to the insurance company the nature of the patient's functional progression. The patient can be encouraged to keep a log of daily activities. Some patients do extremely well with charting their exercise programs and gauging their progress in that manner. Simple computer programs, as well as very expensive mechanical devices, are available on the market to allow more sophisticated methods of functional assessment. It has been our experience that reasonable monitoring of a patient's progress often can be accomplished with relatively inexpensive approaches, including flowcharts, flowsheets, and simple mechanical devices.

Physicians who are not in a situation to spend tens of thousands of dollars on sophisti-

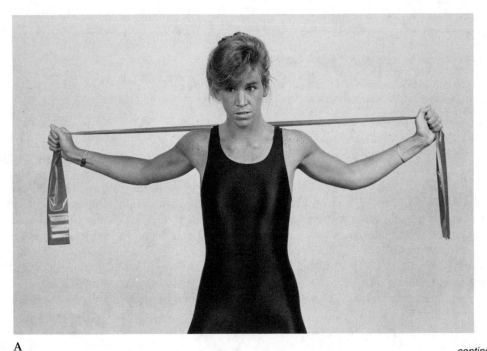

A   *continues*

Figure 8–2 Cervicothoracic muscle stabilization techniques. A: patient working with a Theraband; B: patient doing supine reciprocal arm raises while on a Swiss gym ball; and C: patient doing prone flyes while on a Swiss gym ball. *Source:* A: Courtesy of Spine Care Center, Daly City, California; B and C: Reprinted from Sweeney, T., Prentice, C., Saal, J.A., et al., Cervicothoracic Muscular Stabilization Techniques, *Physical Medicine & Rehabilitation: State of the Art Reviews: Neck & Back Pain*, Vol. 4, No. 2, p. 357, with permission of Hanley & Belfus, © 1990.

Figure 8–2 continued

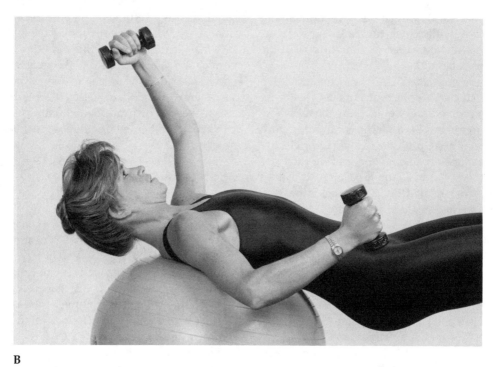

B

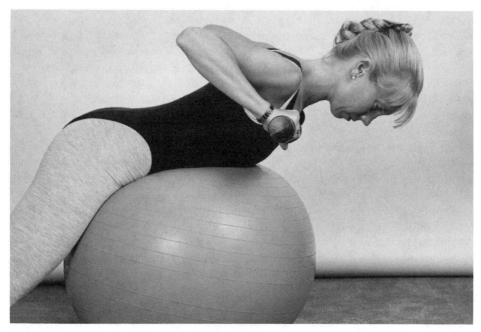

C

cated mechanical testing devices should not be discouraged from being as creative as possible in developing functional assessment methods with which they are comfortable. There is a wide variety of literature available on this subject.

Ergonomic considerations at this point become much more practical. For the patient who has recovered fairly quickly to a level where ergonomic issues are fairly straightforward, little may need to be done. There is a significant percentage of patients who, during the early recovery process, continue to have difficulties with work-related demands, including postural demands in the office related to the sitting position or heavy physical demands that patients are expected to meet. For example, an office worker who spends a good deal of time answering the phone at the same time he or she is working with a computer screen raised above eye-level height might have difficulty attempting to jot down notes on a desk that is set too low for comfortable use.

Patients involved in more physically demanding activities at the workplace, such as lifting and placing objects on shelves, loading and unloading heavy materials, or frequent twisting and turning of the neck and upper back, also are going to require modification at this stage. Careful assessment of what kinds of modified activities might be available for the patient should be discussed. In many cases, discussion with the patient's employer and education about the nature of the patient's difficulties may lead to a more successful resolution of such dilemmas.

Many industries do not allow a patient to return to work unless he or she is at full recovery. It is well accepted, however, that the longer a patient is out of work, the greater the chances that he or she will never return to gainful employment. There must be a give-and-take attitude by all involved at this phase to allow the long-term recovery process to move forward as aggressively as possible. It is during this phase, particularly during the first 1 or 2 months postinjury, that many of the long-term secondary psychosocial sequelae begin to develop. Simple interventions at this stage, such as careful work on posture, limitation of work hours, reduction of the 10% to 20% most demanding activities, or other ergonomic interventions, could make a big difference. The patient who has the opportunity to work with a slant board, raised work surface, or speaker set or headphone oftentimes can get back to higher-level activities much more quickly.

CHRONIC PHASE

At this phase, more aggressive strengthening typically can be initiated. This usually occurs at approximately 4 to 6 weeks postinjury. Treatment frequency for modalities and hands-on therapy can usually be tapered to a much lower frequency at this stage. Aerobic conditioning should be continued, and oftentimes a wider variety of activities can be undertaken in this regard. This is particularly important to prevent generalized deconditioning in the individual who would be returning to work or sports activities that require higher levels of general physical conditioning. Such activities promote confidence, reduce general stress, and encourage independence. All too often, over-restriction leads to a long-term process of deconditioning and higher risk of reinjury.

Stretching at this point usually can be carried out independently by the patient. Typically, the patient is encouraged to stretch early in the morning upon arising, before the exercise program is initiated, and again before bed. Some patients who have difficulty getting comfortable during the night and have stiffness the following morning often can be helped by stretching the affected areas for 5 to 10 minutes just before retiring to bed.

Strengthening at this phase should be moving in the direction of formal cervicothoracic stabilization training. Cervicothoracic stabilization approaches are directed toward both strengthening and conditioning affected areas, as well as developing a proper base of support for the cervical and upper thoracic spine. This process includes more aggressive exercise involving the areas described previously. At this stage, the patient can begin to use higher levels of weight with both endurance and aggressive strengthening types of approaches. A pyramid approach, using one weight for 8 to 12 repetitions and gradually adding on to a higher weight through the third set, can be of particular value in promoting full recovery of strength. Again, when the patient has reached a point when he or she can accomplish 8 to 12 repetitions of a particular exercise, more weight can be added.

Some patients, by their nature, are not going to participate as actively as preferred in aggressive strengthening and conditioning programs. However, there is a general level of strengthening and conditioning at which the patient absolutely needs to participate in order to allow a reasonable level of recovery. Patients need to be followed and encouraged to participate at least to that degree in order to enhance long-term functional tolerance. Many of the exercises can be accomplished at home. This can again be done with Theraband and light weights, depending on the patient's tolerance.

At this stage, more formal gym types of programs, particularly for the patient who requires a greater level of reconditioning and strengthening, can be considered. If the patient does become involved in a gym program, a site visit of 1 to 2 hours to review the proper use of the equipment and the sequence of exercise is essential. All too often, patients begin to work out on exercise equipment that is inappropriate for their particular problems. The types of exercises done for general fitness and conditioning in a gym or health club are not necessarily of benefit to all patients recovering from a whiplash injury. Patients need to be educated in that regard and not allow themselves to fall into the trap of trying to compete with those around them.

These types of programs, however, can be of great benefit, particularly for the patient who requires higher levels of strengthening and conditioning for vocational activities. More formal types of programs, such as work-hardening programs, have also been more readily available and acceptable in recent years. Much of this conditioning, however, can be accomplished with good supervision by the treating chiropractor, assuming that he or she has taken the time to become fully acquainted with the techniques.

There are some patients who simply need to be referred to a health professional who specializes in this particular area. If earlier programs were done properly, however, the percentage of these patients tends to be relatively small. Patients most likely to benefit from this kind of approach are those who have developed weakness from neurologic involvement, surgical interventions, or generalized atrophy of deconditioning who require more intensive supervision. Such a program typically should last approximately 4 to 6 weeks, at which time the patient essentially should be independent. More intensive programs also can be undertaken, but a period of simple recovery and healing should be allowed between exercises so that areas targeted by specific exercises can achieve their full benefit. Careful functional monitoring and assessment of recovery at such centers are paramount to ensure that the money being spent is being used wisely.

There is a percentage of patients at this stage who simply fail to follow through or participate in the active program. These patients should be identified and documented so that it is understood that recovery is reaching a plateau. Unfortunately, some patients, particularly at this stage, begin to attempt to manipulate their medical care; failure to identify such patients can damage the long-term credibility of the treating physician.

Cervicothoracic stabilization training at this point usually can be expected to follow a fairly logical sequence.

Ergonomic issues at this stage typically revolve around assessment of long-term restrictions and modifications that might be necessary to allow the patient to carry out functional tasks that may be difficult into the foreseeable future. Issues such as long-term job modification and restriction from inappropriate physical demands need to be reviewed with the patient and others involved in the patient's vocational situation.

Provision of ergonomic chairs, adaptation of patient workstations, transfer to less physically demanding assignments, or potentially even vocational rehabilitation may be discussed. These issues need to be thoroughly assessed and reviewed with all those involved in as comprehensive a manner as possible. Participation by all concerned parties often will lead to solutions that otherwise might not have been considered because of a lack of understanding of the nature of the patient's functional capabilities.

GENERAL PERPETUATING FACTORS

It has been documented in a variety of studies that general health and habit factors may perpetuate the presence of myofascial/soft tissue patterns of pain. These include nutritional, metabolic, drug, endocrine, and psychologic influences. Following are some of the contributors:

- regular use of alcohol leading to reduced folic acid levels[1]
- more than two cups of coffee per day[1]
- sustained postural demands[2]
- fatigue and poor sleep
- poor body mechanics
- hypothyroidism[3,4]
- hypoglycemia[3]
- psychologic factors, including stress, anxiety, and depression
- nutritional deficiencies, including deficiencies of vitamins B_1, B_6, and B_{12}; folate; vitamin C; potassium; iron; and calcium[1,3,4]

These factors, when identified in the initial patient interview, should be discussed with the patient and general advice offered. Obviously, long-term habits are not easily changed, but such factors should be addressed whenever possible.

GENERAL POSTURAL ADVICE

An area of primary concern in the post-whiplash patient as outlined above is that of prolonged postural stress during the recovery process. The relationship between postural demands and patterns of recovery can be difficult to quantify. There is little doubt, however, that such demands will only serve to impede the general nature of the recovery process for such patients. There is, therefore, a significant advantage to outline for the patient specific areas of postural advice to help facilitate recovery, particularly during the early phase, when there is still so much to be gained and so much to be lost by not acting appropriately and aggressively from the very start.

- Posture should be changed on a regular basis, on average every 30 to 60 minutes.
- Most patients tend toward a head-held-forward type posture, and this should be particularly discouraged.
- The seated posture is generally correct if right angles are found in the ankles, knees, and hip joints.
- Maintenance of a mild lumbar lordosis is generally most effective, but may require significant individual variation. Postures with the neck tilted or held sideways for prolonged periods, such as with the use of the telephone, should be avoided.
- A slanted work surface of approximately 10° to 30° can be of particular value for table-top work.
- Chairs with armrests with adequate arm support can be of help in reducing shoulder and neck muscular tension.
- When necessary, an adjustable backrest in a chair or individual lumbar support

should be considered. Pillows are also of potential benefit.

- Computer monitors should be set at eye level to eliminate unnecessary postural demands.
- Bifocal glasses can cause the patient to tilt the head into positions that increase muscle/joint tension.
- When standing for prolonged periods of time, putting one foot up on a low platform or step can reduce lumbar demands.
- Carrying heavy bags or purses over one shoulder also can be structurally demanding.
- Soft couches and chairs generally should be avoided at home. Proper support during home activities can be every bit as valuable as in the workplace.

HOME MANAGEMENT: FOCUS ON ACTIVE ROLE OF PATIENT

Older injury-management models emphasized a passive role of the patient after a car accident. Many physicians were encouraged to play a very active role during the entire healing process, leaving the patient very dependent on the doctor. With changes in the health care management system, the physician is now encouraged to utilize available family resources. If the physician sees the patient over several weeks, he or she should ask the patient whether the patient has a family member or friend who can help with exercises, stretching, or muscle massage. As the symptomatic patient's condition becomes more chronic, having someone to encourage good postural habits, progressively increase stretching/exercise routines, and follow other recommendations the physician has made can result in many cases in less dependence on the doctor and have the net effect of helping relieve pain and reduce costs associated with these cases.

CONCLUSION

The rehabilitation approach to whiplash types of injuries, in my opinion, must incorporate not only promotion of proper spinal alignment and normal spinal mobility, but also—perhaps more important—provision of an aggressive program of active rehabilitation. This type of approach is absolutely essential to prevent long-term, recurrent problems and relapse of symptoms in the future.

The cornerstone of such a program is progression of the patient from the acute, modality-oriented phase into the active strengthening and reconditioning phase. Modalities are an important part of the initial treatment process. As time passes, however, the patient can be moved to a more active and independent type of program. Patient education about posture, body mechanics, ergonomics, and lifestyle adaptations is essential in this regard. General health maintenance should also be part of the process.

Exercise programs, in general, must progress from lower-level to upper-level activities. Typically, they are done at first with low levels of resistance, such as with Theraband, and with close supervision. They can then progress into workouts with exercise machines, free weights, pulleys, and finally into work- and sports-specific activities. Much of any program can be accomplished by the chiropractor who has made an effort to become familiar with some of the more recent techniques in exercise training and reconditioning. Much of this process can be accomplished fairly inexpensively, both in the office and by the patient at home.

Requiring active participation by the patient in self-rehabilitation not only promotes good health but ensures all involved that the patient's primary goal is enhancement of his or her own recovery. This requirement allows more thorough evaluation of the patient who truly is not putting forth the kind of effort that would be expected.

Exercise programs for whiplash patients in general cannot be carried out in a generic fashion and must be tailored not only to the particular injury that is being treated, but also to the age, general health, and underlying physical capability of the individual patient.

REFERENCES

1. Travell JG, Simons DG. *Myofascial Pain and Dysfunction: The Trigger Point Manual.* Baltimore: Williams & Wilkins; 1983.
2. Bennett M. Current issues concerning management of the fibrositis/fibromyalgia syndrome. *Am J Med.* 1986;81(suppl 3A):15–18.
3. DeMar E. Treatment of myofascial pain and dysfunction. In: Gerhardt JJ, et al., eds. *Interdisciplinary Rehabilitation in Trauma.* Baltimore: Williams & Wilkins; 1987.
4. Simons DG, Travell JG. Myofascial origins of low back pain, part 1: principles of diagnosis and treatment. *Postgrad Med.* 1983; 73:66–77.

SUGGESTED READINGS

Akeson W, Wo S, Amiel D, et al. Connective tissue response to immobility. *Clin Orthop.* 1973;93:356–362.

Cailliet R. *Neck and Arm Pain.* 3rd ed. Philadelphia: FA Davis Co; 1991.

Chamberlain GJ. Cyriax's friction massage: a review. *J Orthop Sports Phys Ther.* 1982;4(1):16–22.

Dale WA. Thoracic outlet compression syndrome. *Arch Surg.* 1982;117:1437–1441.

DeWall M, Van Riel MPJM, Snijders CJ. The effect on sitting posture of a desk with a 10° inclination for reading and writing. *Ergonomics.* 1991;34(5):575–584.

Echternach JL. *Pain.* New York: Churchill Livingstone; 1987.

Hirsch SA, Hirsch PJ, Hiramoto H, et al. Whiplash syndrome: fact or fiction? *Orthop Clin North Am.* 1988;19(4):791–795.

Huffman JD. Electrodiagnostic techniques for and conservative treatment of thoracic outlet syndrome. *Clin Orthop.* 1986;207:21–23.

Jaeger B, Reeves JL. Quantification of changes in myofascial trigger point sensitivity with the pressure algometer following passive stretch. *Pain.* 1986;27:203–210.

Jerrett SA, Cuzzone LJ, Pasternak BM. Thoracic outlet syndrome: electrophysiologic reappraisal. *Arch Neurol.* 1984;41:960–963.

Keane G, Saal J. Sports medicine approach to occupational low back pain. *West J Med.* 1991;154:525–527.

Kenna CJ. The whiplash syndrome: a general practitioner's viewpoint. *Aust Fam Physician.* 1984;13(4):256–258.

Leffert RD. Thoracic outlet syndrome and the shoulder. *Clin Sports Med.* 1983;2(2):439–452.

Linton SJ, Kamwendo K. Risk factors in the psychosocial work environment for neck and shoulder pain in secretaries. *J Occup Med.* 1989;31(7):609–613.

Lowman CL. The sitting position in relation to pelvic stress. *Physiother Rev.* 1941;1:30–33.

McCain GA. Role of physical fitness training in the fibrositis/fibromyalgia syndrome. *Am J Med.* 1986;81(suppl 3A):73–77.

McNab I. The whiplash syndrome. *Orthop Clin North Am.* 1971;2:389–403.

Roos DB. The thoracic outlet syndrome is underrated. *Arch Neurol.* 1990;47:327–328.

Rosomoff HL, Fishbain DA, Goldberb M, et al. Physical findings in patients with chronic intractable benign pain of the neck and/or back. *Pain.* 1989;37:279–287.

Russell IJ, Vipraio GA, Morgan WW, et al. Is there a metabolic basis for the fibrositis syndrome? *Am J Med.* 1986;81(suppl 3A):50–54.

Saal J. Rehabilitation of sports injuries. In: Saal J, ed. *Physical Medicine and Rehabilitation: State of the Art Reviews.* Philadelphia: Hanley and Belfus; 1987:524–525.

Saal J, Saal J. The non-operative treatment of herniated nucleus pulposus with radiculopathy: an outcome study. *Spine.* 1989;14:431–437.

Schüldt K. On neck muscle activity and load reduction in sitting postures. *Scand J Rehabil Med Suppl.* 1988;19.

Seltzer S. Foods, and food and drug combinations, responsible for head and neck pain. *Cephalalgia.* 1982;2:111–124.

Simons DG. Fibrositis/fibromyalgia: a form of myofascial trigger points? *Am J Med.* 1986;81(suppl 3A):93–98.

Smith KF. The thoracic outlet syndrome: a protocol of treatment. *J Orthop Sports Phys Ther.* 1979;1:89–99.

Sweeney T, Prentice C, Saal JA, et al. Cervicothoracic muscular stabilization techniques. In: Saal J, ed. *Physical Medicine and Rehabilitation: State of the Art Reviews.* Philadelphia: Hanley and Belfus; 1990:335–359.

Zohn DA. *Musculoskeletal Pain: Diagnosis and Physical Treatment.* 2nd ed. Boston: Little, Brown & Co; 1988.

Chapter 9

When All Else Fails

Arthur H. White

INTRODUCTION

As in all fields of medicine and most areas of life, when efforts are not bringing forth success, one should examine the premise on which they are based. Therefore, if a patient treated for whiplash syndrome, disc bulge, radiculopathy, and so on does not improve and return to normal function in a reasonable period of time, the doctor should refer this patient to another physician and determine whether the diagnosis was accurate, whether there are other problems present, or whether equipment limitations are restricting proper rehabilitation. Perhaps the patient should be referred to a specialty spine center or a multidisciplinary evaluation program.

Even if the diagnosis is not wrong, there might be some factor present that prevents the condition from stabilizing, or there might be variable factors that require different forms of treatment. By using only one treatment the doctor may be treating one aspect of the condition and may even be aggravating other aspects of the condition. For example, if there is soft tissue injury that would ordinarily respond quite well to manual therapy, but there

is in addition a herniated disc or spinal stenosis, then the manual therapy may be aggravating the underlying disc or stenosis. On the other hand, immobilizing the disc or stenosis may improve symptoms from that source but may create stiffness and symptoms in the area of the soft tissue injury. Most commonly the patient will be put on a temporary trial of no adjustment and later immobilization.

The trick, therefore, is to recognize when adequate progress is not being made. Ongoing unsuccessful treatment may be adding to the burden of the disease process by emotional factors, socioeconomic factors, or physical organic factors. Figure 9–1 illustrates the steps that should be taken when treatment appears to be ineffective.

PROCESS OF MULTIDISCIPLINARY EVALUATION

Multidisciplinary evaluation does not need to be done under one roof, although it is more efficient to do it that way and saves wear and tear on the doctors, the patient, and third-party payers. It is important that there be coor-

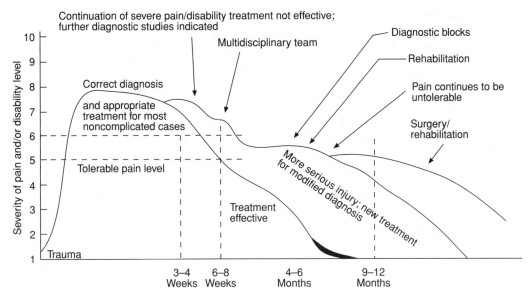

Figure 9–1 Steps that need to be taken to manage a case when severe pain or disability fails to respond to treatment.

dination, open discussion, and communication between the patient and all team members. It is helpful to have all of these individuals in one room at some time during the process if for no other reason than to impress the patient that everything possible is being done for him or her. Collective diagnostic groups of this sort usually work well. There seems to be a positive feedback process in which each member's understanding of the problem and presentation stimulates other members of the panel to new ideas and better solutions.

There can be a tendency, however, to cut corners to save time or for economic reasons and not "start fresh." It is a mistake to have the previous primary doctor prejudice the group with his or her prior unsuccessful experience with the patient. That valuable input can come later, after other members have had an opportunity to develop their independent opinions.

For the sake of time and efficiency it is wise to have an independent data collector who ensures that all previous significant medical information is available and summarized. Each

subspecialist can review such a summary and then go into the extensive details of his or her special field. Standardized patient history forms can help this process.

MULTIDISCIPLINARY EVALUATION

The members of a multidisciplinary team do not always need to be the same, but there is some rationale for the selection of certain specialties. The primary doctor for most whiplash cases will usually be a chiropractor or a generalist. More specialized diagnostic expertise might be provided by an orthopedic surgeon or a neurosurgeon. Because of the chronic nature of these whiplash cases that fail to improve, a psychologist, a psychiatrist, or a specialist in pain disorders is needed. A radiologist is also desirable to better define underlying pathoanatomy through X-rays, scans, discograms, and blocks. From a therapeutic standpoint, the case will probably require specialists such as anesthesiologists, physiatrists, medical pain specialists, and a variety of therapists and trainers.

Other subspecialists who may be called include urologists; neurologists; rheumatologists; endocrinologists; and practitioners of acupuncture, biofeedback, hypnosis, Rolfing, and Feldenkrasis, to name a few fields. Although some of these treatment modalities may have been attempted previously, their use in a multidisciplinary setting as an adjunct (but not as the primary thrust) might be helpful.

It cannot be emphasized enough that these difficult cases have a multiplicity of disability generators, which are likely to require several different therapeutic modalities. Even if surgery is required, it is only one step in the rehabilitation process. Exercise, education, manual therapy, and posture and movement therapy may all be necessary to maintain long-range success.

MULTIDISCIPLINARY EXAMINATION

Subspecialists all have their own favorite examination methods that are determined by their training. Most doctors can do a reasonable neurologic examination and even a reasonable manual examination, but years of experience with manual evaluation or neurologic evaluation bring with it nuances that the generalist cannot begin to appreciate. Similarly, the internist's evaluation of the heart, lungs, liver, eye grounds, and abdominal and pelvic organs requires considerable expertise that is mandatory in some of these complex whiplash cases, which may be associated with neoplasm or metabolic or other systemic disease. For the sake of time, efficiency, and economy the team of specialists will usually do a general examination in concert, saving the detailed subspecialty examination for individual evaluation.

WORKING DIAGNOSIS

We have already established that the previous working diagnosis was either incorrect or correct but incomplete. Some other factor (such as an endocrine disorder) or a multiplicity of factors might have mitigated successful treatment. We therefore arrive at a new working diagnosis that has been made possible by new knowledge. This new working diagnosis may be agreed upon as early as the first general evaluation by the team. It allows us to select further tests and begin treatment to help confirm the working diagnosis. That is, if treatment based on the new working diagnosis brings improvement, that diagnosis is somewhat validated.

DIAGNOSTIC TESTS

Entire books have been written on the subject of scanning diagnoses for spinal problems. Suffice it to say that current imaging techniques for the cervical spine can visualize almost any pathology from syringomyelia to spinal stenosis. The magnetic resonance imaging (MRI) scan is more accurate for soft tissue lesions, and the computed tomography (CT) scan with multiplanar reformatting is better for diagnosing bony lesions. At some imaging centers, one can obtain a combination CT and MRI at no greater expense than that for one test alone. When a working diagnosis is of a very specific nature, an MRI or a CT scan can be selected that has the greatest probability of identifying the suspected pathology. When the working diagnosis is unclear, and we are doing somewhat of an exploratory imaging, the combined study is most appropriate.

ELECTRODIAGNOSTIC TESTS

Electromyograms and somatosensory evoked potentials can be very helpful in confirming diagnoses of neurologic involvement, be it individual spinal nerves or the spinal cord itself. Diagnostic blocks can be helpful, too. There are subspecialists in radiology and anesthesia at this time who spend their entire medical careers placing needles in pathologic areas of the spine for the purpose of provoking and relieving pain for diagnostic as well as therapeutic reasons.

FINAL DIAGNOSIS

All examinations and diagnostic testing can be accomplished in as short a time as a few hours, and at most 2 or 3 days in efficient settings. When all the information is in, the final diagnosis and the ultimate treatment plan seem to simply fall into place. The diagnosis is self-apparent when the quest to find the pain generators is accomplished. If the pain generator is "this disc" or "that nerve," then we need only ask the question, What is happening to the disc or nerve? The images generally show us the herniated disc, bone spur, or other pain-evoking pathoanatomy.

We have, in addition, through our psychosocial evaluation, determined the proportion of emotional input into this pain-disability equation. If there are minimal psychologic factors, then we will not usually include any psychologic treatment measures in the treatment plan. If, however, there is moderately severe or severe psychologic involvement, then the treatment plan will definitely include some psychologic reorientation and possibly even medical-psychologic treatment.

From a strictly organic physical standpoint, the treatment plan follows the pathoanatomy. We need to know how severe the pathology is. If there is severe nerve damage, severe stenosis, or instability, our conservative measures are much less likely to be successful. If there is only minor pathology, we can expect conservative care to be more successful. In some cases the patient has already undergone extensive conservative care, and now, in the face of severe pathology, it may be clear to all evaluators that surgery is the only hope for any improvement.

The team should help the patient develop realistic expectations from any proposed treatment. Statistics allows us to state very clearly to the patient the level of success that can be expected on average with a specific pathologic entity and a combination of other psychosocial and rehabilitation factors.

SURGERY

Surgery is only one step in the rehabilitation process. After all conservative measures have been exhausted and all diagnostic tests unequivocally point to surgery, the surgical consultation is obtained. The surgeon should discuss frankly with the patient the physical and test results that have led him or her to believe that surgery is a reasonable alternative. This author suggests giving the patient a grade or score on each of the items important in surgical decision making: history, physical examination, electrodiagnostic testing, imaging (CT and MRI), diagnostic blocks, discograms, psychologic evaluation, and response to training and physical therapy. If the grades or ratings in these areas are all good to excellent, the surgical outcome statistically is in the 80% to 90% range. If most of these items are below average, the surgery does not have a very good likelihood of success.

The surgeon should also discuss the types of surgery that are available for the underlying pathoanatomic condition. We are mostly talking about disc herniation and spinal stenosis. These conditions are generally approached anteriorly through a discectomy, and a fusion is frequently involved. Rarely is discectomy of more than one or two levels required in whiplash cases. Some of the more severe long-range stenotic problems can become very complex, but that is not a subject for this book.

Surgery is rarely the total answer to whiplash and degenerative cervical spinal problems. The surgery is only one step in the rehabilitation process. The patient will be expected, postoperatively, to continue to participate in self-care, training, self-mobilization, and ergonomic changes. After the offending pain generator is dealt with surgically, the patient should be able to respond better to training, manual therapy, and other physical modalities.

In the immediate postoperative period a patient usually has some form of external immobilization in the form of a collar or brace for several months. After removing such external immobilization there is a degree of disuse, atrophy, and transfer of forces that need to be dealt with. This will require several weeks, if not months, of ongoing rehabilitation. The effects of surgery should reach their maximum benefit by approximately 6 months. Once a patient has reached a plateau in improvement in physical functioning, he or she should be encouraged to adjust to the lifestyle that is reasonable for resultant good rehabilitation. Most

patients can return to normal lifestyles with some prophylactic restrictions for activities that place a heavier burden on the cervical spine.

CONCLUSION

Whiplash does not need to result in long-term disability. When early, reasonable, conservative measures have not returned an individual to normal function, he or she should have a thorough multidisciplinary evaluation in order to establish an unquestionably accurate diagnosis and a very aggressive stabilization training to try to avoid surgery. In the rare case that surgery is necessary, it can have a high level of success when coupled with good rehabilitation.

Chapter 10

Disability after Car Crashes

Lawrence S. Nordhoff, Jr.

INTRODUCTION

This chapter begins by addressing temporary and permanent disability associated with mild to moderate injuries resulting from motor vehicle collision injury (MVCI). This chapter then moves into discussions about human and crash factors influencing disability and the types of functional disorders that result in loss of functional capacity. At the end of the chapter there is a discussion about the independent medical examination process.

The National Safety Council reports that about one of every four permanent impairments due to injuries in the United States occurred in moving motor vehicle crashes.[1] It is estimated that in the United States there are about 1.6 to 2 million disabling injuries, 148 to 157 million restricted-activity days, and 49 to 50 million bed days resulting from MVCIs annually.[1,2] A restricted-activity day is defined as a day during which the person stays in bed for more than half a day, misses work or school for a day, or is unable to perform his or her normal daily activities for a day. The National Safety Council reports that in 1993 the average economic cost in the United States for a nonfatal disabling injury was $32,800.[1]

Discussions about temporary disability guidelines are covered early in this chapter. Many physicians, at some time, deal with the temporary or permanent disability issue. Frequently, the doctor may have to make a statement for the patient, employer, and/or insurance carrier regarding full and partial temporary disability or permanent disability. It may be difficult for some doctors to perform disability evaluations because of limitations of training. A complete evaluation assesses the anatomic, physiologic, functional, biomechanical, psychologic, and rehabilitation issues. Looking at chronic pain solely as a disease is not adequate,[3] since the opinion of the patient is considered less valid than examinations, X-rays, and other tests.

The doctor will have to qualify the amount of disability and make predictions about future disability. For neck and head injuries, less defined rules have been assigned than for injuries in other areas. In some instances, these injuries have been underestimated in terms of significance regarding the amount of disability assigned and subsequent monies awarded. For example, many claims adjusters feel that it is easy to understand why a person with a herniated L-5 disc is unable to return to work. In the eyes of the same carrier, however, a patient with a bulging cervical disc, who has a job using a computer and is unable to perform it because of weakness, pain, or sensory loss, may be considered only partially disabled.

Permanent disability may be difficult to assess because the doctor must consider the person's age, sex, economic status, educational background, and social environment.[4] The professional doing a disability rating evaluation must estimate the injured person's ability to engage in gainful work activity,[5] or determine his or her ability to adjust to an impairment, return to preinjury status at work, and participate fully in society.[6] Disability rating involves several complex issues, such as medical, legal, functional, and societal influences.

DEFINITIONS

The terms *impairment*, *disability*, and *handicap* are sometimes used interchangeably in our society; however, these words do have different meanings.

Impairment

States and Viano describe impairment as the loss of function after an injury heals.[6] Injuries may cause loss of function of a single part or multiple parts of the body, resulting in an impairment.[6] An impairment is a lessening in value or strength. An impairment is independent of the person's age, gender, occupation, or socioeconomic status.[7] An impairment can be observed and measured uniformly and accurately by different examiners. These measurements allow the professional to describe and define the extent of loss of structural integrity and functional capacity, or to use the data in substantiating chronic pain through objective findings.[5] For example, having loss of joint range of motion is an impairment that may cause pain and that then can become a disability.[8] Functional loss includes five major attributes: (1) physical activity, (2) mobility, (3)

work performance, (4) role in family and community, and (5) emotional status. Impairment ratings can be impractical in the personal injury arena.

Disadvantages of Using Impairment Systems

Impairment ratings are not practical in MVCI. One author feels that impairment systems cannot measure dynamic function or adequately describe the functional potential of an individual.[9] Impairment systems assume that there is a typical person. We know in the automotive literature that there is no typical human being or typical crash. We know, for example, that if a general asymptomatic population impairment study was performed, such as measurable loss of neck motion, significant numbers would be found.

Disability (Functional Capacity Loss)

Measurement of disability or functional capacity losses caused by a car crash is a much more practical system to use, as it relates to ability of the individual to adapt to an impairment. Disability is defined here as a reduction in one's ability to participate actively in society in a manner appropriate to the person's age, sex, socioeconomic status, and relationship status prior to the injury.[7] It also has been described as the inability of the patient to perform tasks because of an impairment.[5] Disability limits the individual when competing in the social, personal, or open-labor market. When rating permanent consequences of injury impairments, the professional should include mobility, dexterity, cognition, cosmetic, sensory, pain, and sexual findings.[6] Disability may involve a single impairment or several components, and can be defined as loss of functional ability,[10] the end result of single or multiple impairments of a whole person,[6] or as subjective findings.[8] For example, pain may cause a disability[8] but not an impairment. The role of pain must be considered in order to determine disability.[3]

The physician has a more realistic ability to determine what the victim can do by considering vast elements such as work demands, type of injury, type of pathology, social support systems, educational level, and economic status. Mooney believes that other components should be evaluated, including performance coordination, strength, speed, and endurance.[9]

Handicap

A handicap is one's difficulty in functioning in a social environment, and relates to the internal makeup of the person.[10] It is society's view of the functional loss (hindrance or disadvantage) resulting from an impairment.[7] States and Viano describe a handicap as what the general public recognizes as one in a person, including abnormal appearance, function, and behavior.[6] A handicap exists when a person cannot perform and maintain his or her role in an environment, whether at work, recreationally, or at home, without the presence of some pain, loss of function, or other symptoms.

TEMPORARY WORK DISABILITY

MVCIs frequently cause temporary and permanent disability (time off work) and are in a distinct classification when compared with other injury types, such as sports- and work-related injuries. In a comparative hospital study of neck injuries from traffic accidents versus neck injury from other types of accidents, it was found that the median number of days of sick leave for an auto accident was 31 days and for other accidents was 17 days. Auto accident victims with neck injuries had considerably more sick leave than did victims with neck injuries from other causes.[11]

Several studies have estimated the percentage of crash occupants taking time off work

and the number of days typically lost from work as the result of MVCI. Recent nationwide insurance and consumer studies conclude that 40% to 50% of auto injury claimants will lose some time from work.[2,12] Depending on the study, for outpatient or hospitalized patients the average work time lost may vary from 4 days to 31 days.[13,14] Of those who miss work, one third returned to work within 3 days after the auto accident, over half returned within 7 days, and almost 20% missed more than 30 days of work due to auto accidents.[12] The vast majority of MVCI patients return to work within 2 months.[15] Generally speaking, most MVCI patients should return to work within 6 weeks. Any patient on full disability with intractable pain for more than 1 month should have an orthopedic or neurologic evaluation. Surgical intervention should be considered if severe pain and disability continue for more than 6 months.

The primary responsibility of the physician is to describe objectively the amount of the patient's disability based on symptoms, examination findings, and individual characteristics such as age, physical condition, pain threshold, and job demands. Always ask the patient whether he or she thinks that job duties will make the pain worse. Also ask follow-up questions such as, "What do you do at work that might make the condition worse?" "Is there anything that could be modified at work that would make your pain less?" It is very important to tell the patient that you want to get him or her back to part-time or full-time work as soon as possible. Clarification of your role as a doctor in guidelines for recommending disability leave for the patient often saves time and confrontations.

Initially, the doctor should allocate temporary disability days off work for a short period correlating to pain and injury severity. Most patients with mild to moderate injuries require only 2 to 4 days off work. Patients with severe injuries are usually given a week off and then reassessed to determine whether the time off needs to be extended. If the pain continues to be severe at the end of the first week, there is no problem in extending the time of disability.

Work Restrictions for Temporary Disability and Return-to-Work Guidelines

Work restrictions for temporary disability should be based on the specific job demands of the injured person, as well as the location and severity of the pain. Sending MVCI patients home to be on complete bed rest is usually not advised and has been shown in the literature to be counterproductive. One study that compared outcomes of patients who had rest as the primary method of treatment with those of patients who underwent physiotherapy concluded that the rest group did not achieve any improvement of symptoms, whereas the other group did. The recovery times of patients who were advised to rest lagged 1 month behind those of patients who were mobilized earlier.[16]

The prerequisites for returning to work include the ability to work either part of a day or a full day, fulfilling all job requirements, such as sitting, standing, stooping, lifting, reaching, carrying, and squatting, with no resultant injury or flare-up of symptoms. Getting the patient back to work as soon as possible, and allowing only activities that will not cause further injury, will help speed the recovery. An early return to work has psychologic benefits. In some instances, having the patient start work on a partial day with some restrictions has value. The patient is told to try to work, taking an occasional 20-minute break to lie down to rest the neck. Removing the gravitational forces and postural stress with an occasional break helps speed the return to full-time, unrestricted work. It is important to make the patient's employer aware of the objective of work modification without flare-ups due to overexertion.

In mild head injury (MHI), the goals of allocating temporary disability are primarily focused on educating the employer and family members about normal sequelae. Unlike most neck injury patients whose work can be resumed with no limitations, the MHI patient who returns to work soon after injury always has temporary restrictions. The MHI patient needs to lessen mental stresses and not perform activities that will raise intracranial pressure. Unlike the neck injury patient whose early work resumption will usually be beneficial, in the MHI patient it may be deleterious. The author suggests giving 1 week off work for most MHI cases. The doctor must evaluate the patient in both physical and mental job descriptions. Physical activities that must be excluded include bending forward with the head, lifting, or heavy exertion. Head injury patients, in particular, must be provided with a form to give their employers listing common problems to expect. Exhibit 7–3 illustrates such a form. It is important that the employer support the employee during the early stages of healing.

Doctor's Role in Permanent Disability

The doctor's role during all initial and subsequent patient examinations is to perform an impartial assessment and state the facts as presented.[17] The doctor who is performing the disability examination must be thorough in taking a history and doing a complete evaluation and examination. He or she must render a factual opinion based on objective findings,[17] personal experience, the patient's pain description, and current medical literature. If a patient becomes injured and has pain to the point of being unable to work, or if his or her regular job duties would cause further injury and/or aggravation, the doctor must be able to evaluate work requirements and pain/reinjury-associated risks and then write a disability statement substantiating the injury and length of disability. The doctor must be able to make a determination without measuring the patient's dynamic function[9] during specific activities.

Factors That May Have a Significant Effect on Disability/Impairment

- Age[6,18]
- Gender, females having more frequent and higher disability levels than males[19]
- Use of seat belts (increases neck disability)[18,20]
- Education and training level[6]
- Economic status; those having net worth over $100,000[6]
- Job status at time of injury
- Previous permanent impairment[6]
- Sedentary lifestyle
- Family support[6,21]
- Work and social support[21]
- Fear-avoidance behavior[22]
- Postinjury treatment factors, i.e., delay in treatment, early use of ice
- Drug dependency[23]

Factors That May Have Slight Influence on Disability

- Financial compensation
- Litigation
- Psychologic factors

SOCIOECONOMIC FACTORS AFFECTING DISABILITY

There are several factors that may influence when an injured person returns to preinjury work status. A recent hospital study of 266 traumatized individuals found that important correlates for these patients reaching preinjury work status included educational level, strong social network, severity of injury, type of injury, and economic status.[24] This means that the person's age, sex, desire to return to work, enjoyment of work, and financial motivation all influence outcome.[4] A recent study of 1516 people with lower back injuries concluded that higher educational levels for men resulted in less disability, whereas having low income was related to higher disability over-all. Almost twice as much disability was seen for housewives as for employed women. These variables in the study accounted for up to 15% of the disability variance.[25] A Washington state study on back pain disability and socioeconomic variables concludes that disability frequency will rise when there is job insecurity or economic insecurity, accounting for about one third of the claims.[4]

One report concluded that anywhere from 30% to 50% of patients with chronic pain have a primary drug dependency, which may be an iatrogenic perpetuating factor.[26] Prescription drug dependency can add to the patient's disability by creating the dependency.[23] Other factors may include patient noncompliance with treatment or with frequency of treatment, such as not performing exercises and stretching routines as prescribed. Doctors also may delay or prescribe the wrong type of treatment, or cause the patient to be dependent on drugs. They may authorize too many days off work without any discussion of the patient's work capability. The employer may treat the injured patient with hostility because of the inconvenience or expense, especially if the injury is work related. In addition, if the patient has an attorney, the patient may be told that if he or she has no time off work, the case will not bring in as much money in the settlement. Thus, a person who is employed or is a union member may take five times as much disability time as a self-employed individual.[27] Delays in activity resumption can have harmful emotional effects on the patient.

PREDICTING DISABILITY OUTCOME

Gargan and Bannister[28] found that every patient having intrusive or disabling symptoms at 3 months failed to make full recovery, and they also concluded that the doctor can make a confident assessment of injury outcome at about 9 months, as no patient in their studies changed after that time. Maurette et al.[21] conclude that disability for minor MVCI appears to be fixed at about 1 year after injury and that the moderate to severe injury can continue to improve beyond 1 year. Jennett and Teasdale recommend that for head injuries the best time to assess the outcome is at 6 months after injury.[29]

Typically, for most mild to moderate musculoskeletal injuries, such as injuries to myofascial tissues, ligaments, or discs, or nerve injuries, the disability evaluation should be done as soon as the person's condition has maximally improved and appears to be stabilized. This usually occurs between 3 and 12 months after motor vehicle injury, with the range of time dependent on the severity of the injury and the quality of repair that follows the injury. When the patient has had 6 to 8 weeks of no improvement in the frequency or severity of pain, it is time to perform further patient evaluations. There may be cases, such as those in which patients have injuries that cause permanent disability, when financial matters are treated as immediate priorities and rehabilitation as a secondary concern.

HUMAN FACTORS AND DISABILITY RISK

Table 10–1 reviews the literature on the percentage of MVCI cases having ≥10% disability. Although 40% of all patients have some residual symptoms following MVCI (see Chapter 11), about 6% to 12% of these patients have significant disabling symptoms. Figure 10–1 shows the risk of disability by region of the body. AIS-1 (minor) injuries are predominated by neck disability. A large insurance study found that ≥10 disability risks are related to aging. For occupants aged 15 to 30, the risk was 3.6%; for those aged 31 to 50 the risks were 5.9% for men and 6.7% for women; and for those aged ≥51 years the risks were 8.4% for men and 8.8% for women.[30] Bring and Westman[19] found in their 5-year study of 22 MVCI patients that of 38 listed disabling symptoms women averaged 23.1 symptoms and men 14.6 symptoms; the risk for women was significantly higher than for men. Pre-existing degenerative changes of the cervical

Table 10–1 Frequency of Occupants' Developing ≥10% Disability

Authors	Year	% Having Disability
Ebelin et al.[34]	1981	5.75
Nygren[30]	1984	6.2
Galasko et al.[18]	1986	24
Tunbridge et al.[14]	1990	8.5
Gargan and Bannister[35]	1990	12
Borchgrevink and Lereim[36]	1992	12

spine can increase disability levels.[31] Figures 10–1 and 10–2 illustrate the risk for occupants having developed a permanent disability of 1% and 10%.[32,33]

VEHICLE AND CRASH FACTORS AND DISABILITY

Nygren found that 10.5% of those with no head restraint, 11.8% with adjustable head restraints, and 6.1% with fixed head restraints had ≥ 10% disability.[30] Seat belt use has been shown to increase neck disability as well.[18,20] Nygren[30] reports that the 9.6% of rear-end occupants and 3.8% of side- and frontal-impact occupants will have permanent medical disability from neck injury. Galasko et al.[18] found that 20.5% of occupants who wore seat belts had disability at 6 months, compared with the non–seat belt wearers, who had 7.7% disability. Deans et al.[20] found about two times the risk for chronic pain developing from rear-end crashes as compared to side or frontal collisions. Other factors include vehicle crashworthiness, vehicle size, and velocity of crash. Figures 10–3 and 10–4 show how occupant position may affect the level of disability.

INITIAL INJURY/SYMPTOM SEVERITY AND DISABILITY

Disability risks have been related to the initial injury severity and the number of the presenting symptoms. Watkinson et al.[31] found that groups of patients having initial presenting moderate to severe disruptive symptoms,

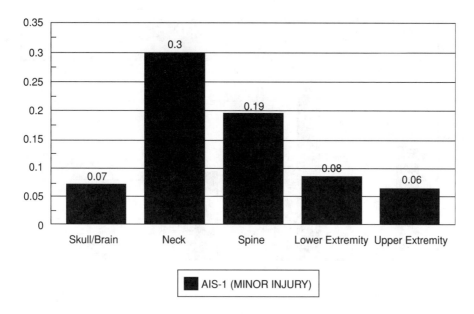

Figure 10–1 Risk for occupants' developing ≥1% disability by body region. *Source:* Data from Koch, M.V., Korner, J., Norin, H., et al., Injury Severity Assessment for Car Occupants Using Disability Scaling, in 36th Proceedings, Association for the Advancement of Automotive Medicine, Portland, Oregon, 1992.

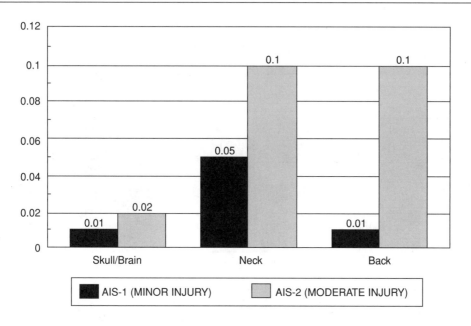

Figure 10–2 Frequency of occupants' developing ≥10% disability for minor and moderately severe injuries by region of body. *Source:* Data from Krafft, M., et al., Values for Permanent Medical Disability Comparing Injury Severity and Region of the Body, Swedish Folksam Insurance Co. Study from 1976–1989, for 12,000 MVCI with Five Year Follow Up, International Conference on the Biomechanics of Impacts, Berlin, 1991.

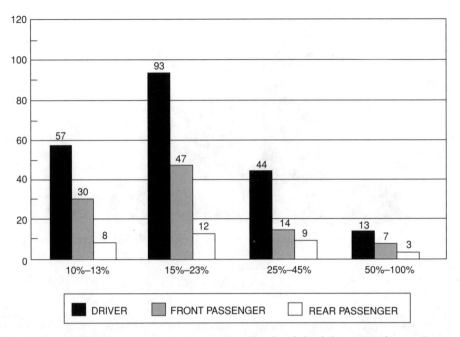

Figure 10–3 Percentage of occupants having various levels of disability ≥10% by seating position. *Source:* Data from Nygren, A., A Study of a Five-Year Material from an Insurance Company, *Acta-Laryngologica* Supplement, No. 395, pp. 1–164, 1984.

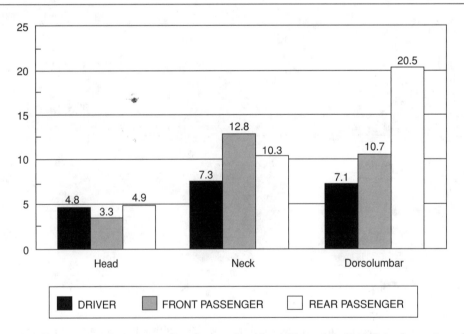

Figure 10–4 Percentage of occupants developing chronic ≥10% ratable disabilities by region of body and seating position. *Source:* Data from Nygren, A., A Study of Five-Year Material from an Insurance Company, *Acta-Laryngologica* Supplement, No. 395, pp. 1–164, 1984.

such as radicular symptoms, interscapular pain, low back pain, and occipital headaches, had significantly higher levels of disabling problems 10.8 years after MVCI. Other authors found that initial injury severity scores have been found to have little value in predicting disability.[18] The opposing findings about injury severity and subsequent disability arise because of study flaws. There was failure to document symptoms typical for poor prognosis, outlined in Chapter 11, such as early radicular pain and management strategies.

It is the author's opinion that it is impossible to predict all cases by depending on injury severity and types of symptoms. In biomechanical terms, every patient's response to trauma is different. In addition, some symptoms that are very common disabling problems for the auto accident victim frequently begin to develop several weeks to months after trauma. Delays in upper-extremity radiating pain, numbness and tingling, and headache development have been reported in the literature. In addition, more recent studies show more disabling headaches in the minor head injury victim and not in the severe head injury victim. See Chapter 1 for correlation between head impact severity and headache development.

DISABILITY RISKS AND SPECIFIC CONDITIONS

Cervical Spine Disability

A large insurance company study concluded that mild injuries to the neck could lead to ≥10% disability and that cervical spine injuries were predominant in cases having ≥50% ratable disabilities.[30] One emergency department study concludes that up to 24% of all persons who had been involved in a car crash developed a disability that lasted at least 6 months, with neck injuries having the highest incidence of residual disability. One of the most important areas of concern in the field of car crash biomechanics, injury prevention,

and rehabilitation is neck injury, because of the extreme disability it may produce and the limited functional restoration currently available.[37] It is well recognized that neck injuries have a high incidence of disability associated with motor vehicle collisions.[33]

Fibromyalgia Disability

Posttraumatic fibromyalgia or myofascial pain syndromes are one of the more common problems that lead to chronic disability following trauma. Wolfe's recent report[38] summarizes fibromyalgia disability well. Wolfe believes that there is a reasonable hypothesis for the link between trauma and the development of chronic symptoms and disability related to fibromyalgia. One of the primary difficulties for the physician who has a MVCI patient who develops fibromyalgia is face validity: these patients do not look ill.[38] The physician needs to elicit information from the injured patient to support causation. Fibromyalgia usually begins locally and then spreads slowly from one location to another, before it becomes generalized. In most MVCI patients the pain distribution should have a unilateral presentation or unilateral predominance. Research also shows that most fibromyalgia pain symptoms are relatively stable over time.[39]

According to Monsein, the current disability system demonstrates its bias against the myofascial pain syndrome, the most common cause of lost work, by excluding it from the ratable area of disability.[3]

Headaches and Disability

Balla's retrospective analysis of 5000 whiplash cases[15] showed that about 25% of these cases developed chronic disability, with most reporting headaches. Packard and Ham[40] have a proposed criterion for posttraumatic headaches; they use the mnemonic *IMPAIRMENT:* Intensity, Medication use, Physical signs/symptoms, Adjustment (coping ability), Incapacitation, Recreation, Miscellaneous activity of daily living, Employment, Number (frequency) of attacks, and Time (duration) of attacks. They then modify the scores based on patient treatment motivation, overexaggeration, and litigation interest. These authors also believe that, since headaches are rarely continuously severe or incapacitating, headache impairment should rate no higher than 15% to 20%.

Chest Wall/Thoracic and Lumbar Region Disability

Although minor- to moderate-level chest wall injury disability is rarely reported in the literature, these cases do exist. A study of 22 MVCI patients found that more than half had pain and tenderness related to chest wall and rib regions, with 3 patients having disabling symptoms.[19] There are also rare reports of thoracic disc protrusions. I have seen several cases of patients (drivers) involved in higher-speed crashes who had been in either frontal or rear-end crashes; these patients sustained substantial chest wall injury from the steering column and later developed severe disabling syndromes. These patients typically have demanding occupations and, with development of severe myofascial adhesions in the subscapular and intercostal muscles, report frequent bouts of their backs freezing up.

Lumbar injuries are well recognized for causing high levels of pain and permanent disability. A large insurance study found that the body region having the highest frequency of disability was thoracolumbar spine in rear-seated occupants, this injury having 20.5% permanent disability.[30] This study also found that 7.1% of the drivers and 10.7% of front passengers had permanent disability. Dorsolumbar injuries are particularly common because these occupants interact and flex over a seat belt.

Mild Head Injury Disability

A large insurance company study found that even mild head injury (MHI) could lead to ≥10% permanent disability.[30] Long-term studies showed that 22 of 26 patients with closed head injuries were unemployed an average of 2.8 years after settlement of litigation.[41] The postconcussion syndrome is diagnosed by a constellation of findings persisting beyond 3 to 6 months after trauma (see Chapter 1).

Disability from MHI includes residual problems from scar tissue in the scalp, leading to site-of-impact headaches, associated neck problems, cognitive and personality changes, headaches, and cranial nerve symptoms, and symptoms typical for sympathetic nerve irritation such as auditory and visual symptoms. Determination of a baseline for each MHI patient is essential for all physicians. The examiner needs to request records from any prior treating doctors to see whether any MHI symptoms were present. Unfortunately, most forms used by physicians are inadequate. In many cases the doctor assumes that the MHI will resolve by itself, and no baseline history is taken. (See Chapter 11 for MHI prognosis.)

Every MVCI patient initially should be given a questionnaire (see Chapter 2) that includes questions about cognitive symptoms. Many MHI patients have forgotten the initial symptoms by the time the doctor realizes that a postconcussion syndrome has developed. In many MHI patients the initial symptoms may either subside or intensify. Some symptoms may develop as a function of time and the patient's having to adapt to the neurologic dysfunction.

Once the treating doctor determines that the head injury victim has a disability resulting from a direct head impact or from inertial loading in a noncontact car crash, the physician needs to send the patient to a neuropsychologist who specializes in head injury to evaluate the disability. It is impossible for a nonspecialist to evaluate properly these patients having prolonged symptoms. It takes a minimum of 6 hours to do a proper neuropsychologic evaluation. The examiner must evaluate the MHI patient for memory, learning, motor skills, constructive tests, language, problem solving, and administrative skills.

Once the written and verbal tests are completed by the patient, the examiner compares the outcome with information in the prior history and with normal values. The interpretation of this complex case takes both specialized training and experience. Many MHI patients may appear normal in brief examinations. It usually takes some fatiguing effort or stress to intensify the symptoms to a diagnostic level.

TYPES OF DISABILITY RATING SYSTEMS

There are several guides or scales currently available to the physician, including the American Medical Association guidelines; those published by the National Highway Traffic Safety Administration[7]; hospital studies such as the Oswestry system; the Neck Disability Index[42]; and other systems that focus on areas such as function, work capacity, pain, pain drawings, and psychologic factors. It is impossible to show that one system is better than all others, and this is primarily due to human variables such as tolerance level and motivation level, different crash types and severities, and varying work environments and demands. To add to the confusion, some impairment/disability scales commonly used in MVCI cases in fact focus on low back regions and do not properly address the upper body and neck and head regions. As a result the physician is stuck trying to adapt one or many systems to the patient. This is why there is frequent disagreement among examiners. With the multitude of disability systems currently available, the physician needs to familiarize himself or herself with several systems and adapt them to the individual patient. It is essential that the process adequately address the specific problems of the patient. Exhibit 10–1 illustrates a sample form that can be used to determine whether specific activities are causing functional problems. It does not give a ranking system and therefore is less useful for monitoring progress over time.

Suggested Multiple Injury Functional Capacity Questionnaire

The following recommended two-page functional capacity questionnaire (Exhibit 10–2) modifies the original Oswestry[43] low back pain disability scale into a system that addresses the patient having multiple injuries. As described in Chapter 1, most patients seen after a car crash have two or more injuries. To address adequately the functional capacity loss specific to the personal injury field, a reliable scale must include the most common types of problems associated with MVCIs. These problems include neck, upper extremity, low back, lower extremity, and head injury symptoms and related loss of function. The reader will also note that the proposed questionnaire does not include the term *disability* in its heading. The patient may be confused as to the intent of the questionnaire since he or she often does not know the difference between pain and other symptoms and what *disability* means. The heading of functional capacity is less negative and should focus the patient on function instead of pain.

One of the problems facing the Oswestry scale[43] and the Neck Disability Index[42] is that two sections that address pain intensity look only at the pain and do not address how the pain affects the patient's ability to function; therefore they do not relate to disability. The Neck Disability Index also includes headaches, but again looks only at intensity and frequency and not at the effect the headaches have on functional capacity. Although these and other indexes have been found to have reliability in studies, further refinement will aid in more sensitive measures of outcome.

Scoring for Functional Capacity Loss

The first portion of determining functional capacity loss includes a 10-part questionnaire marked by the patient (Exhibit 10–2). The doctor gives each of the 10 categories a score of 0 to 5. The point system works as follows: The

Exhibit 10–1 Activity Questionnaire

Patient Name: _____   Date: _____

Check only the activities below that affect you currently. Be specific and indicate whether your pain, weakness, stiffness, or other symptoms while doing the activity annoy you, slow you down, make the activity hard to do, or prevent (unable to do) your ability to perform the activity.

ACTIVITY DESCRIPTION	ANNOYS ONLY	SLOWS DOWN	HARD TO DO	UNABLE TO DO	INDICATE HOW SOON (MINUTES OR HOURS) THE ACTIVITY TAKES TO AFFECT YOU
Bending head downward or upward					
Working at computer station					
Driving car					
Sitting					
Working at desk					
Lifting/reaching hands over level of shoulder					
Lifting/reaching hands over level of head					
Doing reaching activities					
Combing/brushing hair					
Typing on a keyboard					
Carrying objects in hand					
Gripping objects or using wrist or hands					
Sleeping					
Recreational/sports/hobby activities					
Doing housework or gardening					
Stooping/bending					
Twisting					
Crouching/kneeling					
Walking					
Standing					
Pushing/pulling					
Lifting at work/home					
Having sex					

continues

Exhibit 10–2 Multiple Injury Functional Capacity Questionnaire

Name: _____ Date: _____ Age: _____

Patient: Fill out Sections 1 to 10. In each category, check one box that best applies to your current condition.

1. CURRENT PAIN INTENSITY

- ☐ I have no pain currently.
- ☐ I have occasional pain that mildly disturbs me at work and at home.
- ☐ I have frequent annoying pain with an occasional pain that slows me down.
- ☐ I have frequent moderate level pain and occasional severe pain that stop me from performing an activity.
- ☐ I have some degree of pain at all times with frequent bouts of severe pain that prevent me from performing many activities.
- ☐ I have pain all of the time, mostly severe, because of which I am unable to do most activities for myself. Medications don't help.

2. WORK ABILITY

- ☐ I am currently able to work full time with no pain.
- ☐ I work full time and have slight (annoying) symptoms that occasionally may slow me down, thus taking slightly longer to perform an activity.
- ☐ I work full time. My work output quality and/or quantity are reduced 10%–20%. Symptoms vary from slight to moderate levels, which cause intermittent halting. I require assistance occasionally at work.
- ☐ I am able to work part time. I am not able to work at a normal pace beyond 2 hours and at a slower pace beyond 4 hours. My performance output quality and/or quantity are reduced by 30%–60%.
- ☐ I am able to work part time. I am not able to work at a normal pace for more than 30–60 minutes at a time. I can work at a slower pace beyond 2 hours. My ability to perform in output is reduced by over 70%.
- ☐ I am not able to work at a normal or a slower pace at all. Job quality and quantity output are reduced by more than 90%. I am unable to work on part-time status even with a flexible work schedule.

3. SPORTS, HOBBIES, AND SOCIAL ACTIVITIES

- ☐ I can perform normal sports, hobby activities, and social activities with my friends, family, or business acquaintances.
- ☐ My sports, hobby, and social life is normal, but pain slows me down occasionally.
- ☐ Pain or other symptoms limit my more energetic or competitive sports, hobbies, and social activities such as dancing and running.
- ☐ Severe pain or other symptoms limit moderate energetic sports, hobbies, and social activities. I do not go out as often.
- ☐ Pain or other symptoms limit me to only minimal sports, hobbies, and social activity. I usually stay at home.
- ☐ I am unable to participate in any sports, hobbies, or social activity due to pain.

4. HOME ACTIVITIES

- ☐ I can perform normal home activities such as vacuuming, cooking, cleaning, mowing the lawn, and doing laundry with no pain.
- ☐ I am able to do all normal home duties, but pain slows me down occasionally with very strenuous activities.
- ☐ Pain prohibits very strenuous home activities. I am able to do light to moderately strenuous home activities.
- ☐ Severe pain or other symptoms limit moderate and strenuous home activities. I need help doing some activities.

Exhibit 10-2 continued

❑ I am able to do only light home activities. I am unable to vacuum the floor, do dishes, sweep, mop, and do laundry.
❑ I am unable to do any home activities due to pain or other symptoms. I need help putting on clothes and taking a bath.

5. SLEEPING
❑ I normally have no difficulty sleeping due to pain or other symptoms.
❑ I have occasional difficulty sleeping due to pain or other symptoms. I wake up at night, resulting in 30-minute loss of sleep.
❑ I have occasional difficulty sleeping due to pain or other symptoms. I lose 10%–15% of normal sleeping hours a night.
❑ I have frequent difficulty sleeping due to pain or other symptoms. I am restless most of the night. I lose 25% of normal sleeping hours a night.
❑ My sleeping hours are reduced about 50%. I usually need medications to sleep well.
❑ I have no normal sleeping hours. I am never able to sleep more than 2–3 hours without heavy medication. I never feel rested.

6. SITTING
❑ I can sit at my desk or drive my car normally with no pain.
❑ I can sit at my desk or drive my car with occasional annoying pain. I need to take breaks on long trips.
❑ Sitting or driving causes frequent annoying pain. Pain becomes severe if I sit for more than 2 hours and I need to change position.
❑ I can sit or drive for 3–4 hours, but I need frequent breaks to change my body position. I am unable to sit constantly over 1 hour.
❑ I cannot sit or drive for more than 30 minutes at a time due to pain severity.
❑ I cannot sit at my desk, chair at home, or drive my car at any time due to pain severity.

7. UPPER BODY FUNCTION (neck and arms)
❑ I am able to use my neck, shoulders, arms, and hands in all normal activities with no pain.
❑ I am able to use my neck, shoulders, arms, and hands in all normal activities with occasional annoying pain.
❑ I am able to lift and move my head and neck, lift arms over my head, reach over my head, carry objects, and grip objects with my hands. I have occasional pain when lifting heavy objects over my head, which causes me to stop. Occasionally, I will have difficulty feeling or gripping objects with my hands due to either weakness or numbness. I am limited to light to moderate weights in my hands.
❑ I am able to lift my arms up to the height of my shoulder for short periods but not over my head, carry light to moderate weight objects, and grip objects with my hands. I get occasional pain when lifting heavy objects over my head. Occasionally, I will have difficulty typing, feeling, or gripping objects with my hands due to either weakness or numbness. I drop objects two or three times a week. I have to use two hands for some activities that I could do with one hand before. I am limited to moderate weights.
❑ I am able to carry and grip light weight objects only. I get frequent pain when lifting any object above my waist and sometimes I am unable to lift to the height of my shoulder. I am not able to lift my arms up to the height of my shoulder and lift over my head. I frequently have difficulty feeling or gripping objects with my hands due to either weakness or numbness. I drop objects daily unless I am very careful. I have to use two hands for most activities that I could do with one hand before. I have frequent difficulty typing, using a computer, and writing letters. I am limited to light weights. I have lost 75% of hand-lifting ability.
❑ I am able to lift my arms to the level of my shoulders only, and just lifting my arms above my waist causes severe pain. I am unable to lift any object over the height of my waist. Every time I lift my arms I get severe pain in my neck, shoulders, or arms, and I have to lower my arm or arms immediately. I am unable to write letters. I am unable to lift 5 lbs in my hands.

8. LOWER BODY FUNCTION (low back and legs)
❑ I can sit, drive, stand, squat, stoop, walk, bend my knees, use my feet, and lift normal heavy weights with no low back/leg pain.

continues

Exhibit 10–2 continued

☐ I can sit, drive, stand, squat, stoop, walk, bend my knees, use my feet, and lift normal heavy weights with occasional annoyance of mild pain. I can do all of these activities, but more slowly if demands are high.

☐ Moderate levels of low back/leg pain happen if I do prolonged or repeated sitting, driving, standing, stooping, walking, or bending. I can lift heavy objects if properly positioned. Pain limits me to walking to 1/2 mile. I am unable to stand for more than 45 minutes at a time. Repeated stooping or bending for more than 20 minutes will cause me to slow down.

☐ Moderate to severe levels of low back/leg pain happen if I do prolonged or repeated sitting, driving, standing, stooping, walking, or bending. I can't lift heavy objects at all and am able to lift moderately heavy objects (1/4 my body weight) if properly positioned. Pain limits me to walking to 1/4 mile. I am unable to stand for more than 30 minutes at a time.

☐ I experience severe levels of pain if I do short-term sitting, driving, standing, stooping, walking, or bending. I can't lift moderate or heavy objects at all and am able to lift light objects only (10–15 lbs). I need lumbar belt support and/or a cane for support to walk. Pain limits me to walking to one block. I am unable to stand for more than 10 minutes at a time.

☐ I experience severe levels of pain if I do sitting, driving, standing, stooping, walking, or bending. I am able to walk only with use of a cane, crutches, or a wheelchair. I need to lie down frequently to relieve pain. I am unable to lift or carry any object over 5 lbs. I need lumbar belt support and/or a cane for support to move about in my home. During the daytime I lie down for 3–4 hours.

9. HEADACHES

☐ I have no headaches normally.

☐ I have headaches occasionally, which only annoy me at work or at home.

☐ I have occasional headaches that are intense enough to slow me down at work and at home.

☐ I have occasional headaches that cause me to stop and rest for short periods of time.

☐ I have frequent headaches that stop all of my activity. I frequently lose time at work or have delays in work production due to pain.

☐ I have frequent headaches that cause my not being able to go to work, school, or home, or participate in recreational activities.

10. MENTAL ABILITY

☐ My memory and mental function are normal. I have no difficulty with work or home demands.

☐ I am able to perform most mental activities and am able to function at work, at home, and in society. I have occasional slight difficulty with complex tasks, memory, and math.

☐ I am able to function normally in most work, home, and society activities. Complex tasks, multiple tasks, and intense concentration tasks are difficult, often resulting in mistakes. I have noticed about a 10%–25% memory loss and a job performance decline recently.

☐ I am not able to handle difficult or complex tasks. I have notable memory loss and difficulty making decisions. My friends, family, and I have noticed recent personality changes. It takes much longer to do work and home tasks. I can handle one simple task at a time. I have to write down my daily tasks to remember. My job performance ratings are poor. I have noticed about a 26%–50% memory loss and a job performance decline recently.

☐ I am able to handle only simple tasks one at a time. I am unable to keep a full-time job. My job performance ratings are poor. My reaction times have slowed down a lot. I have noticed about a 51%–75% memory loss and a job performance decline recently.

☐ I am unable to hold any job at all. I am unable to balance my checkbook and need help. I am unable to shop without a shopping list. I have severe performance difficulties. I am unable to remember instructions.

TOTAL SCORE (1–10): _____ × 2 = _____

Source: Adapted from Fairbanks, J.T.C., Couper, J., Eisenstein, S., et al., The Oswestry Low Back Pain Disability Questionnaire, *Physiotherapy,* Vol. 66, No. 8, pp. 271–273, Chartered Society of Physiotherapy, 1980.

top box gets a 0 score, and the score for each following box goes up in single increments from 1 to 5. A score of 1 indicates a mild annoyance only, with less than 10% rating. A score of 2 equals a slight disability of about 10%. A score of 3 equals a moderate disability. A score of 4 equals a serious disability. A score of 5 equals a severe disability that totally incapacitates an individual.

With 10 sections rated there is a total possible score of 50 points. Multiply the patient's total score by 2 for the total score. For example, if the patient scores 15, multiply by 2. The result shows the patient having a 30% loss of functional capacity. This modified Oswestry disability score[43] interpretation recommends the following: 0% to 10%, minimal to mild disability; 10% to 19%, slight disability; 20% to 40%, moderate disability; 40% to 60%, serious disability; 60% to 80%, crippling; and 80% to 100%, bed bound. Figure 10–5 illustrates a type of graph that can be used easily by the doctor's staff. Once the patient completes the functional capacity questionnaire the scores and pain levels are plotted at appropriate intervals. This is a useful tool for evaluating subjective factors, and by plotting them over time, the clinician is able to produce objective evidence of treatment responses. This system aids treatment credibility.

Modifiers in Functional Capacity Loss Rating

As every clinician knows, it is impossible to fit every patient into simple categories. Disability rating is a complex matter and many factors come into play. Individuals with similar functional capacity losses have different levels of disability. General questions in this section discuss educational and socioeconomic factors that correlate with the person's ability to compensate for the disability and become a productive part of society. Section two looks at the confidence level of the person and whether the fear of doing work or whether the activity or exertion that causes the pain to in-

tensify to greater than moderate levels by itself is causing the disability. In addition, the patient's subjective complaints; the doctor's objective examination findings; diagnostic exam (magnetic resonance imaging [MRI], computed tomography, somatosensory evoked potentials) findings; and the patient's response to treatment, injury severity, pre-existing conditions, and factors that indicate poor prognosis must be considered. In this section, the doctor must be able to correlate the information on the questionnaire, looking at the patient's social and family resources and ability to cope with the disability, and compare this information with injury severity, treatment type, response to treatment, examination findings, and radiologic and neurodiagnostic findings. Recent evidence shows that persons with higher educational degrees, close family support, and net worths of over $100,000 have significantly less difficulty in handling disabilities.[6] Pre-existing complicating factors also must be evaluated. The doctor must consider pain-related activity observed in the patient during the course of treatment or during the examination process. Examples are facial grimacing, holding onto fixtures for support, ease or restriction of mobility, stationary motion, and verbal responses to questions about what causes or stimulates symptoms. The duration, threshold, and amount of pain must also be considered. Patients who have an organic basis for pain usually use fewer words when describing their symptoms than those who have no organic basis.

PROBLEMS WHEN DOING DISABILITY EVALUATIONS

Many problems can be avoided by the doctor's explaining his or her office policy on disability to the patient during the first office visit. Nevertheless, the following three situations can pose difficulty for the doctor:

1. The patient's attorney has informed him or her that taking long periods off work will strengthen the case when the

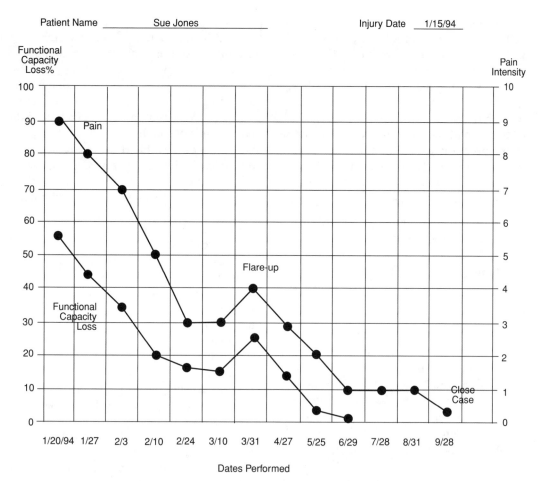

Patient Name _____ Sue Jones _____   Injury Date ___ 1/15/94 ___

Figure 10–5 Functional capacity outcome graph. The doctor can document each assessment and chart the treatment outcome as illustrated.

time comes to settle, resulting in a larger settlement for both the patient and the attorney.

2. The patient sees disability as an opportunity for a vacation. The doctor's authorization to take time off from work is seen not as a specific recommendation to prevent further injury, but as a chance to substitute work with home projects such as rebuilding cars, painting, planting gardens, or cleaning house. The excuses for more time off are numerous, and often indicate a person who is trying to manipulate the symptoms and the doctor or is simply overexerting at home.

3. The patient may be self-employed, with a disability insurance policy that pays for time off from work. Occasionally, these patients ask to extend disability time past the 30-day waiting period, then when more than 30 days elapse, they have conveniently been given 6 weeks' more disability time by the doctor.

Ultimately, establishing a diagnosis of disability is an administrative decision[4]; unlike impairment, which is easily measured, disability is a complex process that is not easily measured. There are no true objective methods for evaluating pain intensity and functional loss for spinal injuries. Frequently the examiner must rely on questionnaires or look for behavioral modifications, such as awkward movements, limps, motion delays, or facial expressions or sounds indicating pain (e.g., groans), in order to see the effects of pain. Methods of evaluating disability include the following:

- In-depth questionnaires regarding injury, pain, activity level, limitations, and so forth
- Strength, endurance, and flexibility tests. These tests have been used for lower back strength typically, but for neck and shoulder problems no adequate system exists today. If the patient has unilateral arm symptoms, the affected arm can be compared with the normal side, taking into account the dominant arm and hand. For example, have the patient abduct both arms 90° and rapidly open and close both hands until both fatigue and drop, and measure time differences. The examiner can then show that there was a certain percentage of loss time on the affected side. If both sides of the body are affected, the examiner must call on normal values or the experience of persons of similar size, gender, and age. In testing for strength, the examiner must look for fatiguing effects. Single muscle strength tests frequently miss subtle problems.
- Duplicate specific activity and environment functional testing. Have patients perform the specific activity that they say they are unable to perform, and observe. If computer use bothers them, have them document, in writing, the time before pain, the degree of pain, and how the pain restricts them.
- Psychologic testing

The patient's subjective complaints are reviewed first, to determine the severity of the complaints and the extent of restricted activities due to pain, weakness, paresthesia, or loss of motion. The physical examination findings are compared with patterns of complaint, watching for possible overexaggeration on the part of the patient. The more the doctor knows about anatomy, pain referral patterns, methods of testing inconsistent findings, and what the test findings indicate, the less likely the doctor will produce inaccurate disability reports.

In the report, the doctor should include the following: history, examination findings, diagnosis, job/home/recreational activity descriptions, correlation between disability and activity, prognosis, and how much disability there is.[4] Additionally, the report should contain the causes of the disability and residual complaints or functional impairments.

The doctor must correlate the history of the patient, pre-existing conditions, type of injury, factors influencing repair, and job description. He or she must also consider the injury severity, age of the injured, educational level, amount of social support, other medical problems, other tests such as MRI, types of treatment, number of flare-ups, and response to previous treatment. The doctor's perception of the patient's motivation to function in society must be considered.

INDEPENDENT MEDICAL EXAMINATION

Nationwide, according to a 1987 All-Industry Research Advisory Council study,[2] 7% to 10% of all personal injury claims are sent to an independent medical examination (IME) doctor for evaluation, depending on the state and its type of insurance system. There has been a definite trend to utilize IMEs or paper reviewers more in the past 10 years. Ethical problems with IMEs are widespread, affecting every field of medicine, due to their frequent pro–

insurance company bias, lack of knowledge about MVCI, and unsupportive and predictable reporting. There has been a trend in the past 2 to 3 years to have paper file reviews of patient cases done, in which a doctor is paid to collect and review a patient file, without actually seeing or touching the patient. The reviewer renders an opinion as to whether prior treatment has followed an appropriate course to diagnosis and whether billing is excessive, evaluates the patient's permanent stationary status, and estimates the need for future care. The paper review process is inadequate and sometimes harmful in determining MVCI musculoskeletal disability. In reality, paper reviewers are management consultants. They have similar licenses and have the ability to request and review records and suggest courses of action. The treating or examining doctor is essential and more accurate than a paper reviewer in feeling for joint play, muscle spasm, and soft tissue texture, and then correlating symptoms and disability with the findings.

The current disability system offers little means to account for the severe chronic pain syndromes (such as myofascial pain) that frequently cause prolonged disability and pain outside the normal spectrum of severity. Current disability/impairment standards deal with most industrial injury cases, but they do not adequately address neck and head injury cases following automobile crashes. This failing is primarily due to the focus of the medical, chiropractic, insurance, and research community in the past decade on low back disability systems. A recent practical guideline has been developed for IMEs that covers many of the issues confronting the physician.[44]

MVCIs account for the vast majority of the worst cervical spine injuries in our society. Yet medical schools and chiropractic colleges do not adequately educate their students about car crash trauma, with traditionally more educational focus being given to less common disorders. The workers' compensation courses for IME doctors similarly do not cover the subject of MVCIs adequately, resulting in few doctors in the personal injury field having even a minimal understanding of the mechanisms of injury, and fewer still understanding prognosis factors. Some IME doctors who have never had a single course on whiplash injury or neck injury are determining the fates of injured victims.

The author has found that the IME process is more effective if the examination appointment is made 2 to 3 weeks ahead. The person having the examination is sent several pages of paperwork to fill out prior to the examination. The forms cover much of the detail covered in the interview process. The primary concern is having the patient complete the sections on the injury event, names of doctors or therapists seen, treatment types, and current work and home activity level restrictions, if any. When the doctor meets the person having the IME, it is important for the doctor to explain the process, answer questions, and not rush into the examination. The doctor needs to ensure that adequate time has been set aside for the examination and interview. The appointment-setting office staff should ask in the initial phone call where the patient is having pain. If the case looks complex, that is, pain in three or more areas, more time should be made available for the doctor.

The patient being evaluated may be resistant to this additional intrusion upon his or her time. He or she may not understand why the examination is being performed, or may feel bothered by the insurance carrier. Some patients are told by the treating doctor that the IME doctor works for the insurance company and opposing attorneys, and is out to disprove any basis for continued pain, disability, or treatment. Doctors who perform IMEs should mail the patient a packet of information to be filled out and brought to the appointment. This saves a lot of time, and gives the patient time to consider the questions without the pressure of the receptionist.

REFERENCES

1. National Safety Council. *Accident Facts*. Chicago, 1994.

2. All-Industry Research Advisory Council. *Compensation for Automobile Injuries in the United States*. Oak Brook, Ill; March 1989.

3. Monsein M. Soft tissue pain and disability. In: Fricton JR, Awad E, eds. *Adv Pain Res Ther*. 1990; 17:183–200.

4. Vasudevan SV. Clinical perspectives on the relationship between pain and disability. *Neurol Clin*. 1989;7:429–439.

5. Petrucelli E. Injury scaling and some considerations of disability consequences. In: Aldman B, Chapon A, eds. *The Biomechanics of Impact Trauma*. Amsterdam: Elsevier Science Publishers; 1984.

6. States JD, Viano DC. Injury impairment and disability scales to assess the permanent consequences of trauma. *Accid Anal Prev*. 1990;22:151–160.

7. Luchter S. Impairment resulting from motor vehicle crashes. In: *12th International Technical Conference of Experimental Safety Vehicles*. National Highway Traffic Safety Administration. Washington, DC: US Dept of Transportation; 1989:1157–1184.

8. Levine RS. A review of the long-term effects of selected lower limb injuries. In: *Biomechanics and Medical Aspects of Lower Limb Injuries*; paper 860501. Detroit, Mich: Society of Automotive Engineers; 1986:143–160.

9. Mooney V. Impairment, disability, and handicap. *Clin Orthop*. 1987;221:14–25.

10. Joynt RL. Rehabilitation of lower limb injuries. In: *Biomechanics and Medical Aspects of Lower Limb Injuries*. paper 861931. Detroit, Mich: Society of Automotive Engineers; 1986:137–142.

11. Björnstig U, Hildingsson C, Toolanen G. Soft-tissue injury of the neck in a hospital based material. *Scand J Soc Med*. 1990;18:263–267.

12. Insurance Research Council. *Paying for Auto Injuries: A Consumer Panel Survey of Auto Accident Victims*. Oak Brook, Ill; 1994.

13. Kahane CJ. *Evaluation of Head Restraints, Federal Motor Vehicle Safety Standard 202*. National Highway Safety Administration. Washington, DC: US Dept of Transportation; 1982:HS 806 108.

14. Tunbridge RJ, Murray PA, Kinsella AM, et al. *The Cost of Long-term Disability Resulting from Road Traffic Accidents: Interim Report*. Transport and Road Research Laboratory Report 212. Washington, DC: US Dept of Transportation; 1990.

15. Balla JI. The late whiplash syndrome. *Aust N Z J Surg*. 1980;50:610–614.

16. McKinney LA, Dornan JO, Ryan M. The role of physiotherapy in management of acute neck sprains following road-traffic accidents. *Arch Emerg Med*. 1989;6:27–33.

17. Gordon EJ. Independent medical evaluations. *Orthop Rev*. 1985;14(4):109–114.

18. Galasko CSB, Murray P, Hodson M, et al. *Long-term Disability following Road Traffic Accidents*. Transport and Road Research Laboratory Report 59. Washington, DC: US Dept of Transportation; 1986.

19. Bring G, Westman G. Chronic posttraumatic syndrome after whiplash injury. *Scand J Prim Health Care*. 1991;9:135–141.

20. Deans GT, Magallierd JN, Kerr M, et al. Neck sprain: a major cause of disability following car accidents. *Injury*. 1987;18:10–12.

21. Maurette P, Masson F, Nicaud V, et al. Posttraumatic disablement: a prospective study of impairment, disability, and handicap. *J Trauma*. 1992; 33:728–736.

22. Waddell G, Newton M, Henderson I, et al. A fear-avoidance questionnaire (FABQ) and the role of fear-avoidance beliefs in chronic low back pain and disability. *Pain*. 1993;52:157–168.

23. Zohn DA. *Musculoskeletal Pain, Diagnosis and Physical Treatment*. 2nd ed. Boston: Little, Brown & Co; 1988.

24. MacKenzie EJ, Shapiro S, Smith RT, et al. Factors influencing return to work following hospitalization for traumatic injury. *Am J Public Health*. 1987;77(3):329–333.

25. Deyo RA, Tsui-Wu Y-J. Functional disability due to back pain: a population-based study indicating the importance of socioeconomic factors. *Arthritis Rheum*. 1987;30:1247–1253.

26. Halpern L. Substitution-detoxification and its role in the management of chronic benign pain. *J Clin Psychiatry*. 1982;43:8(sect 2):10–14.

27. Trunkey DD. Trauma. *Sci Am*. 1983;249(2):28–35.

28. Gargan MF, Bannister GC. The rate of recovery following soft tissue injury of the neck. Paper presented at the British Cervical Spine Society Meeting, Bowness-on-Windermere, November 7, 1992.

29. Jennett B, Teasdale G. *Management of Head Injuries*. Philadelphia: FA Davis Co; 1981.

30. Nygren Å. A study of a five-year material from an insurance company. *Acta Laryngol Suppl*. 1984; 395:1–164.

31. Watkinson A, Gargan MF, Bannister GC. Prognostic factors in soft tissue injuries of the cervical spine. *Injury.* 1991;22(4):307–309.

32. Koch MV, Korner J, Norin H, et al. Injury severity assessment for car occupants using disability scaling. In: Proceedings of the 36th Annual Conference, Association for the Advancement of Automotive Medicine, Portland, Ore, 1992.

33. Krafft M, Kullgren A, Lie A, et al. Car model safety rating based on real life accidents. In: Proceedings of International Research Committee on Biomechanics of Impacts, Berlin, September 11–13, 1991: 25–39.

34. Ebelin M, Furno P, Patel A. Functional sequelae of benign cervical spine sprains from whiplash injuries: report on 61 cases. *J Traumatol.* 1981;2(2): 77–81.

35. Gargan MF, Bannister GC. Long-term prognosis of soft-tissue injuries of the neck. *J Bone Joint Surg [Br].* 1990;72:901–903.

36. Borchgrevink GE, Lereim I. Symptomer hos pasienter med nakkeskade etter bilkollisjon. *Tidsskr Nor Laegeforen.* 1992;112:884–886.

37. McElhaney J, Roberts V, Paver J, et al. Etiology of trauma to the cervical spine. In: Ewing CL, Thomas DJ, Sances A Jr, et al., eds. *Impact Injury of the Head and Spine.* Springfield, Ill: Charles C Thomas; 1983:41–71.

38. Wolfe F. Disability and the dimensions of distress in fibromyalgia. *J Musculoskel Pain.* 1993;1:65–87.

39. Hawley DJ, Wolfe F, Cathey MA. Pain, functional disability, and psychological status: 12-month study of severity in fibromyalgia. *J Rheumatol.* 1988;15:1551–1556.

40. Packard RC, Ham LP. Impairment ratings for post-traumatic headaches. *Headache.* 1993;33:359–364.

41. Kelly R, Smith BN. Post-traumatic syndrome: another myth discredited. *J Roy Soc Med.* 1981;74:275–277.

42. Vernon H, Mior S. The neck disability index: a study of reliability and validity. *J Manipulative Physiol Ther.* 1991;14:409–415.

43. Fairbank JCT, Couper J, Eisenstein S, et al. The Oswestry low back pain disability questionnaire. *Physiotherapy.* 1980;66(8):271–273.

44. Clark W, Haldeman S. The development of guideline factors for the evaluation of disability in neck and back injuries. *Spine.* 1993;18:1736–1745.

Chapter 11

Prognosis after Car Crash Injuries

Lawrence S. Nordhoff, Jr.

INTRODUCTION

One of the more challenging aspects of the minor to moderate injury following car crashes is determining factors that influence long-term prognosis. The prognostician becomes, in fact, a forecaster of the natural course and probable outcome of this specific injury. This forecast includes the chances of further recovery, the benefits of continued or alternative treatment, factors that support opinion, and any effects of this injury on the work/social/recreational quality of life. Patients, insurance companies, and attorneys all want the doctor to discuss this aspect of the injury. Knowledge of the various prognostic factors that have been found in literature should help the doctor. Human and vehicular factors, such as vehicle size ratio, collision speed, head restraints, age, injury severity, and underlying pre-existing human factors must all be considered when evaluating whether the long-range prognosis is good or bad. Chapters 15 and 16 cover this information in detail. When compiling prognosis factors for this chapter, the author reviewed many crash studies, held discussions with

other treating physicians, evaluated articles and books on clinical experience, and used personal observations of a patient base of approximately 800 motor vehicle collision injury (MVCI) cases over the past 10-year period.

PROGNOSTIC LITERATURE REVIEW

Several resources are available to determine whether MVCIs result in prolonged symptoms. These include insurance company studies, clinical research, automotive crash studies, and epidemiologic research. Numerous studies have been published that evaluated a MVCI group over time to determine the percentage of patients with initial injury complaints who subsequently had symptoms. At a specified time after the initial injury, anywhere from 6 months to 15 years later, the occupants' symptoms and other clinical findings were reassessed. Every study from 1980 to 1994 that was reviewed showed significant numbers of occupants having long-term symptoms of some type. Of the 32 studies found, the average percentage of persons having long-term persistent symptoms was about 40%. Table 11–1 shows such studies from 1980

Table 11–1 Prognosis for Automotive Collision Injuries (1980–1994)*

Authors	Study Year	Study Size (n)	Study Period	% Having Long-Term Symptoms	Where Study Done	Type of Crash
Balla[1]	1980	300	6 mo–2 y	40–73	Australia	Mixed
Ebelin et al.[2]	1981	61	10 y	62	UK	Rear
Norris and Watt[3]	1983	61	2 y	37–90	UK	Rear
Balla[4]	1984	5000	>6 mo	27	Canada	Mixed
Larder et al.[5]	1985	53	>6 mo	8	UK	Mixed
Deans[6]	1986	137	1–2 y	20–34	N Ireland	Mixed
Galasko et al.[7]	1986	695	6 mo	24	UK	Mixed
Gore et al.[8]	1987	205	15± 5 y	32	USA	Mixed
Maimaris et al.[9]	1988	102	2 y	26–89	UK	Mixed
Su and Su[10]	1988	55	>6 mo	25	USA	Mixed
Miles et al.[11]	1988	73	2 y	28	UK	Mixed
McNamara et al.[12]	1988	351	25 ± 20 wk	43	USA	Mixed
McKinney[13]	1989	247	2 y	23–46	N Ireland	Mixed
Dvorak et al.[14]	1989	207	4–7 y	24	Switzerland	Mixed
Hodgson and Grundy[15]	1989	40	10–15 y	62	UK	Mixed
Pearce[16]	1989	100	1 y	35–100	USA	Mixed
Gargan and Bannister[17]	1990	61	10 y	88	UK	Rear
Olsson et al.[18]	1990	33	>1 y	36	Sweden	Rear
Hildingsson and Toolanen[19]	1990	93	2 y avg	58	Sweden	Mixed
Tunbridge et al.[20]	1990	333	1 y	44	UK	Mixed
Watkinson et al.[21]	1991	35	10.8 y	86	UK	Rear
Radanov et al.[22]	1991	78	6 mo	35	Switzerland	Mixed
Kischka et al.[23]	1991	56	2 y	44	Switzerland	Mixed
Pennie and Agambar[24]	1991	151	5 mo	13	UK	Mixed
Burgess[25]	1991	100	1 y	12–22	USA	Mixed
Cornes[26]	1992	521	2 y	71	UK	Mixed
Dies and Strapp[27]	1992	149	1–10 y	40	Canada	Mixed
Borchgrevink and Lereim[28]	1992	139	>60 mo	63	Norway	Rear
Parmar and Raymakers[29]	1993	100	1–3 y	18–44	UK	Rear
Robinson and Cassar-Pullicino[30]	1993	21	13.5 y	86	UK	Mixed
Radanov et al.[31]	1993	117	6 mo	27	Switzerland	Rear
Radanov et al.[32]	1994	117	1 y	24	Switzerland	Rear

*Summary of 32 studies performed for 6 months to 15 years and published from 1980 to 1994 demonstrating that about 43% of all MVCI patients will develop chronic disorders.

to 1994. Although this chapter does not cover pre-1980 literature, consistent data were found from the 1950s through the 1970s. These averages do not take into account issues such as gender, age, collision vector, and other human and crash variables. Another method of determining whether MVCI results in long-term pain is to look at studies published by chronic pain centers and note the percentages of those patients who had trauma from car crashes as the precipitating event. A third valuable resource, although not as scientific when each opinion is considered individually, involves the numerous clinical editorials on neck pain and trauma, headaches, extremity pain, and head injury. The consensus of opinion in clinical research confirms the specific studies that follow patients over time.

STUDIES COMPARING SPECIFIC INITIAL AND CHRONIC SYMPTOMS

To understand the complexity of Table 11–1 it may help the reader to review the percentages of specific types of symptoms that MVCI patients have initially and then compare them with symptoms found in chronic studies. Of interest is that some complaints, such as headaches and upper-extremity symptoms, are under-reported in the initial findings because of their common delays in onset. Tables 11–2 and 11–3 illustrate the types of symptoms that arise initially and then develop into chronic syndromes. When comparing these two tables, we find that upper-extremity radiating symptoms do not appear in some patients until several months after injury.

NECK INJURY PROGNOSIS

Many authors have concluded from clinical experience that patients having mild (AIS-1) neck injuries continue to have significant long-term pain and/or disability following car crashes.[6,12,34–51] A recent study by Radanov et al.[48] of 51 patients averaging 27 months postinjury found that two different syndromes often develop: (1) the cervico-encephalic syndrome, and (2) the lower cervical spine syndrome. In addition, several studies of chronic, intractable neck pain show that for 69% to 89% of these patients a motor vehicle crash or an industrial injury was the precipitating event.[34,52]

COMPARISON OF NECK PAIN IN MVCI AND GENERAL POPULATIONS

There are two methods of looking at the prevalence of neck pain in the population. First, compare the MVCI population with control groups, the population not involved in a previous auto crash; second, look at the incidence of neck pain in control groups, studies of the general population not having a prior history of automobile crashes, with reports of 7.2%[53] to 8%.[17] Another study looks at the percentage of people in the entire population having neck pain, with auto accidents mixed into the studies. The incidences of neck pain in the population reported were 13.5% for women and 9.5% for men.[54] A recent report (44 patients 8 to 12 years after MVCI) compares these groups.[55] The researchers found that the subjects in the control group reported symptoms as follows: neck pain, 8%; paresthesia, 2.5%; back pain, 24%; simultaneous neck and back pain, 1%; and occipital headaches, 2.5%. Eight to 12 years after injury, the MVCI group was compared with the control: 83% reported neck pain, 41% reported paresthesia, 27% reported back pain, 32% reported neck and back pain, and 27% reported occipital headaches.

MILD HEAD INJURY PROGNOSIS

Kay[56] defines mild head injury (MHI) as trauma in which the head is struck or moves violently, resulting in a transient alteration of consciousness for which the person typically is discharged with no formal treatment program. The term *mild head injury* refers to persons having initial Glasgow Coma Scale scores of 13 to 15 without subsequent neurologic deterioration, and excludes those with skull fractures, intracranial hematomas, and neurosurgical pathology.[57] The MHI involves (1) less than 30 minutes of loss of consciousness, (2) any loss or memory (less than 24 hours) before or after the crash (anterograde or retrograde amnesia), and (3) any indication of altered mental status immediately follow-

Table 11-2 Percentages of Patients Having Initial Symptoms following MVCI

Authors	Study Year	Neck Pain (%)	Neck Stiffness (%)	Headache (%)	Shoulder and Interscapular Pain (%)	Lumbar Pain (%)	Arm Symptoms (%)	Visual and Auditory Symptoms (%)*	Dizziness (%)	Fatigue or Weakness (%)
Ebelin et al.[2]	1981	45	37	37			16	9–14	16	
Norris and Watt[3]	1983	100		48–80			43	7–30		
Gore et al.[8]	1987	92		37	54					
Maimaris et al.[9]	1988	100	86	63	49		6			
Dvorak et al.[14]	1989	90			75	45	50			
Hildingsson and Toolanen[19]	1990	82	64	50	37		13	4–8		
Kischka et al.[23]	1991									37
Radanov et al.[31]	1993			80			16	21		
Dies and Strapp[27]	1992	49		36		40	10.7	5.4		
Average %		**80**	**65**	**52**	**54**	**43**	**22**	**13**		

*Visual symptoms include blurry vision and diplopia. Auditory symptoms include tinnitus and loss of hearing.

Table 11–3 Percentages of Patients Having Chronic Symptoms following MVCI

Authors	Study Year	Neck Pain (%)	Neck Stiffness (%)	Headache (%)	Shoulder and Interscapular Pain (%)	Lumbar Pain (%)	Arm Symptoms (%)	Visual and Auditory Symptoms (%)*	Dizziness (%)	Fatigue or Weakness (%)
Ebelin et al.[2]	1981	73	60	60			26	23–26	26	
Balla[4]	1984	98	85	97			39			
Gore et al.[8]	1987	50		23	38		25			
Maimaris et al.[9]	1988	89	40	26	66		40			
Pearce[16]	1989	100	78	43			35		15	
Gargan and Bannister[17]	1990	74		33		42	45	2–14	19	
Hildingsson and Toolanen[19]	1990	27	23	14	16	25	8	10		
Kischka et al.[23]	1991	44		61						
Oosterveld et al.[33]	1991	92		87	16	34	90	43	4	
Watkinson et al.[21]	1991	75		17		34	51	7		12
Average %		**72**	**57**	**46**	**34**	**34**	**40**	**19**	**13**	

*Visual symptoms include blurry vision and diplopia. Auditory symptoms include tinnitus and loss of hearing.

ing the crash (feeling dazed, disoriented, or confused).[58] A concussion has been described as a neurobehavioral reaction to a traumatic brain injury that is followed by lack of a demonstrable focal neurologic deficit and a clinical course of apparent recovery.[58]

The postconcussion syndrome (PCS) following an automotive crash for the purpose of this book refers to a large number of single or multiple symptoms that persist beyond 3 months after head injury. The patient must exhibit the classic symptoms seen in Table 11–3. Even with head injuries in which no loss of consciousness was documented, long-term deficits may result.[56] The authors suggest that all persons hitting their heads in car crashes have had a concussion until it is ruled out. Both concussion and the postconcussion syndrome can occur in whiplash patients having no head impact, although collision speeds need to be 2 to 3 times higher to produce these injuries.

It is estimated that out of more than 300,000 annual MVCI-related head/brain injuries in the United States, about 60,000, or 20%, will have long-term impairment and disability.[59] A report by Alves[60] shows that a substantial proportion of adult patients, possibly as high as 50%, are at risk for posttraumatic syndrome at some time after minor head injury. The majority of all head injuries (concussions) are mild, but many patients nevertheless suffer long-lasting complaints.[35,56,60–71] A recent report by Luchter estimates that those people who suffer a partially disabling brain injury will have a 5-year reduction in life span and a 20% disability for the remaining life span. He estimates the total lost life span time to be 12.6 years.[59]

A significant number of MHI patients in one study did not return to previous levels of work, especially when the nature of the person's work was such that it required complex attention, creative thinking, learning, memory, and mental speed.[56] In a study by Rimel et al.[69] of 538 MHI patients who were gainfully employed before the MHI, 34% were still unemployed 3 months later. About 17%

reported difficulty with household chores and activities of daily living at 3 months after MHI.[69] Rimel et al.[69] believe that there are two significant factors for the high unemployment rates: (1) organic brain damage as evident in neuropsychologic testing demonstrating attention, concentration, memory, or judgment problems, and (2) psychologic (emotional stress) response to injury. Vocational dysfunction may include those who are unemployed following MHI. One area needing research is the number of MHI patients who stay employed, but lose advancement or are demoted to lesser jobs after MHI. Table 11–4 describes common symptoms after head injury.

When taking the history, it is important to involve the spouse or someone close to the MHI patient. The added insight may be useful. It has been reported that "significant others" indicate greater memory problems in MHI patients than the patients themselves, who either do not recognize or are unwilling to admit the memory deficits.[69]

COMMON LONG-TERM SYMPTOMS AFTER MVCI

A vast range of injuries and symptoms may present themselves after a car crash injury. A recent large consumer survey found that the most common (70.4%) and serious (27.3%) injuries were soft tissue neck and back strains and sprains.[77]

The extensive list of common MVCI-related symptoms reminds me somewhat of reading the *Physicians' Desk Reference* (*PDR*) for side effects of a medication. The diversity and unpredictability of these symptoms quickly confirm that there is no typical human in biomechanical, neurologic, or biochemical terms. Until proven otherwise, the physician should consider any of the following as legitimate problems that in fact have an organic basis. As pharmacists have reported over the years many diverse, consistent side effect symptoms, so have automotive and clinical studies shown consistent MVCI symptoms. Most doc-

Table 11-4 Percentages of Patients with Persistence of Symptoms following MHI

Authors	Study Year	Study Size (n)	Study Period	Headache (%)	Dizziness (%)	Memory Loss (%)	Cognitive Function Loss (%)	Visual Symptoms (%)*	Auditory Symptoms (%)†
Rimel et al.[69]	1981	424	3 mo	78		59			
Alves[60]	1986	1151	1 y	29	13	21		6	
Colohan et al.[72]	1986	1216	3 mo	41	26	22		9	
Edna and Cappelen[73]	1987	569	3–5 y	23	19	20	14		12
Schoenhuber et al.[74]	1988	103	1 y	34	21	44	30		13
Yarnell and Rossie[71]	1988	27	>1 y				85		
Leininger et al.[75]	1990	53	1–2 y				32–78		
Kischka et al.[23]	1991	52	2 y		72		50	38	
Radanov et al.[48]	1992	51	27 mo			50	73	33	
Uomoto and Esselman[76]	1993	104	26 mo	89					

* Visual symptoms include blurry vision and diplopia.
† Auditory symptoms include tinnitus or hearing loss.

tors do not assume that a side effect of a drug (consistent with *PDR*) is based on monetary gain. If most MVCI cases were based on financial gain, why does the literature consistently find that patients in rear-end crashes have more pain and disability than any other vector of crash?

Significant numbers of MVCI patients have experienced long-term effects on their work status and leisure activities. One retrospective study of more than 5000 MVCI patients concludes that about 25% of these patients develop chronic disability of some type.[78] Hodgson and Grundy showed that in patients who had continued symptoms 12 years after MVCI, 44% had permanently changed their jobs to lighter work, and 62.5% had modified their leisure activities.[15] Another study of 93 patients injured in car crashes found that 43% had discomfort sufficient enough to interfere with their capacity to work an average of 2 years after injury.[19]

Common Chronic Symptoms

- Neck pain and stiffness
- Headaches and migraines (all types)
- Arm pain or paresthesias
- Interscapular pain
- Low back and hip pain
- Myofascial pain syndrome
- Myofascial trigger points
- Thoracic outlet syndrome
- Intercostal pain and subscapular pain
- Shoulder pain
- Dizziness
- Visual and auditory symptoms
- Temporomandibular joint pain
- Upper- and lower-extremity joint pain and stiffness
- Carpal tunnel syndrome
- Double crush syndrome
- Fatigue
- Cervical and lumbar disc bulging with compression symptoms

- Cognitive and memory difficulties (postconcussion syndrome)

Less Common Chronic Symptoms

- Guillain-Barré syndrome
- Other cranial nerve syndromes
- Reflex sympathetic dystrophy
- Posttraumatic seizures or tremors
- Posttraumatic stress disorders
- Horner's syndrome

STABILIZATION OF INJURY SYMPTOMS

There are varied opinions as to when most MVCI patients' symptoms become stable and they have reached maximal therapeutic recovery. Patients will experience most of the symptom improvement within 3 to 4 months after injury and then will taper off with a slower, gradual lessening of symptoms until their conditions stabilize at about 6 months to 1 year. "Viewed simplistically, the outcome for an individual patient is dichotomous: either the neck pain will resolve in the first few months, or it will persist indefinitely."[79] Bannister and Gargan[80] conclude in their review of the literature "that the vast majority of patients reach their final state within a year." See Chapter 10 for more information.

DETERMINING PROGNOSIS

Prognosis is best determined after observing the patient's response to treatment and time, usually 3 to 6 months after injury or when the symptoms have stabilized. The patient's pre-existing physical and psychologic condition, pain sensitivity, and reparative capability also must be considered. A multidimensional disability questionnaire, as seen in Chapter 10, is useful in correlating all factors that may lead to the injured person's inability to return to preinjury home and work status.

Prognosis is determined by doing or evaluating the following:

- Correlation of history of incident and crash factors
- A detailed symptom questionnaire filled out by the patient
- Clinical assessment of types of chronic symptoms
- Examinations and radiologic and special tests to confirm opinion
- Correlation of pertinent literature, as well as clinical experience
- The patient's motivation to return to work and home/social activities, the patient's educational level, and resources available

INFLUENCE OF LITIGATION ON PROGNOSIS

At issue is whether pending litigation or settlement has any influence on prognosis. The majority of patients entering litigation do, in fact, have organic, anatomic, and physiologic causes for their chronic pain, rather than a neurotic basis, even though few objective findings exist to substantiate pain. The vast majority of MVCI prognostic studies show that litigation does not have a significant effect on the degree or frequency of long-term postsettlement disability or other related symptoms.[3,15,80,81] One excellent review of medical literature, evaluating 18 prognostic studies, concluded that only three studies favor the view that claimants improve after settlement.[82] Hodgson and Grundy make a valid point: if litigation is a factor, why are patients involved in rear-end crashes so much more highly symptomatic than those involved in frontal and side crashes?[15]

Unlike neck injury, there is more debate about MHI prognosis. Many of the conflicting perceptions of head injury in our society stem from the movie industry and have profound effects on juries, attorneys, and doctors. The mythologic portrayal in the movies, that most people return to life as it was before the blow on the head, creates an unrealistic viewpoint. However, most recent scientific research shows that litigation and compensation have only a slight role in the persistence of these MHI symptoms.[69] Fee and Rutherford[83] in their pre- and postsettlement study found that there was only a small further improvement (5%) among patients 1 year after settlement.

DELAYS IN ONSET OR WORSENING OF SYMPTOMS OVER TIME

It is common for upper-extremity symptoms or headaches to start several weeks or months after trauma. The delays in upper-extremity paresthesias are often due to the classic nature of thoracic outlet syndrome. Balla and Karnaghan[78] report that 14% of whiplash headaches have onset beyond 1 week, and Radanov et al.[48] report that 29% of patients have onset of neck pain within a few days. These delays frequently account for some of the problems encountered when interpreting studies that document patients' prognosis.

Many patients continue to suffer the same, or lessened, symptom severity as experienced at the original injury, but some studies show that in some MVCI cases the postinjury symptoms worsen over time. A recent 10.8 year follow-up study concludes that 23% had worse or more intrusive symptoms.[21] Most of the symptoms that worsen over time include the upper-extremity referring symptoms, headaches, and the failed back syndromes. Several possibilities account for the increase in severity. In contrast to those who believe that most MVCI claims stem from seeking financial gain, there is more evidence supporting the opposite findings—many patients get worse. The worsening of complaints may be due to chronic musculoskeletal biomechanical dysfunction, myofascial trigger point syndromes, acquired hypersensitivity, or psychologic factors. To date there is no study that evaluates this issue.

INJURY SEVERITY CORRELATING TO CHRONIC PAIN

In many cases the initial injury severity can be correlated to the development of chronic pain. This is frequently seen in neck injury studies, which relate more severe injuries to more severe symptoms at a later date. However, this correlation does not apply to all types of symptoms that either commonly have onset delays or may have inverse relationships between injury severity and symptom frequency and/or severity. Headaches are the most common symptom after head injury that persists in follow-up studies. A recent study[76] compared the frequency of headaches after mild head injuries with the frequency after moderate and severe head injuries; the study found that the mild head injury group had more severe symptoms than the moderate/severe head injury group (Figure 11–1). There appears to be an *inverse relationship* between headaches and injury severity.

FACTORS THAT AFFECT MUSCULOSKELETAL INJURY PROGNOSIS

Several significant factors that play a role in the prognosis for postcollision neck injuries have been documented in the literature. The following lists are based on automotive research and clinical studies, as well as the author's clinical experience. These variables are categorized into factors that influence injury and prognosis before the crash takes place; factors during the crash, such as the car interior or type of crash; and events after the injury. Figure 11–2 illustrates several variables that may benefit or harm MVCI prognosis.

Precrash Prognostic Factors

- Female gender[50,80,84]
- Occupant age over 50 to 65[80,85–87]
- Cumulative effects of previous whiplash injury[50]

- History of head injury and headaches[32]
- Prior cervical spine fusion[88]
- Seating position. Ebelin et al.[2] found that 72% of drivers and 42% of passengers developed chronic symptoms.
- Occupant in a minicar or subcompact[89]
- Horizonal distance between head restraint and occupant's head, 12% having neck symptoms over 1 year if distance is less than 10 cm and 67% if distance is 10 cm or more[18]
- Pre-existing degenerative changes shown on X-ray[3,11,14,21,50,88,90]; reversal of neck curve[3,23,84,88]
- Alcohol intoxication[91,92]
- Cigarette smoking.[54,93] One study showed that smoking 1 year prior to onset of symptoms increases the incidence of prolapsed cervical disc. Each added 10 cigarettes per day prior to onset increases risk by about 30%.[93]

Crash Prognostic Factors

- Low or absent head restraints in rear-end collisions[18]
- Involvement in a rear-end crash.[3,15,18,46,50,53,94–96] Otremski et al.[97] found that the highest incidence of neck pain occurred in middle-aged women wearing a seat belt, in the front seat, and subjected to a rear-end crash.
- Wearing a seat belt[50,53,88]

Postcrash Prognostic Factors

- Early radicular symptoms[3,9,18,32,42,84]; early symptoms other than neck pain[21]; initial loss of consciousness[50]; arm numbness and pain later in time[50]; thoracic and lumbar pain[80]
- Severe injury[32] or severe pain initially[8,32]
- Interscapular pain at the time of the first examination; about 30% of these patients will experience long-term pain[9,42]

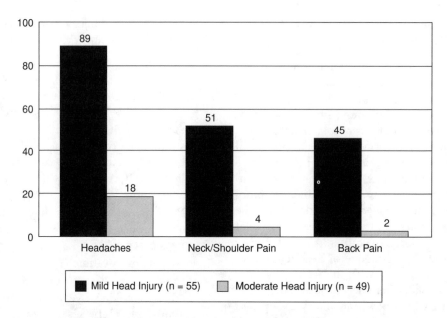

Figure 11–1 Inverse relationship between head injury severity and the development of posttraumatic pain. *Source:* Data from Uomoto, J.M., and Esselman, P., Traumatic Brain Injury and Chronic Pain: Differential Types and Rates by Head Injury Severity, *Archives of Physical Medicine and Rehabilitation*, January 1993, pp. 61–64, American Congress of Rehabilitation Medicine, 1993.

- Early sleep disturbances[32]
- Prior history of head trauma or pretraumatic headaches[32]
- Delay in appropriate treatment; need to resume treatment for more than one flare-up of pain[42,84]
- Collar use for more than 2 weeks[42,50]
- Symptoms persisting beyond 6 to 12 months[9,80]
- Psychosocial factors may have no effect on recovery.[80] The study by Radanov et al. of 78 whiplash patients for 6 months found that psychosocial factors had little role in the recovery from these injuries.[48]
- Clinically significant nutritional or endocrine disorders, e.g., diabetes

FACTORS THAT AFFECT MHI PROGNOSIS

Several factors have been implicated for prolonging MHI symptoms and affecting long-term prognosis, including those listed below:

Precrash MHI Prognostic Factors

- Intoxication at time of crash[63]
- Female gender[57,73]
- Low socioeconomic status[63]
- Repeated head injury[57]
- Occupants over age 40[57]
- Less reserve capacity of brain[98]
- Preinjury psychologic disorders[98]

Postcrash MHI Prognostic Factors

- Injury severity
- Management strategies that include family and work education and support[99]
- Persistence of symptoms beyond 3 months[60]
- Smoking and alcohol consumption after MHI[63]

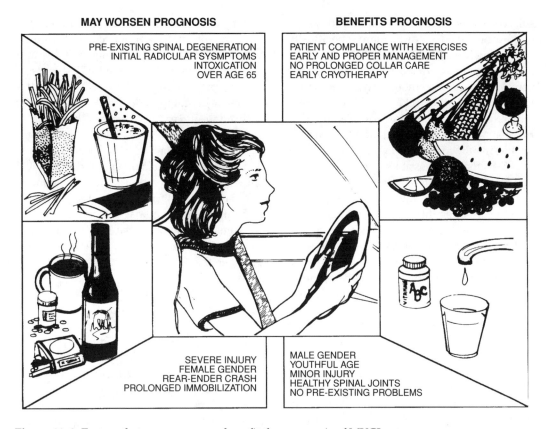

MAY WORSEN PROGNOSIS

PRE-EXISTING SPINAL DEGENERATION
INITIAL RADICULAR SYSMPTOMS
INTOXICATION
OVER AGE 65

SEVERE INJURY
FEMALE GENDER
REAR-ENDER CRASH
PROLONGED IMMOBILIZATION

BENEFITS PROGNOSIS

PATIENT COMPLIANCE WITH EXERCISES
EARLY AND PROPER MANAGEMENT
NO PROLONGED COLLAR CARE
EARLY CRYOTHERAPY

MALE GENDER
YOUTHFUL AGE
MINOR INJURY
HEALTHY SPINAL JOINTS
NO PRE-EXISTING PROBLEMS

Figure 11–2 Factors that may worsen or benefit the prognosis of MVCI cases.

- Only a slight role shown by pending litigation and postlitigation studies[69,83]
- Time off work[100]
- Emotional stress caused by persistent symptoms

TYPES OF DYSFUNCTIONAL DISORDERS SEEN IN MVCI VICTIMS

Four major functional areas are involved in the development of chronic symptoms after MVCI: (1) the neuromusculoskeletal system, which is affected by neck pain, headaches, nerve compression syndromes, and the like; (2) the cognitive system, which is affected by symptoms typical of the postconcussion syndrome (see Chapter 1); (3) the psychologic system, which can suffer anxiety and depression; and (4) employment and social interaction ability systems. When documenting persisting symptoms in the patient progress records or narrative reports, the physician must consider the interaction or overlap of any of these systems. For patients having head injury, by direct impact or by inertial loading, the reader should refer to Chapter 1 under postconcussional syndromes for further clarification. A large insurance company MVCI study concludes that the highest frequency of disability to an individual body region was found among rear-seat passengers with injuries to the thoracolumbar spine, about 21% having permanent disability.[68]

EFFECT OF SPINAL INJURY ON DEGENERATIVE JOINT CHANGES

Spinal injury and its potentiating effect on early synovial joint degeneration have been subjects of much debate over the decades. Several authors and studies, many specifically addressing MVCI, have concluded from either clinical experience or postinjury studies that spinal injury may promote early degenerative joint changes in the neck.[21,36,38] There are long-term effects of neck and lower-extremity injuries that do not become evident until years after the insult, for example, osteoarthritis.[101] Pike feels that one possible long-term sequela to spine joint injury is a higher incidence of arthritis, which may manifest itself as pain for many years after the injury.[102] Schmidek believes that neck trauma damages the disc,[103] and that once the disc is damaged, alterations may progress into the surrounding tissues. Jeffreys and McSweeney believe that annular tears from hyperextension neck injuries may predispose the cervical disc to degeneration, prolapse, and (later) osteophytes.[90] Another study concludes that decreased disc space may cause alteration in the biomechanics of facet joints, changing their motion, contact surface area, and pressures, and eventually leading to degenerative changes. Oegema and Bradford[104] also conclude that minimal disc narrowing over prolonged periods of time leads to osteoarthritis of the facets.

A recent radiologic study concludes that patients who had experienced neck trauma and had normal X-ray findings initially, and who underwent comparative X-ray studies an average of 15 years later, had 65% degenerative changes, compared with 49% for patients with nontraumatic neck pain.[8] Watkinson et al. performed a 10.8 year average postinjury study showing that 68% of follow-up cases had degenerative changes in the cervical spine, significantly more than the control population.[21] Brower concludes that the larger bridging marginal spinal osteophytes are often seen in postinjury cases.[105] Another author feels that if osteoarthritis is seen in persons younger than age 40, trauma is usually related.[106]

It seems that there is little disagreement about lower-extremity traumatic arthritis, but when the area of the spine comes into focus, many find it more difficult to quantify because spinal degeneration usually has slower progression and is more difficult to assess. Another major problem is simply a lack of studies comparing large, normal populations with post–MVCI groups. Most cases are settled before degenerative changes can be discerned by X-ray examination.

REFERENCES

1. Balla JI. The late whiplash syndrome. *Aust N Z J Surg.* 1980;50:610–614.
2. Ebelin M, Furno P, Patel A. Functional sequelae of benign cervical spine sprains from whiplash injuries: report on 61 cases. *J Traumatol.* 1981;2:77–81.
3. Norris SH, Watt I. The prognosis of neck injuries resulting from rear-end vehicle collisions. *J Bone Joint Surg [Br].* 1983;65:608–611.
4. Balla JI. Report to the Motor Accidents Board of Victoria on whiplash injuries. Victoria, Australia; 1984.
5. Larder DR, Twiss MK, Mackay GM. Neck injury to car occupants using seat belts. In: Proceedings of the 29th Annual Conference of the Association for the Advancement of Automotive Medicine; Washington, DC; 1985:153–165.
6. Deans GT. Incidence and duration of neck pain among patients injured in car accidents. *Br Med J.* 1986;292:94–95.
7. Galasko CSB, Murray P, Hodson M, et al. Long-term disability following road traffic accidents. Transport and Road Research Laboratory. Washington, DC: Department of Transportation. Research report 59; 1986.
8. Gore DR, Sepic SB, Gardner GM, et al. Neck pain: a long-term follow-up of 205 patients. *Spine.* 1987;12:1–5.
9. Maimaris C, Barnes MR, Allen MJ: Whiplash injuries of the neck: a retrospective study. *Injury.* 1988;19:393–396.
10. Su HC, Su RK. Treatment of whiplash injuries with acupuncture. *Clin J Pain.* 1988;4:233–247.
11. Miles KA, Maimaris C, Finlay D, et al. The incidence and prognostic significance of radiological

abnormalities in soft tissue injuries to the cervical spine. *Skeletal Radiol.* 1988;17:493–496.

12. McNamara RM, O'Brien MC, Davidheiser S. Post-traumatic neck pain: prospective and follow-up study. *Ann Emerg Med.* 1988;17:906–911.

13. McKinney LA. Early mobilisation and outcome in acute sprains of the neck. *Br Med J.* 1989;299:1006–1008.

14. Dvorak J, Valach L, St Schmid. Cervical spine injuries in Switzerland. *J Manual Med.* 1989;4:7–16.

15. Hodgson SP, Grundy M. Whiplash injuries: their long-term prognosis and its relationship to compensation. *Neuro-orthopedics.* 1989;7:88–91.

16. Pearce JMS: Whiplash injury: a reappraisal. *J Neurol Psychiatry.* 1989;2:1329–1331.

17. Gargan MF, Bannister GC. Long term prognosis of soft tissue injuries of the neck. *J Bone Joint Surg.* September 1990:901–903.

18. Olsson I, Bunkertorp O, Carlsson G, et al. An in depth study of neck injuries in rear end collisions. In: Proceedings of the International Research Committee on Biomechanics of Impacts, Bron, France; 1990:269–280.

19. Hildingsson C, Toolanen G. Outcome after soft-tissue injury of the cervical spine: a prospective study of 93 car-accident victims. *Acta Orthop Scand.* 1990;61:357–359.

20. Tunbridge RJ, Murray PA, Kinsella AM, et al. *The Cost of Long-Term Disability Resulting from Road Traffic Accidents: Interim Report.* Transport and Road Research Laboratory, Report 212. London: Her Majesty's Stationary Office; 1990.

21. Watkinson A, Cargan MF, Bannister GC. Prognostic factors in soft tissue injuries of the cervical spine. *Injury.* 1991;22:307–309.

22. Radanov BP, DiStefano G, Schnidrig A, et al. Role of psychosocial stress in recovery from common whiplash. *Lancet.* 1991;338:712–715.

23. Kischka U, Ettlin R, Heim S, et al. Cerebral symptoms following whiplash injury. *Eur Neurol.* 1991;31:136–140.

24. Pennie B, Agambar L. Patterns of injury and recovery in whiplash. *Injury.* 1991;22:57–59.

25. Burgess J. Symptom characteristics in TMD patients reporting blunt trauma and/or whiplash injury. *J Craniomandib Disord.* 1991;5:251–257.

26. Cornes P. Return to work of road accident victims claiming compensation for personal injury. *Injury.* 1992;23:256–260.

27. Dies S, Strapp JW. Chiropractic treatment of patients in motor vehicle accidents: a statistical analysis. *J Can Chiro Assn.* 1992;36:139–145.

28. Borchgrevink GE, Lereim I. Symptoms of patients with neck injury after a car crash. *Tidsskr Nor Laegeforen.* 1992;112:884–886.

29. Parmar HV, Raymakers R. Neck injuries from rear impact road traffic accidents: prognosis in persons seeking compensation. *Injury.* 1993; 24:75–78.

30. Robinson DD, Cassar-Pullicino VN. Acute neck sprain after road traffic accident: a long term clinical and radiological review. *Injury.* 1993; 24:79–82.

31. Radanov BP, Sturzenegger M, De Stefano G, et al. Factors influencing recovery from headache after common whiplash. *Br Med J.* 1993;307:652–655.

32. Radanov BP, Sturzenegger M, De Stefano G, et al. Relationship between early somatic, radiological, cognitive and psychosocial findings and outcome during a one-year follow-up in 117 patients suffering from common whiplash. *Br J Rheumatol.* 1994;33:442–448.

33. Oosterveld WJ, Kortshot HW, Kingma HA, et al. Electronystagmographic findings following cervical whiplash. *Acta Otolaryngol (Stockh).* 1991; 402:201–205.

34. Abbott P, Rounsefell B, Fraser R, et al. Intractable neck pain. *Clin J Pain.* 1990;6:26–31.

35. Aldman B. An analytical approach to the impact biomechanics of head and neck injury. In: Proceedings of the 30th Annual Conference of the Association for the Advancement of Automotive Medicine; Montreal; 1986:439–454.

36. Ameis A. Cervical whiplash: considerations in the rehabilitation of cervical myofascial injury. *Can Fam Physician.* 1986;32:1871–1876.

37. Dooley JA. Psychological impact of chronic pain and disability resulting from motor vehicle accidents. In: *Crash Injury Impairment and Disability: Long Term Effects.* International Congress and Exposition; paper 860503. Detroit, Mich: Society of Automotive Engineers; 1986:81–85.

38. Dunn EJ, Blazar S. Soft-tissue injuries of the lower cervical spine: instructional course lectures. *Am Acad Orthop Surg.* 1987;36:499–512.

39. Foret-Bruno JY, Dauvilliers F, Tarriere C. Influence of the seat and head rest stiffness on the risk of cervical injuries in rear impact. In: Program of the 13th ESV Conference. Paris, France; 1991.

40. Gustafsson H, Nygren Å, Tingvall C. Rating system for serious consequences (RSC) due to traffic accidents risk of death or permanent disability. In: Proceedings of the 10th International Conference on Experimental Safety Vehicles, Oxford, UK; 1985.

41. Juhl M, Scemp KK. Cervical spine injuries: epidemiological investigation, medical, and social con-

sequences. In: Proceedings of the International Research Committee on Biokinetics of Impacts. Bron, France; 1981:49–58.

42. Kenna CJ. The whiplash syndrome: a general practitioner's viewpoint. *Aust Fam Physician.* 1984;13:256–258.

43. Lewis RC Jr. *Primary Care Orthopedics.* New York: Churchill-Livingstone, Inc; 1988.

44. MacNab I. Acceleration extension injuries of the cervical spine. In: Rothman RH, Simeone FA eds. *The Spine.* Philadelphia: WB Saunders; 1982:647–660.

45. McLean AJ, Simpson DA, Cain CMS, et al. *Head and Neck Injuries in Passenger Cars: A Review of the Literature.* NH & MRC Road Accident Research Unit, University of Adelaide, Report No CR 59. Adelaide, Australia: Federal Office of Road Safety; September 1987.

46. Nilsson S. *Injury Biomechanics.* Government/Industry Meeting and Exposition. Washington, DC: Society of Automotive Engineers; 1987; SP-731:25–26.

47. Nunn PJ, Greenwood MT. Whiplash syndrome: a transformational approach. In: *Pain* (suppl 5). Abstracts of the 6th World Congress on Pain. Adelaide, Australia: Elsevier Science Publishers BV; 1990.

48. Radanov BP, Dvorák J, Valach L. Cognitive deficits in patients after soft tissue injury of the cervical spine. *Spine.* 1992;17:127–131.

49. States JD. Discussion of "neck injury to car occupants using seat belts." In: Proceedings of the 29th Annual Conference of the Association for the Advancement of Automotive Medicine; Washington, DC; 1985:166–168.

50. Teasell RW, McCain GA. Clinical spectrum and management of whiplash injuries. In: Tollision DC, Satterthwaite JR, eds. *Painful Cervical Trauma: Diagnosis and Rehabilitative Treatment of Neuromusculoskeletal Injuries.* Baltimore: Williams & Wilkins; 1992.

51. Wickstrom J, LaRocca H. Head and neck injuries from acceleration-deceleration forces. In: Ruge D, Wiltse LL, eds. *Spinal Disorders, Diagnosis and Treatment.* Philadelphia: Lea & Febiger; 1977.

52. Rosomoff H, Fishbain D, Goldberg M, et al. Physical findings in patients with chronic intractable benign pain of the neck and/or back. *Pain.* 1989;37:279–287.

53. Deans GT, Magalliard JN, Kerr M, et al. Neck sprain: a major cause of disability following car accidents. *Injury.* 1987;18:10–12.

54. Mäkelä M, Heliövaara M, Sievers K, et al. Prevalence, determinants, and consequences of chronic pain in Finland. *Am J Epidemiol.* 1991;134:1356–1367.

55. Gargan MF, Bannister CG. The comparative effects of whiplash injuries. Presented at the British Cervical Spine Society Meeting, Bowness-on-Windermere; November 7, 1992.

56. Kay T. *Minor Head Injury: An Introduction for Professionals.* Framingham, Mass: National Head Injury Foundation; December 1986:1–12.

57. Evans RW. The postconcussion syndrome and the sequelae of mild head injury. *J Neurotrauma.* 1992;10:815–848.

58. Katz R, Deluca J. Sequela of minor traumatic brain injury. *Am Fam Physician.* November 1992:1491–1497.

59. Luchter S. Traffic related disabilities and impairments and their economic consequences. In: *Crash Injury Impairment and Disability: Long Term Effects.* International Congress and Exposition; paper 860505. Detroit, Mich: Society of Automotive Engineers; 1986; SP-661:93–113.

60. Alves WM. Motor vehicle head injury: damage and outcome. In: *Crash Injury Impairment and Disability: Long Term Effects.* International Congress and Exposition; paper 860423. Detroit, Mich: Society of Automotive Engineers; 1986; SP-661:167–176.

61. Alves WM, Colohan ART, O'Leary TJ, et al. Understanding posttraumatic symptoms after minor head injury. *J Head Trauma Rehabil.* 1986;1:1–12.

62. Auerbach SH. The postconcussive syndrome: formulating the problem. *Hosp Pract.* October 30, 1987:9–11.

63. Carlsson GS, Svärdsudd K, Welin L. Long-term effects of head injuries sustained during life in three male populations. *J Neurosurg.* 1987;67:197–205.

64. Cartlidge NEF, Shaw DA. *Head Injury.* Philadelphia: WB Saunders; 1981.

65. Gennarelli TA. *Mechanistic Approach to the Head Injuries: Clinical and Experimental Studies of the Important Types of Injury, Head and Neck Injury Criteria, A Consensus Workshop.* Washington, DC: US Government Printing Office; July 1983:20–25.

66. Gronwall D. Cumulative and persisting effects of concussion on attention and cognition. In: Levin HS, Eisenberg HM, Benton AL, eds. *Mild Head Injury.* New York: Oxford University Press; 1989: 153–162.

67. Jane J, Rimel RW, Pobereskyn LH, et al. Outcome and pathology of minor head injuries. In: Grossman R, ed. *Seminars in Neurologic Surgery.*

Proceedings of 4th Conference on Neurotrauma. New York: Raven Press; 1982.

68. Nygren Å. Injuries to car occupants—some aspects of the interior safety of cars: a study of a five-year material from an insurance company. *Acta Otolaryngol Suppl (Stockh).* 1984;395:1–164.

69. Rimel RW, Giordani B, Barth JT, et al. Disability caused by minor head injuries. *Neurosurgery.* 1981;9:221–228.

70. Siegel JH, Mason-Gonzalez S, Cushing BM, et al. A prospective study of injury patterns, outcomes, and costs of high speed frontal versus lateral motor vehicle crashes. In: Proceedings of the 34th Annual Conference of the Association for the Advancement of Automotive Medicine; Scottsdale, Ariz; 1990:289–313.

71. Yarnell PR, Rossie GV. Minor whiplash head injury with major debilitation. *Brain Injury.* 1988; 2(3):255–258.

72. Colohan ART, Dacey RG, Alves WM, et al. Neurologic and neurosurgical implications of mild head injury. *J Head Trauma Rehabil.* 1986;1:13–21.

73. Edna T-H, Cappelen J. Late postconcussional symptoms in traumatic head injury: an analysis of frequency and risk factors. *Acta Neurochir.* 1987;86:12–17.

74. Schoenhuber R, Gentilini M, Orlando A. Prognostic value of auditory brain-stem response for late postconcussion symptoms following minor head injury. *J Neurosurg.* 1988;68:742–744.

75. Leininger BE, Gramling SE, Farrell AD, et al. Neuropsychological deficits in symptomatic minor head injury patients after concussion and mild concussion. *J Neurol Neurosurg Psychiatry.* 1990;3:293–296.

76. Uomoto JM, Esselman P. Traumatic brain injury and chronic pain: differential types and rates by head injury severity. *Arch Phys Med Rehabil.* January 1993:61–64.

77. Insurance Research Council. *Paying for Auto Injuries: A Consumer Panel Survey of Auto Accident Victims.* Oak Brook, Ill: IRC; 1994.

78. Balla J, Karnaghan J. Whiplash headache. *Clin Exp Neurol.* 1987;23:179–182.

79. Barnsley L, Lord S, Bogduk N. The pathophysiology of whiplash. *Spine State Art Rev.* 1993;7:329–353.

80. Bannister G, Gargan M. Prognosis of whiplash injuries: a review of the literature. *Spine State Art Rev.* 1993;7:557-569.

81. Elkind AH. Headache and facial pain associated with head injury. *Otolaryngol Clin North Am.* 1989;22:1251–1271.

82. Mendelson G. Follow-up studies of personal injury litigants. *Int J Law Psychiatry.* 1984;7:179–188.

83. Fee CRA, Rutherford WH. A study of the effect of legal settlement on post-concussion symptoms. *Arch Emerg Med.* 1988;5:12–17.

84. Hohl M. Soft-Tissue Neck Injuries. In: Cervical Spine Research Society Editorial Committee. *The Cervical Spine.* Philadelphia: JB Lippincott Co; 1989:436–441.

85. Baker SP, O'Neill B, Karpf RS. *The Injury Fact Book.* Lexington, Mass: DC Heath and Co; 1985.

86. McGee DL, Rhodes P. Estimating trends in the effectiveness of seat belts in saving lives. *Stat Med.* 1989;8:379–385.

87. Pike JA. The elderly and vehicle-related injury. In: *Effects of Aging on Driver Performance.* paper 762, 881753. Warrendale, Pa: Society of Automotive Engineers; 1988.

88. Hirsch SA, Hirsch PJ, Hiramoto H, et al. Whiplash syndrome: fact or fiction? *Orthop Clin North Am.* 1988;19:791–795.

89. Cerrelli EC. Relative risk of fatal injury in vehicle to vehicle impacts involving cars of different sizes. In: Proceedings of the 29th Annual Conference of the Association for the Advancement of Automotive Medicine; Washington, DC; 1985: 199–212.

90. Jeffreys E, McSweeney T. *Disorders of the Cervical Spine.* London: Butterworth; 1980.

91. Fell JC, Hertz ES. The effects of blood alcohol concentration on time of death for fatal crash victims. In Proceedings of the 34th Annual Conference of the Association for the Advancement of Automotive Medicine; Scottsdale, Ariz; 1990:69–81.

92. Stewart JR. Estimating the effects over time of alcohol on injury severity. In: Proceedings of the 32nd Annual Conference of the Association for the Advancement of Automotive Medicine; Seattle, Wash; 1988:319–326.

93. Kelsey JL, Githens PB, Walter SD, et al. An epidemiological study of acute prolapsed cervical intervertebral disc. *J Bone Joint Surg [Am].* 1984; 66:907–914.

94. Addison RG. Cervical pain syndrome. In: Lipton S, et al, eds. *Advances in Pain Research and Therapy.* New York: Raven Press; 1990;13:227–230.

95. Dunsker SB. Hyperextension and hyperflexion injuries of the cervical spine. In: Dunsker SB, ed. *Cervical Spondylosis: Seminars in Neurological Surgery.* New York: Raven Press; 1981:135–144.

96. Patrick LM. Neck injury incidence, mechanisms and protection. In: Proceedings of the 31st Annual Conference of the Association for the Ad-

vancement of Automotive Medicine; New Orleans; 1987:409–431.

97. Otremski I, Marsh JL, Wilde BR, et al. Soft tissue cervical spinal injuries in motor vehicle accidents. *Injury*. 1989;20:349–351.

98. Binder LM. Persisting symptoms after mild head injury: a review of the postcussive syndrome. *J Clin Exp Neuropsychol*. 1986;8:323–346.

99. Levine AM. Minor head injury: a not so minor problem. *J Neurol Orthop Med Surg*. 1987;8:381–382.

100. Wrightson P, Gronwall D. Time off work and symptoms after minor head injury. *Injury*. 1981;12:445–454.

101. Aldman B, Mellander H, Mackay M. The structure of European research into the biomechanics of impacts. In: *27th Stapp Car Crash Conference Proceedings with International Research Committee on Biokinetics of Impacts*; paper 831610. San Diego, Calif: Society of Automotive Engineers; 1983:129–136.

102. Pike JA. *Automotive Safety: Anatomy, Injury, Testing, and Regulation*. Warrendale, Pa: Society of Automotive Engineers; 1990.

103. Schmidek HH. Cervical spondylosis. *Am Fam Physician*. 1986;33:89–99.

104. Oegema TR, Bradford DS. The inter-relationship of facet joint osteoarthritis and degenerative disc disease. *Br J Rheumatol*. 1991;30(suppl 1):16–20.

105. Brower AC. *Arthritis in Black and White*. Philadelphia: WB Saunders; 1988.

106. Altman RD. Osteoarthritis: differentiation from rheumatoid arthritis, causes of pain, treatment. *Postgrad Med*. 1990;87:66–78.

Chapter 12

Medicolegal Reports

Lawrence S. Nordhoff, Jr.

INTRODUCTION

Narrative reports are usually requested by the patient's attorney when the patient's status has stabilized or when treatment is concluded. The doctor or patient will usually notify the attorney that the case has reached the point where the patient is being released from active curative treatment. At the time of case closure, the patient usually has reached maximal medical improvement and has reached one of the following three status levels: he or she (1) has reached preinjury status with no residual symptoms, (2) has residual symptoms that are not ratable (less than 10%), or (3) has not returned to preinjury status and has ratable (≥10%) factors of disability. This legal report must be clear, concise, and easy to read. The insurance company and defense attorney will review the report and evaluate the case for its credibility. If the case looks weak because of a poor report or other factors, settlement may be delayed or the case might be settled for less than it was worth. It is suggested that only pertinent data be included in the report.

The concluding report is primarily for the legal benefit of the patient. The doctor should perform this medicolegal report in a timely manner. A timely report lets the attorney, the insurance company, and patient know that the doctor is concerned about the patient; once the report is finished, the attorney can immediately begin negotiations with the insurance company. The sooner the case is settled, the better. Once the legal case is concluded, the patient can return to normal life activities. As long as the case is open the patient has a constant focus on the pain or discomfort. Some doctors wait several months before completing the report. This delay is inconsiderate of the patient who is waiting for settlement. The personal injury (PI) practice is not for the doctor who hates writing reports.

TIPS IN WRITING REPORTS

The doctor should avoid using prognostic terms such as *fair*, *guarded*, or *poor*. These descriptive terms tell the insurance carrier or attorney nothing about the actual functional status of the injured person.

If the doctor wants to use medical literature to support his or her opinion, it is suggested that it be limited and as specific as possible.

Depositions and trials are the place where literature is more useful and can be a powerful tool to substantiate injury and treatment claims.

For the sake of keeping the paperwork simple and easy for the attorney to review, include only the positive examination findings. Most attorneys focus their attention on medical bills, diagnosis, and prognosis.

After page 1, each additional page should be numbered with the patient's name and date of injury (DOI).

BEGINNING THE REPORT PROCESS

The closing report should be initiated by the doctor once the patient's status has stabilized, usually 3 to 6 months after injury. By this time most doctors can evaluate a motor vehicle collision injury (MVCI) case, determine the level of pain, and quantify any residual objective and subjective findings. Since most PI cases take several months to process and negotiate, the patient who requires further supportive treatment can still be under care. A simple, short, updated report about any changes in the patient's status and any new opinions or factors influencing prognosis can be sent to the attorney 2 to 3 months later without impeding the negotiation process. In most cases the attorney will have a paralegal subpoena all medical and police records. Although medical literature currently shows that litigation does not significantly alter the long-term prognosis of posttraumatic pain, it does show that prolonged litigation can keep these patients focused on pain.

When the doctor feels that the patient's condition has stabilized, the author suggests that a letter should be sent to the attorney advising him or her that the case is closed, along with a brief notation about the patient's current symptom and treatment status and a request that the attorney begin the settlement process. A brief closing report of one to two pages can be offered for the cost of X dollars, or a more complex report of four to five pages for an additional cost of X dollars, payment due in advance. Many PI attorneys do not know what type of report to request. It is suggested that most uncomplicated cases that resolve with no ratable factors of disability be short reports. Complicated cases, those having residual ratable factors of disability such as severe myofascial pain syndromes, disc syndromes, or other forms of radiculopathies or neuropathies, should have longer reports. If the doctor's office has not received the attorney request for report within 2 weeks, the doctor's office should call the attorney to find out why delays are occurring. It is just as important for the attorney to do his or her job in a timely fashion.

A comprehensive report must allow the physician to be flexible and thorough. The following report is a sample of only one style. The author uses a variety of report styles, depending on the type of case, the prognosis, and settlement difficulties, and does not intend that all reports should follow this style. Generally, all reports should include all of the following information:

Report Identification

- Report heading from originating office
    1. Office name, office title, address, and phone number
    2. Doctor's state license number and tax ID number
- Name and address where report is being sent
- Patient's name
- Patient's age
- Date of first office visit and date of report
- Date of injury

Review of Prior Medical History, Account of Collision, and Injury History

- Pertinent prior medical and injury history

- History of crash and subsequent injury
- Review of prior records/tests/reports
- Review of prior treatment and whether beneficial
- Immediate postinjury patient complaints
- Symptoms patient felt 1 to 2 days later
- Presenting patient complaints

Examination Findings and Diagnosis

- Physical examination findings
- X-ray views taken and findings
- Initial diagnosis
- Special examination or testing
- Concluding diagnosis

Management Discussion

- Treatment methods used
- Appliance/brace use
- Exercise/stretching recommendations
- Patient recovery pattern
  1. Flare-ups
  2. Complicating recovery factors

Time Off Work during Course of Care

- List dates off work

Permanent Disability/Impairment

- Concluding subjective and objective findings
- Consistency among crash, concluding symptoms, and findings

- Permanent disability rating
  1. Apportionment issues
  2. Ratable factors of disability
  3. Concluding work, lifestyle, recreational, and social activity limitations

Prognosis

- Concluding diagnosis
- Prognosis
  1. List any crash factors influencing injury severity or correlating with poor prognosis.
  2. Note any pre-existing complicating human factors.
  3. List factors influencing recovery.
  4. List psychologic factors influencing recovery.
- Future management recommendations
  1. Future treatment and home/work recommendations or modifications (exercises/restrictions)
  2. Ergonomic changes at work and home
  3. Vocational retraining recommendations

With the Report, Be Sure To Send

- Two report originals, both signed
- Copies of all specialized testing reports
- Photos
- Current curriculum vitae of the doctor
- Glossary of nonstandard terminology

NARRATIVE REPORT

Dr. Brent Backbone
400 Neck Street, Suite 911
Pane, CA 90000 (000) 444-4444
SSN 900-90-9000
State Lic 000000

June 12, 1992

Report on Susie Jones

Report sent to:
Seymore Suits, Esq
911 Collision Valley Road
Pane, CA 90000

Patient name: Susie Jones
Patient age: 33
Date of injury: 11-28-91
Date of first office visit: 12-14-91

PERTINENT MEDICAL/OCCUPATIONAL HISTORY

The patient has a history of neck pain 5 years ago, when, she states, she had pain for 2 days after going on a roller coaster ride. The pain was mild in nature and resolved itself without any treatment. She has no history of any other neck pain, back pain, or injuries. She reports no significant illnesses, fractures, or surgeries. The patient's occupation at the time of injury was full-time secretary, for 5 years.

HISTORY OF INJURY

Ms. Susie Jones came into my office for an initial evaluation on 12-14-91. History, examination, and treatment were done at my office. She relayed the following information: On 11-28-91 she was driving a 1988 Toyota Corolla (compact size). She was stopped at a light with her foot on the brake. She relates that she had her head turned to the right talking to the front passenger in the car when, suddenly, and to her surprise, her car was hit from the rear. Her car was pushed into the middle of the intersection. Her head jerked rapidly backward and forward, hitting the steering wheel. The next thing she remembers is opening her eyes and seeing several people looking in her car, asking her if she was okay. She estimates that she blacked out for approximately 15 to 20 seconds. The head restraint was the movable type and was at its lowest position, around mid-neck in height, and about 6 inches back from the head. The vehicle that hit her was a large tow truck that was going approximately 25 mph, according to the police report.

REVIEW OF PRIOR TREATMENT AND TESTS

After the injury a Valley Regional ambulance took her to Valley Hospital, where the emergency department doctor had skull X-rays taken, did an examination, and released her home with pain pills and muscle relaxants. Review of the hospital records shows that she was advised by the emergency department doctor (Jack Smith, MD) that she had suffered a concussion, that she would probably be okay in 2 to 3 days, and if not to see her family doctor. X-rays included a skull series, and Dr. Cran, a radiologist, reported normal film results. The patient relates that the muscle relaxants made her too drowsy to work and she opted to stop taking them. She has had no other treatment since the crash. She was hoping that the pain would go away. Instead the pain has persisted and has gotten significantly worse in the past 2 days, which is why she then presented herself to this office.

IMMEDIATE POSTINJURY SYMPTOMS

Right after the accident on 11-28-91, the patient had the following complaints:

- Severe pain in the front of her head, where her head hit the steering wheel
- Moderate, constant dizziness/lightheadedness
- Severe neck stiffness

SYMPTOMS 24 TO 48 HOURS AFTER INJURY

- Severe, constant pain in the front of her head, where her head hit the steering wheel
- Slight, occasional dizziness/lightheadedness
- Severe neck pain and stiffness

CURRENT SYMPTOMS

- Severe, constant, right-sided neck pain that shoots sharp, stabbing pain down the right arm to the lower arm and fourth and fifth fingers. This symptom started 3 days after injury. She has occasional numbness in the right fourth and fifth fingers.
- Memory loss; loss of concentration ability; inability to handle multiple tasks
- Daily, severe, constant headaches, primarily in suboccipital and frontal regions. Recently, she has begun to feel head pain during all waking hours.
- Upper back pain, between shoulder blades; it hurts to breathe deeply.

PHYSICAL EXAMINATION FINDINGS

The physical examination was performed by Dr. Backbone on 12-14-91. Ms. Jones is 65 inches tall, weighs 122 lbs, and has a blood pressure of 124/82.

Neurologic Examination

Extremity sensory examination showed hypoesthesia in the right lower arm and right fourth and fifth fingers. Other neurologic tests were within normal limits.

Orthopedic Examination

Foraminal compression test was positive on the right side, making fingers numb, indicating right-sided nerve root compression. Arm abduction-relief test showed relief of arm numbness, indicating that the C-5 to C-6 nerve root is the most likely site of irritation, consistent with a disc bulge. Digitized cervical range-of-motion testing showed 25° of right lateral flexion with severe pain noted in middle to end ranges of motion, indicating a muscular and ligamentous component on the right side. The left side was 35°. Cervical rotation motion was limited to 60° on the right side, and 75° on the left. Neck flexion motion range was within normal limits, but she has moderate pain at end of motion in extension. Thoracic outlet syndrome tests were negative.

Palpation Examination

Palpation neck and upper back examination showed generalized muscle spasm on the entire right side of the neck to the T-3 to T-4 region. The muscle felt boggy and was very sensitive to pressure. The sternocleidomastoid muscle was very sore and boggy on the right side, and the following muscles were also sore: levator scapulae, anterior scalenes, trapezius, rhomboids, pectoralis minor, and pectoralis major. Right side of the neck motioning elicited a boggy end-feel, indicating fluid buildup within the joints and joint capsules.

Functional Capacity Testing

Multiple-region functional capacity testing was performed. This two-page form (see Chapter 10) modifies the Oswestry disability system for the car crash injury patient. The patient initially reported a 59% loss of functional capacity.

X-RAY FINDINGS

The patient had APOM, lateral, and flexion-extension cervical views and anteroposterior/lateral dorsal X-rays taken at my office. These films were sent out to a chiropractic radiologist for review. The X-ray report is enclosed. Findings include a moderate loss of cervical lordosis, a mild disruption of George's line between C-5 and C-6. Flexion-extension cervical stress views showed significant loss of joint motion when stressed in flexion in the C-4 to C-6 complex. All other findings were normal.

INITIAL DIAGNOSIS

- Mild concussion, healing
- Severe, constant, posttraumatic cervicalgia secondary to paraspinal muscle spasm and inflammatory responses to injury

- Subacute, severe cervical-dorsal sprain with attendant muscle spasm
- Early right arm radiculitis possibly due to C-5 to C-6 disc protrusion and C-6 nerve rootlet irritation
- Cephalgia secondary to suboccipital muscle strain and muscle spasm

SPECIAL TESTS

Because of the persistence of her pain and severity levels, special diagnostic tests were indicated. She was referred to Valley Diagnostics Center for magnetic resonance imaging (MRI) evaluation of the neck and nerve conduction velocities. See enclosed report. In summary, a moderate right disc bulge shown on MRI at the C-5 to C-6 level was found; this diagnosis was further confirmed by abnormal nerve conduction velocity findings at the same level.

TREATMENT

As a direct result of the motor vehicle collision injury, the above complaints required the following treatment for Ms. Jones. Her treatment began in the subacute stage of repair because there had been more than a 2-week delay of treatment from injury onset. Treatment consisted of neck and upper back paraspinal myotherapy, gentle soft tissue and spinal manipulation, and mobilization of restricted right-sided lower cervical joints. It also involved cryotherapy for 2 weeks at a frequency of two to four times a day, manual supine lower cervical spine traction beginning at the third week, and postural and exercise recommendations starting from the first week of treatment and progressively getting more demanding as her condition improved. She was advised to avoid any prolonged forward head bending for 2 to 3 months.

EXERCISE RECOMMENDATIONS

Exercise recommendations began during the first week of care and involved gentle, smooth, isotonic neck exercises in all neck motions in the pain-free level and range of motion. Initially the patient pushed against hand pressure four or five times a day for 2 to 3 minutes, but never into pain. These exercises led progressively to heavier loading. In addition she was shown how to do shoulder rolls and torso stretching and exercises using a Swiss exercise ball. Exercises progressed to heavy workouts three times a week and daily stretching routines.

PATIENT RECOVERY PATTERN

The patient responded to treatment slowly during the first 2 weeks of care, then rapidly made progress for the next 2 months. Starting at 3 months her symptoms began to taper, and very slight gradual improvement was noted. She had one flare-up of severe neck pain on 1-2-92 while she was brushing her hair, resulting in 2 weeks of intensive treatment, which resolved the pain. Weekly functional capacity tests and pain intensity forms were given to her for the first month and then biweekly afterward for 2 months so that I could measure her outcome responses to treatment and repair. Initially she had a 59% loss of functional capacity with a level 9 pain intensity. At the close of her case she had an 18% loss of functional capacity with a level 3 pain intensity.

TIME OFF WORK DURING COURSE OF CARE

The patient was able to work at full capacity during treatment of this injury except for two occasions: she took 2 days off, 11-29-91 and 11-30-91, and 3 days off, 1-2-92 to 1-4-92, during one painful flare-up. She is currently working full time at her same job. She has had some partial disability during the entire course of treatment. See below for details.

PERMANENT DISABILITY

There are no apportionment issues in this case. She had no prior related problems. There is consistency among her history of incident, symptoms, and examination findings. Her concluding symptoms and disability are consistent with those of my experience and the medical and automotive literature. Ms. Susie Jones has permanent ratable factors of disability that will affect her future home and work activity. It is reasonably certain that she will have future pain and disability solely from the residual musculoskeletal dysfunction she suffered in this motor vehicle collision.

Work Restrictions

After working at a computer for more than 45 minutes she can't feel the keys with her fingers. She frequently drops objects because of weakness in the fingers or loss of sensation. She estimates that she is able to keep her job only by working an average of 1½ hours extra per day. She is unable to maintain her previous typing speed. Neck pain frequently bothers her, but it is usually just an annoyance. One or two times a month the neck pain gets bad enough that she has to take Motrin to ease the pain.

Home Restrictions

She has difficulty doing tasks that require forward head bending, such as ironing, doing dishes, and vacuuming. It takes her twice as long to complete some household tasks, and she has to take frequent breaks.

Recreational Activity Restrictions

She was an active volleyball player before the injury, but has had to drop out of the sport entirely because of right hand weakness, difficulty feeling the ball, and difficulty lifting her hands over her head.

Social Activities

No changes in social activities have been noted.

PROGNOSIS

Concluding Diagnosis

- Residual intermittent, mild-to-moderate, neck pain secondary to healed myofibrosis of repair; posttraumatic cervical myofascial pain syndrome
- Dizziness, resolved
- Persistent, severe, posttraumatic headaches, three or four times a week, with associated trigger points in masseter, temporalis, anterior scalenes, and suboccipital muscles
- Persistent postconcussive syndrome, confirmed by three persistent classic postconcussion symptoms beyond 3 months (See second item under Current Symptoms.)
- Persistent right arm numbness and pain secondary to moderate right disc bulge shown on MRI at the C-5 to C-6 level; diagnosis further confirmed by abnormal nerve conduction velocity testing (MRI report and nerve conduction report are included.)
- Upper back pain, resolved

Factors That Complicated This Case

Several factors resulted in this patient's having this severe injury and having persisting symptoms and disability, and they include the following:

- She is female. Women have been shown in the automotive and medical literature to have significantly more injuries and worse prognoses in rear-end collisions than men do.
- She was unaware of the impending crash, so there was no time to brace herself. Recent literature slows that occupants who do not brace themselves at the time of impact are 15 times more likely to develop chronic neck problems than those who do brace themselves.[1]
- The head restraint was positioned abnormally low, which has been shown to worsen prognosis. The low head restraint allowed her head to move backward, up and over the head restraint, acting as a fulcrum, which caused the acceleration to be two or three times faster than if she had a high, fixed head restraint.
- Her head was turned at the time of collision, which adds a great amount of rotational injury to the cervical spine ligaments and disc fibers, causing worse annular disc tearing.
- Mass ratios between her car and the truck that struck her vehicle were of a magnitude to make injury extent worse.

FUTURE MANAGEMENT RECOMMENDATIONS

At this time her condition has stabilized with residual arm radiculopathy and headaches three or four times a week. She has been advised to continue exercises as previously shown on a daily basis. She has also been told to avoid prolonged forward head posture, to avoid carrying her purse on her shoulder, to avoid carrying heavy objects in her arms, and to take frequent breaks from her work. In my opinion, she will continue to have persistent long-term problems in her arm because of the residual damage and the fact that the symptoms are still severe 1 year after injury, indicating that further repair probably will be minimal if any. She wants to avoid surgery, but I told her that eventually she may have to undergo the procedure. She was advised of pathologic symptom changes about which she is to call me immediately, possibly alerting me to refer her to a surgeon. Examples of such changes are loss of bladder control and lower-extremity problems indicating cord involvement.

INCLUDED WITH THIS REPORT

- One original signed copy of the report
- Copies of all specialized test reports
- Current curriculum vitae of the doctor

If you have any questions about this patient's case or this report, please feel free to contact my office.

Sincerely,

Brent Backbone, DC

REFERENCE

1. Ryan GA, Moore VM, Dolinis J. Crash severity and neck strain in car occupants. In: International Conference on the Biomechanics of Impacts, Lyon, France; 1994.

Chapter 13

Going to Court?

Shawn Steel

TYPES OF AUTO INSURANCE COVERAGE

The Insurance Research Council reports on 1992 data from more than 61,934 insurance claims reported from 61 insurance carriers in the United States. As of 1992, 14 states had no-fault insurance laws.[1] Twenty-seven states are tort liability/fault states and nine states are add-on states (no-fault benefits added onto tort laws). Georgia and Nevada recently repeated their no-fault statutes because of its failure to lower insurance premiums. No-fault states use personal injury protection (PIP) coverage, whereas fault states use bodily injury (BI), MedPay, uninsured motorist, and underinsured motorist coverage. A 1989 report on uninsured motorists concludes that approximately 13% of all crashes involve uninsured motorists.[2] The number of injury claims per 1000 cars can vary dramatically between states.

ATTORNEY INVOLVEMENT IN THE UNITED STATES

A recent nationwide insurance study shows that about 42% to 46% of auto injury victims use attorneys in the United States.[1,3] Attorneys represent 31% of cases in states that use no-fault systems and 57% in bodily injury states.[1] It is known that the percentage of claimants using attorneys varies by the type of community (i.e., urban or rural) and by the state.[3] It is apparent that attorneys are used more as the seriousness of the personal injury economic costs rise (Figure 13–1).

How Claimants Fare with and without Representation

An estimated $2.5 billion was spent in legal fees and $4.2 billion was spent on insurance administrative expenses.[4] How much more money will the represented motor vehicle collision injury (MVCI) victim net after everything settles? Positive gains of $612 and $101 were seen in 1987 and 1992, respectively, for represented cases in the United States with a striking decline in 1992.[1,2] A recent insurance industry–financial study is also in agreement in that the average case has little cost gain, if any, with the use of an attorney.[3] See Table 13–1 for a breakdown of the most serious types of injuries and the average net payment to claimants.

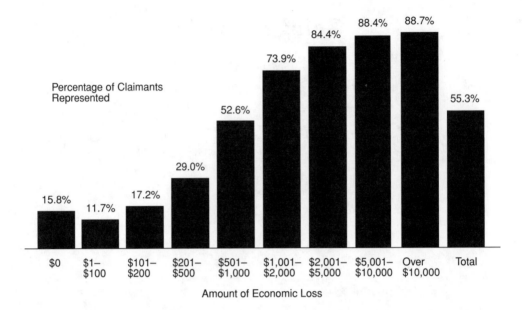

Figure 13–1 Attorney representation by amount of economic loss. *Source:* Reprinted from *Compensation for Automobile Injuries in the United States* with permission of the Insurance Research Council, © 1989.

Represented claimants generally have higher medical costs, more time lost from work, and more serious injuries than unrepresented claimants.[1-3] The insurance study concluded that attorney-represented claimants incurred $14,718 in economic costs, including medical costs, compared with $4,123 for claimants not using attorneys.[3] Consumers and claims review panelists report that 16% to 18% of attorneys advised their clients as to which doctor or clinic to use.[1,3] Claimants with attorneys will generally receive gross settlements higher than those without attorneys, for each dollar of economic loss reported.

One frequently asked question that the patient will ask is, "Should I settle this case now with the money offered by the insurance company or should I go to court and try to collect more money in the settlement?" The attorney should make the patient aware of the settlement statistics so the patient can make an informed decision. One factor to consider is the trial expertise and knowledge of the plaintiff's attorney and the case credibility. The Insurance Research Council found in a limited study that only about 16% of all awards by trial verdict were equal to or greater than the plaintiff's last demand.[1] Table 13–2 shows the comparison between pretrial and posttrial settlements.

Why Auto Accident Victims Seek Attorneys

A large consumer study reports that claimants talk to attorneys primarily to determine coverage protection or because of delays in settlement or insufficient money in settlement offers. Figure 13–2 outlines the various reasons.

Average Total Settlement Amounts

Consumers report that the average total settlement is $19,482, with the average attor-

Table 13–1 How BI Claimants Fared with and without Attorneys in the United States

Most Serious Injury	No. of BI Claimants	Average Economic Loss	Average Gross BI Payment	Average Net Payment after Fees and Expenses*	% of Extra Gross Payment Delivered to Represented Claimants
Neck Sprain/Strain					
Attorney	7,119	$4,098	$7,918	$1,207	
No Attorney	5,035	1,237	2,480	1,243	
Difference		2,861	5,438	(36)	−1%
Back Sprain/Strain					
Attorney	5,285	5,208	9,342	1,051	
No Attorney	2,652	1,541	3,074	1,533	
Difference		3,667	6,268	(482)	−8
Other Sprain/Strain					
Attorney	665	5,074	9,322	1,172	
No Attorney	707	1,258	2,328	1,070	
Difference		3,816	6,994	102	2
All Sprains/Strains					
Attorney	13,359	4,577	8,537	1,143	
No Attorney	8,511	1,339	2,665	1,326	
Difference		3,238	5,872	(183)	−3
Fracture of Weight-Bearing Bone					
Attorney	559	23,842	39,397	2,554	
No Attorney	146	10,685	19,105	8,420	
Difference		13,157	20,292	(5,866)	−29
Other Fracture					
Attorney	591	10,566	24,317	5,726	
No Attorney	321	4,708	9,895	5,187	
Difference		5,858	14,422	539	4
All Fractures					
Attorney	1,150	17,019	31,647	4,184	
No Attorney	467	6,576	12,774	6,198	
Difference		10,443	18,873	(2,014)	−11
Minor Lacerations					
Attorney	619	2,021	4,771	1,175	
No Attorney	1,236	688	1,166	478	
Difference		1,333	3,605	697	19
All Injuries					
Attorney	18,135	6,391	11,939	1,608	
No Attorney	12,049	1,755	3,262	1,507	
Difference		4,636	8,677	101	1%

Note: Excludes permanent total disability and fatality claimants. Excludes claimants with zero or missing economic loss.

*Net payment represents payment after deducting economic loss. For represented claimants, the net payment reflects an additional 33% reduction to the gross payment, the average amount absorbed by legal expenses (31% for attorney fees and 2% for court costs). Source of legal expense estimates: Insurance Research Council, *Paying for Auto Injuries,* May 1994.

Source: Reprinted from *Auto Injuries: Claiming Behavior and Its Impact on Insurance Costs* with permission of the Insurance Research Council, © 1994.

Table 13–2 Percentage of Cases Having Lawsuits Filed, Going to Court, and Verdict Settlements

Status of Lawsuit	No. of BI Claimants	% of Total
No Lawsuit Filed	26,871	81.4%
Lawsuit Filed	6,133	18.6
Lawsuit Settled before Trial	5,803	17.6
Lawsuit Settled during Trial	118	0.4
Suit Tried to Verdict	212	0.6
Total	33,004	100.0%

Outcome of Verdict	No. of BI Claimants	% of Total	% of Suits Tried to Verdict
Verdict Less than Last Offer	54	0.2%	27.1%
Verdict Equal to Last Offer	16	*	8.0
Verdict More than Last Offer but Less than Last Demand	98	0.3	49.2
Verdict Equal to Last Demand	9	*	4.5
Verdict More than Last Demand	22	0.1	11.1

*Percentage lower than 0.05%.

Source: Reprinted from *Auto Injuries: Claiming Behavior and Its Impact on Insurance Costs* with permission of the Insurance Research Council, © 1994.

ney fee being about 31% of the total settlement amount, or $6,039 (Figure 13–3). Consumers generally do not advance fees or costs when retaining counsel.

PERSONAL INJURY EVALUATION FACTORS

The modern family doctor needs to adopt a comprehensive approach when he or she first sees a patient who is a personal injury victim. Not only must the doctor seek a thorough diagnosis and determine an appropriate health management strategy, but he or she needs to consider the kind of legal case the patient may have. Important factors include the nature of the patient's injury, the severity of the condition, mechanisms of the injury, whose negligence caused the injury, the patient's likely residual pain/disability, loss of earnings, treatment length and frequency, and extent of the medical bills.

Doctors get minimal training about liability and other legal factors involving their pa-

tients' injuries, because their primary concerns are accurate diagnosis, treatment, and recovery. Doctors who treat personal injury victims need to become sensitive to the realities of the personal injury case. The doctor, in effect, needs to "evaluate" the personal injury case with a short checklist in order to get an accurate sense of the patient's legal position. The more the doctor knows about the legal aspects of the case the better, because payment for services rendered and the time it takes to close the case with the insurance carrier will be affected by the insurance carrier–doctor–attorney relationship. A delayed settlement may even have a negative influence on the patient's recovery. The doctor therefore can play a significant role in these cases. The following issues help determine the evaluation process.

Patient's Pre-Existing Condition

Matters that must be addressed at the first examination include whether the patient's

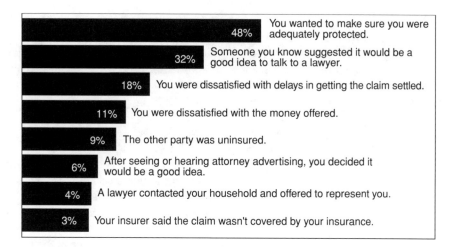

48%	You wanted to make sure you were adequately protected.
32%	Someone you know suggested it would be a good idea to talk to a lawyer.
18%	You were dissatisfied with delays in getting the claim settled.
11%	You were dissatisfied with the money offered.
9%	The other party was uninsured.
6%	After seeing or hearing attorney advertising, you decided it would be a good idea.
4%	A lawyer contacted your household and offered to represent you.
3%	Your insurer said the claim wasn't covered by your insurance.

Figure 13–2 Reasons claimants talk to attorneys about claims. *Source:* Reprinted from *Auto Injuries: Claiming Behavior and Its Impact on Insurance Costs* with permission of the Insurance Research Council, © 1994.

pre-existing history may have an impact on his or her current complaints. Any prior significant trauma or surgery must be considered. Merely asking the patient about such events without explaining the consequences of forgetfulness can be devastating. The Index Bureau (a nonprofit agency of liability carriers) keeps accurate records of all persons' claims. The patient may "forget," but the insurance carriers never do. The doctor who writes a patient's history and fails to mention a previous auto accident risks being asked at deposition whether he or she was covering up the prior trauma or took an incompetent history. A good history form is essential to avoiding this trap. The patient's age and relative health prior to the trauma are critical to determining the degree of pain he or she will suffer. If the patient has an fragile frame, then even a slight trauma may cause significant damage. Elderly patients suffer the most. Jurors usually have much more sympathy for elderly trauma victims.

Car Damage

Many doctors would rather not know anything about how much it costs to fix the patient's car. This approach is no longer appropriate. With the burden of car insurance rates increasing, jurors want to know about the connection between the cost of the damage to the car and the extent of the patient's trauma. Indeed, these issues are closely related in the minds of most people (although falsely, based on physical laws). The doctor

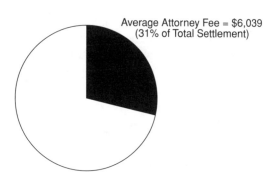

Average Attorney Fee = $6,039 (31% of Total Settlement)

Average Total Settlement = $19,482

Figure 13–3 Average attorney fees in the United States. *Source:* Reprinted from *Paying for Auto Injuries: A Consumer Panel Survey of Auto Accident Victims* with permission of the Insurance Research Council, © 1994.

needs to know not only the cost of repairing the patient's car, but also the extent of damage to the other vehicle. The size and weight of the vehicles are important. Was the patient's vehicle moving at the time of the crash? What part of the patient's car was struck? The mechanics of the injury are verified by knowing where the car sustained the unwelcome impact. Even the angle of collision may be critical toward explaining how the patient got hurt (see Chapters 1 and 14).

Liability

Liability is classic lawyer's turf. But a common-sense approach to determining "who did it" will help clarify whether the case is a personal injury case (with negligence by another) in those states where there is liability for fault. If liability is uncertain, then it is probably a troublesome case.

Patient's Residual Health Problems

The victim's residual symptoms may count substantially in the settlement value of a personal injury case. If the patient will require future surgery or is likely to have a lifelong physical disability (i.e., wheelchair bound), the value of his or her legal recovery escalates dramatically. Merely mentioning that the soft tissue injury "could" have a deleterious impact on the musculoskeletal system, without a firm foundation and specific application of the case, is useless.

Loss of Earnings

Most doctors omit this vital information. Today's trauma doctor is charged with the responsibility for knowing his or her patient's physical injury and disabilities. It is undeniable that any patient requiring treatment is to some extent disabled, that is, incapacitated from doing work, deprived of or having reduced power of acting, walking, etc. When the doctor omits documenting the patient's absence from work or fails to account for the suf-

fering the patient endured while at work, the value of the case is diminished. The doctor should note specifically partial or full disability and mention what specific restrictions should apply and what activities aggravate pain.

Medical Bills

Medical bills are a crucial factor toward establishing settlement value or as a basis for the jury to award. But the quality of the bills is what really matters. Unscrupulous doctors try to provide huge billings that will be taken seriously. Overutilization is easy to spot by anyone in the insurance community. By thorough attention to the foregoing elements, the doctor should derive a relatively sound feeling about the extent of treatment and the time necessary to assist the patient's recovery.

APPROPRIATE ATTORNEY REFERRAL: ETHICAL CONSIDERATIONS

No question touches the ethical behavior of a doctor or a lawyer as to when a referral from a doctor to a lawyer is appropriate. Clearly, for any form of monetary gain, such a referral must be considered unethical, if not illegal. Minor musculoskeletal injuries rarely require intervention of counsel. Generally, most trial attorneys would not accept small cases involving minor injuries with miniscule bills. It simply isn't worth the trial lawyer's time or effort to proceed with a case that may be very expensive to litigate with very little prospect of recovery for the client.

If the case involves significant injuries, prolonged recovery, major trauma, or objective neurologic and orthopedic symptoms, then an attorney's intervention may be essential. A tort victim cannot be expected to represent himself or herself effectively against an insurance company for a favorable outcome. An insurance company always has a conflict of interest when attempting to "buy out" a claim against an unrepresented MVCI victim. Usually, the mere intervention of counsel may not only safeguard the victim's right for appropriate restitution, but also see to it that all medical providers are adequately paid.

Appropriate ethical behavior suggests that a chiropractor or other general practitioner should refer all patients with serious to severe MVCIs to counsel; those with minor to moderate injuries usually require no referral, unless complicating matters arise, such as persistent intractable pain, severe disc protrusions, or conditions needing surgery.

PERSONAL INJURY DOCUMENTATION

The Chart Is the Soul of the Practice

The patient's chart is the cornerstone for the attorney and physician. In today's personal injury practice the physician must utilize paperwork that adequately covers a thorough crash history and examination, prior history, injury symptoms, prior treatment, and other related factors. In addition to the initial records, a treatment plan must be developed and progress notes need to be taken during each visit, indicating treatment methods and relevant findings. Periodic SOAP (subjective, objective, assessment, plan) notes or similar systems should be utilized in reasonable time increments or when situations arise that dictate the need for detailed notes and treatment plans. These SOAP red flags may include test results that affect management strategy, referral indicators, flare-ups, unusual symptoms, new injuries, or abnormal responses to treatment. Typically SOAP notes are done more frequently in the acute and subacute stages, tapering off in the chronic phases. Good records will help the doctor and the patient defend themselves from the defense attorney.

Canned Computer-Generated "Report"

These modern-day timesavers obviously lessen the doctor's credibility. The jury will know it when the defense attorney can show that the doctor always uses the same format and the same language for all patients with soft tissue injuries, often repeating notations and the language used for prognosis.

Doing It Right

Handwritten SOAP Charts

This is the most time-consuming, but also the most credible, form of record keeping. However, in a busy practice it may be unduly burdensome. Doctors are required to keep copious charts when in a school clinic, but the pressure of daily practice may force them to resort to shortcuts.

Dictation

Some doctors dictate their findings well. If the doctor has sufficient transcription backup, this protocol will give great credence to the clinic.

Lasar SOAP Transcriptions

This is a relatively new innovation in which a bar code reading device, which takes seconds to use, gives great detail in the patient's chart. The software and flexibility of several companies that produce it continue to improve.

Voice-Activated Dictation

Currently used at some hospitals for certain surgical procedures, this procedure promises to be the most revolutionary means for keeping detailed, accurate charts. Imagine merely dictating your patient's SOAP and then letting the computer process your transcription.

Patient's Diary Documentation

A valuable tool is encouraging the patient to keep a personal diary for the injury. The diary should be kept at home. Information should include details about any activities that cause pain, frequency of pain, severity, time of day, and other relevant details, as well as an account of whatever physical hardships are suffered by the patient during the recovery period.

Pain Diagram

The pain diagram, in which the patient diagrams his or her injuries on an outline of the human body, is useful.

PATIENT'S DISABILITY DOCUMENTATION

Workstyle Disability

Often the full impact of an injury on everyday routine is overlooked, and the doctor ought to seek greater understanding of the patient's abrupt accident disability. Many patients are forced to go to work to maintain their jobs, even if doing so prolongs healing. A doctor who documents clearly what impact the MVCI had on the patient's workstyle and lifestyle provides a valuable service for the patient.

Temporary Total Disability

Any loss of time from work must be documented by the doctor. That includes whole days missed and the hours missed by the patient even when required to visit the doctor.

Partial Disability at Work

Most patients, to keep their jobs, work through their pain. Patients are still "disabled" from their preaccident status. Documentation of these problems may have great influence with the jury—establishing critical credibility for the patient's daily suffering. For example, a waitress accustomed to carrying up to 20 lbs of food at a time may, because of her pain, be "transferred" to the dinner-hour shift. In fact, not only does she lose *time* from work, but she may lose income because of her injuries, by servicing the less-busy dinner hour. When the doctor carefully documents the patient's workstyle disability, he or she shows great concern and knowledge about the patient's recovery.

Lifestyle Disability

Most of the time, doctors fail to mention salient examples of lifestyle disabilities in their legal reports. Such examples of real situations often provide the best evidence of suffering: the father who returns home after work, unable to pick up his 4-year-old daughter because of a low back injury; the housewife with three children who is unable to go to the store for a month; or the blue-collar worker who is forced to drop out of a bowling league. Activities of daily living (ADLs) need to be noted by the doctor. Simple ADLs checklists can be periodically completed by the patients.[5]

THE ZEN OF BILLING: AVOIDING THE SIX RED FLAGS

Insurance adjusters are carefully trained to examine all billings for diagnostic and radiologic procedures, treatment, and rehabilitation programs, and to look for basic flaws. Some of the more obvious ones, which are red flags to an adjuster, are listed below.

Erroneous Dates

With sloppy billing, a doctor may have billed for treatment on Christmas, Easter, or a Sunday. Insurance adjusters are justifiably suspicious of any billing for treatment rendered on a holiday. This error is easy to avoid by checking bills before they are mailed.

Siamese Twin Syndrome

No two people in the same accident have exactly the same symptoms, should receive exactly the same treatment, or should have exactly the same prognosis. So, why do some doctors bill identically for two or more parties who were involved in the same accident? It doesn't make sense, and payment of such bills will be delayed and scrutinized by senior adjusters.

Overuse of or Duplicative X-Rays

Overuse, duplications, or inappropriate timing of X-rays may be professionally questionable and unnecessarily expensive. See Chapter 6 for guidelines. Once a patient has undergone extensive X-rays at an emergency department, for example, or at the office of an orthopedist, careful justification must be given before subjecting the patient to a new series of diagnostic radiation.

Duration of Treatment

At some point, the patient must achieve maximum medical improvement, and no additional work by the doctor will improve measurably the patient's condition. The great majority of musculoskeletal injuries are resolved within 9 months of the trauma. Treatment of longer duration is questionable and requires diagnostic justification. Doctors who treat patients three times a week for 3 months without recognizing different stages of repair are usually abusing the patient and the insurance system. Most patients require more frequent office treatment early, but as their condition improves, the frequency of treatment should be reduced. If a reasonable limitation is exceeded, it raises a red flag.

Average Daily Fee

The average daily fee is perhaps the most obvious red flag. The adjuster simply divides the total bill by the number of visits. Some doctors are actually surprised by how much they charge per visit, as this single calculation will reveal.

Diagnostic-Treatment Ratio

Jurors will give compensation to hands-on treatment. But jurors and adjusters are skeptical of overutilized diagnostic procedures and the charges for them. Generally, if more than 25% of the treating doctor's bill is for diagnos-

tic tests, it is considered an unnecessary part (diagnostic work done outside the clinic is not part of the doctor's diagnostic-treatment ratio). There are exceptions to these guidelines in complicated cases.

Understanding the methodology of adjusters when they review doctors' bills will provide a solid foundation for a proper approach to billing in personal injury cases. Payment of suitable billing should not be reduced or delayed.

LITIGATION

If the case did not settle, why not? To find out, a doctor should always be able to identify the adjuster, carrier, and claim number of the adverse party (third party). When opening the file, the doctor's staff should always get this information—usually from the patient's lawyer or insurance company. With this information, the doctor's staff has independent means of learning the status of the third-party case.

Liability and Bills

Two issues usually force a third-party case into litigation. Either there is a dispute as to who caused the accident (the issue is called "liability") or whether the medical bills (i.e., for the treatment given) were reasonable and necessary ("damages"). In either case, you may be called upon to testify for your patient. Your testimony is critical for the success of the patient's case.

Human Contact between the Doctor and the Adjuster

Often the contact between the doctor and the adjuster is an advisory relationship; it is important that doctors make a genuine effort to communicate personally with insurance adjusters. It is recommended that doctors not only discuss the patient's condition (with appropriate authorization) with the adjuster, but also seek to discuss personally with the adjuster the doctor's philosophy with regard to treating patients. Some doctors even offer to speak before groups of adjusters, explaining the purpose and the mission of the doctor's clinic. This type of proactive reaching-out can greatly enhance the communication between the doctor and the insurance adjuster.

Monitoring Early Litigation

Today's doctor will want to be aware of the status of his or her litigation cases. Records must be up to date and maintained properly. Keep track of the patient's residence and periodically bill the patient for any outstanding balance on an account that is open and payable, although your payment is protected by a lien. Often, the first notice you receive that the case is in litigation is when a copy service unexpectedly shows up at the clinic, demanding to copy your patient's records. Always cooperate with the copy service if they have provided you with notice of an appointment, a reasonable fee to your staff for locating the file, and either the patient's authorization or a subpoena.

Defense Medical Examination

In 1992, 7% of bodily injury states and 14% of no-fault states used defense medical examinations, also called independent medical examinations (IMEs).[1] Defense attorneys routinely use a stable of "insurance" doctors to generate predictably legal reports. The credibility of the IMEs would be greatly enhanced if the treating doctor and the defense could agree on using a panel of reputable nonbiased doctors. Treating doctors should assist their patients to prepare for IMEs by encouraging the patients to cooperate and seek counsel from their attorneys. Some patients like to bring a tape recorder to monitor the examination. Never discuss liability or how the accident happened with the insurance doctor or the staff. The IME doctor should inquire only into injuries.

Paper Reviews

A controversial and possibly illegal approach by certain insurance companies is to review the treating doctor's records and bills to determine whether excessive fees are charged and whether treatment type, frequency, and duration are appropriate. Commonly, the health care professional (physician or nurse) reviewer will dramatically cut the treating doctor's bill or demand treatment limitation or termination. The legal and ethical issues confronting the physician paper reviewer are these: Are the reviewer's statement and authority contained within the physician's scope of practice? Do medical and chiropractic educational institutions teach or advocate that a patient's diagnosis, access to treatment or provider, appropriateness of duration and frequency of care, and disability and prognosis can be evaluated solely on the basis of a few records? How can a paper reviewer make these determinations without ever seeing, touching, or verbally communicating with the patient directly? Outside an administrative role, such as recommending IMEs, and clarification of records of treatment and billing, the paper reviewer has no credibility and may in fact be acting outside the oath to serve the patient and do no harm.

Professional Contact with the Patient's Attorney

Nothing is more discouraging to a patient's attorney than a doctor who will not cooperate. Some doctors have told me that they would rather forego their fee for treatment than testify because they are afraid. One doctor claims to have quit practice rather than subject himself to testifying at trial. The doctor who handles a personal injury case indirectly consents to cooperate in the preparation of the case. However, even if the doctor is cooperative, the patient's attorney may need organization in trial preparation.

Three suggestions are offered to prepare properly with counsel, as follows:

1. Insist that your office be given immediate notice of potential trial dates, even though these dates are routinely continued, because of limited courtrooms, by telephone and by mail.

2. At least 30 days prior to the trial dates, the attorney should make an appointment with you, in your office, to review the patient's chart. The attorney should be prepared to pay you for your time and should bring the check to the office at the time of the consultation.

3. Within 48 hours of the trial, the attorney should once again meet with you, in your office, to review the substance of your testimony and to go over the chart once again. Often the attorney will have new ideas or questions that came up during the last month of preparation. Once again, the attorney pays for the doctor's time.

Using a Chiropractor in Court

The well-known tort attorney Melvin Belli broke ground for chiropractors in 1973 by writing:

> Lawyers are reluctant to use chiropractors in court against orthopods. They make a mistake. They also make a mistake if they voir dire a jury on the use of a chiropractor. I find, then, on every jury some prospective jurors, if not themselves, their relatives, have used, and successfully, chiropractors so there is inherent goodwill at that jury box, not animosity.[6]

For more than a generation, the use of chiropractors in court has been debated in trial attorney circles. As chiropractic has long been licensed in all 50 states, the profession now dominates musculoskeletal care.[7] Tired invectives against chiropractic for imagined lack of credibility no longer are viable. The chiropractor's educational background, in terms of arriving at diagnoses of musculoskeletal injuries, meets or exceeds that of a medical school graduate in the fields of physiology, neurology, orthopedics, and radiology. Today's newly licensed chiropractors have better undergraduate educations than their predecessors. The Council on Chiropractic Education governs chiropractic education under the authority of the United States Department of Education. Chiropractic students qualify for student loans from the Department of Education.

The practical considerations on whether to use a chiropractor as an expert witness is whether the chiropractor and the lawyer are fully prepared to work as a team for the maximum advantage of the MVCI patient. Some neurologists, internists, and chiropractors make good witnesses; others do not. It depends on the individual. If the lawyer adequately prepares and works with the chiropractor as the expert witness, then the chiropractor can make a formidable witness in proving the musculoskeletal injuries of the MVCI patients.

THE TRIAL

The Doctor As Expert Witness

In some states, the treating doctor is not considered an expert. Rather, the doctor is deemed a percipient witness, having knowledge simply of what was seen and heard. That description gives some unscrupulous attorneys the opportunity to try to pay a minimal fee for the doctor's testimony. Where legally permitted, experienced doctors know how to handle this abuse. First, if the attorney tries to pay only a nominal fee and not a reasonable, hourly "expert" fee, then the doctor should insist on expert fees. If the defendant attorney still insists on the nominal fee, then the doctor during trial should not answer questions about diagnosis or prognosis, which clearly call for expertise. The doctor then may turn to the trial judge and state in open court that he or she believes those questions call for the doctor's expertise and ask the judge to determine a reasonable fee before testimony continues.

Depositions

Most doctors whose practice involves personal injury cases have their depositions taken regularly. A deposition is pretrial testimony under oath, and every word is transcribed by a court reporter. Attorneys for the insurance company and the client should be present. The deposition helps frame the issues for the trial. Often, cases are settled following depositions if the weight of evidence favors one side. Almost always, the insurance attorney calls for the deposition from the patient's doctor. There are three basic rules to follow when a doctor receives a notice of deposition. Have your assistant call the secretary for the attorney with the following requests.

Location

Ask that the deposition be taken in your clinic. Most attorneys will agree to this, in that they get paid while traveling. It is important that the doctor be comfortable in his or her own environment. Naturally, the defense attorney will be tempted to pick up any office literature and may ask questions about suspicious claims for treatment benefits. Generally, the defense law firm will send its most junior attorney to a doctor's office. Oftentimes, the doctor will have more deposition experience than the attorney taking the deposition.

Time and Date

Ask that the time and date of the deposition be set at a time convenient for you. Attorneys regularly change deposition times and dates. Most attorneys have the flexibility that a busy doctor in practice does not. For example, if the clinic is closed Thursday mornings, that might be a convenient deposition time, with less negative impact on the practice.

Fees

Once again, have your assistant ask how much time is required for the deposition. If le-

gally permitted, the assistant should ask that a check be sent promptly to reserve the appointment time for the deposition. Generally, a doctor should be paid more if he or she has deposition experience. Otherwise, the fee should be moderate, as the doctor's "expertise" has not fully matured.

Trial Time: The Doctor in the Center Stage

Preparation

A doctor who wants to be successful should plan to spend several hours preparing, becoming thoroughly acquainted with the patient's chart, the records of other institutions or doctors, and his or her reports and billing. The doctor should write some questions to discuss with the patient's attorney. The attorney should "rehearse" the trial scene by asking and getting answers to all questions that the attorney plans to ask. The patient's attorney and the doctor should anticipate together what questions to expect from the defense attorney, and the best way to answer them. After good preparation, the doctor will be able to handle 95% of questions that may be asked. Thorough preparation will help the doctor to be a more confident and comfortable witness.

Demeanor and Delivery

Tools. Along with careful preparation, the doctor should also plan to use as many props, skeletal models, medical illustrations (although these should be brought to the courtroom by the attorney), and X-rays (with a view box). Not only must the members of the jury be educated in the body mechanics of the injury, they need to be entertained and kept interested with visual presentation.

Qualifications. As the doctor begins to testify (in deposition or at trial), the first series of questions will examine his or her credentials. The doctor's entire professional and academic history may be examined. A current curriculum vitae should be available.

Critical Evidence and Issues

Causal Connection

The plaintiff's doctor must be able to say, under oath and with reasonable certainty, that the plaintiff's injury was directly caused by the accident in question. Otherwise, there is no personal injury case, and unless it is dismissed, the plaintiff will lose at arbitration or trial.

Pre-Existing or Subsequent Injury

Most mature patients have suffered several prior traumas. If there was a pre-existing injury and it was still active at the time of the accident in question, the doctor must be prepared to apportion the degree to which the new accident contributed to the injury. This is done in percentages, based on the patient's history, prior records, current examination, and the doctor's own expertise.

Reasonable Medical Certainty for Diagnosis

The doctor must be able to testify that the diagnosis presented is seriously based on the plaintiff's history and physical examination and is accurate to a reasonable medical certainty in the doctor's expert opinion.

Disability of the Patient

Any patient requiring care is to some extent "disabled." Often overlooked, but critical at trial, is a description of how the patient was able to cope with work, once he or she was permitted to return to work. Did the patient require lighter duty, a desk job, or lose promotion opportunities? How long did the patient suffer after returning to work? At home, was the patient's lifestyle changed? Did he or she have undue trouble with household duties, with children or a spouse? Did the patient have to drop out of sports activities? These losses, more than ever, show the specific damages incurred, in addition to whatever must be secured for musculoskeletal pain and suffering.

CONCLUSION

Successful testimony at trial may be a professional highlight for the modern doctor. Simply following the suggestions provided above will make the litigation experience less frightening and more satisfying and successful. Generally, we fear what we do not know. The experience will enrich you and earn great benefits for your patient. If the Personal Injury community knows that you keep accurate records and that you are professionally prepared, just your availability may contribute to early settlement. In this way, you will have found another way to serve all of your patients involved in a personal injury dispute.

REFERENCES

1. Insurance Research Council. *Auto Injuries: Claiming Behavior and Its Impact on Insurance Costs.* Oak Brook, Ill: IRC; 1994.

2. All-Industry Research Advisory Council. *Compensation for Automobile Injuries in the United States.* Oak Brook, Ill: AIRAC; March 1989.

3. Insurance Research Council. *Paying for Auto Injuries: A Consumer Panel Survey of Auto Accident Victims.* Oak Brook, Ill: IRC; 1994.

4. Miller TR, Luchter S, Brinkman CP. Crash costs and safety investment. *Accid Anal Prev.* 1989;21(4):303–315.

5. Haldeman S, Chapman-Smith D, Peterson DM. *Guidelines for Chiropractic Quality Assurance and Practice Parameters: Proceedings of the Mercy Center Consensus Conference.* Gaithersburg, Md: Aspen Publishers; 1993.

6. Belli MM. Chiropractors as expert witnesses. *Dig Chirop Econ.* May–June 1973.

7. California Department of Insurance. CCA memo dated February 12, 1992. Sacramento, Calif.

Chapter 14

Motor Vehicle Collision Facts

Lawrence S. Nordhoff, Jr.

INTRODUCTION

It is useful for the physician to be aware of the various statistics relating to motor vehicle collision injuries (MVCIs). This chapter is intended to serve as an informational compendium on that subject.

ANNUAL INCIDENCE

In the United States in 1993, for all types of motor vehicles the National Safety Council (NSC) reports approximately 11.9 million accidents, with about 21 million vehicles involved in car crashes.[1] The estimated total number of MVCIs varies depending on the report. Various studies estimate that there were about 4 million reported nonfatal injuries in 1981,[2] and about 5 million from 1982 to 1992 nonfatal injuries annually.[1,3] Of the 5 million reported injuries, the NSC reports that MVCIs account for about 2 million disabling injuries, including 900,000 work-related auto disabling injuries in 1990.[1] A 1990 National Highway Traffic Safety Administration (NHTSA) study reports that about 28% of occupants incur minor to moderate injury and 6% severe to fatal injury.[4] Figure 14–1 illustrates collision frequency and risk of injury seen by collision velocities. The NHTSA[4] reports that in 1990 there was one police reported crash every 5 seconds, one reported minor to moderate injury every 17 seconds, one person killed or injured every 10 seconds, and one multivehicle collision every 7 seconds.[4] It has been estimated that about 50% of all crashes are reported by the police.[4] A recent US Department of Transportation guide estimates that the average driver will have a near crash one to two times a month, concluding that every American will be in a collision of some type every 6 years.[5]

ANNUAL MVCI COSTS

A 1993 report by Miller,[6] evaluating comprehensive costs, concluded that the entire cost for MVCIs in the United States was over $333 billion in 1988. These figures include medical and ancillary costs, property damage, loss of wages, workplace disruption, legal fees, emergency services, administrative fees, and lost quality of life. Miller also concludes that in 1986 dollars the average comprehensive cost for a minor injury according to the abbreviated injury scale (AIS-1) was $13,801.[6] See Chapter 1 for AIS system review.

266

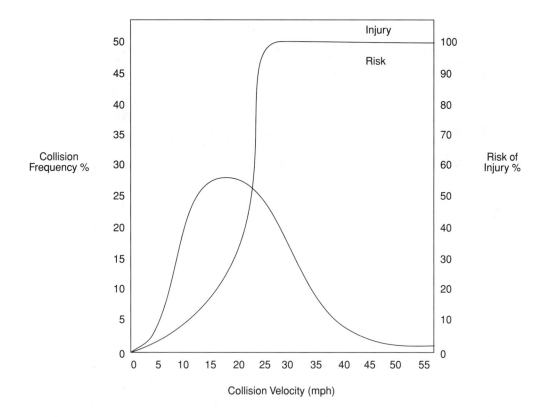

Figure 14–1 Collision frequency and risk of injury seen by crash velocity. *Source:* Data from National Highway Traffic Safety Administration, General Estimates System 1990, A Review of Information of Police-Reported Traffic Crashes in the United States, 1991, and Traffic Safety Facts, A Compilation of Motor Vehicle Crash Data from the Fatal Accident Reporting System and the General Estimates System, 1992.

A 1985 committee on trauma research felt that indirect and direct MVCI costs in the United States account for about half of the total costs to our society from all forms of injury.[7] This is why minor accident analysis, treatment, and data collection must be addressed, although most past and current research has focused only on preventing the serious to fatal injury.

MINOR INJURY AND ITS PORTION OF TOTAL COST

There is consistent agreement that the minor injury accounts for the majority of total costs to our society. Although the more serious to fatal injuries cost more per case, the majority of car crashes cause injuries averaging between mild and moderate in severity. Minor injuries (injuries having no risk of fatality) have been reported to account for anywhere from 50% to 83% of all MVCI costs to our society.[8,9] Luchter's study concludes that minor MVCI costs are 3.5 times higher than critical MVCI costs.[10] Another study by the NHTSA concluded that nonfatal injury costs accounted for 78% of the total economic MVCI costs.[11] The National Safety Council describes in Table 14–1 the nature of MVCI injuries by region of the body and nature of the injury.

Table 14–1 Automobile Occupant Injuries by Nature of Injury and Part of Body, 1991

Part of Body	All Injuries	Nature of Injury						
		Contusion	Laceration	Abrasion	Strain	Fracture	Concussion	Other, Unknown
All injuries	100.0%	42.5%	15.5%	14.4%	10.4%	7.0%	4.1%	6.1%
Total	100.0%	100.0%	100.0%	100.0%	100.0%	100.0%	100.0%	100.0%
Head, skull	11.2	7.4	13.4	5.2	0.0	4.7	100.0	13.6
Face	19.6	16.1	45.2	22.9	0.0	23.5	0.0	12.9
Neck*	8.6	1.2	1.3	2.5	68.6	1.9	0.0	3.2
Shoulder	5.0	6.3	0.7	3.8	1.9	8.4	0.0	14.5
Arm, upper	1.6	2.2	1.6	1.3	0.2	2.2	0.0	0.7
Elbow, forearm	4.4	5.3	4.5	7.3	0.0	4.2	0.0	2.1
Wrist, hand	5.1	3.0	9.1	7.1	0.2	8.1	0.0	13.0
Upper limb*	1.1	1.0	1.3	2.8	0.1	0.2	0.0	1.0
Back*	4.1	1.1	0.6	2.1	26.7	3.8	0.0	3.1
Chest	7.7	12.9	1.6	3.2	0.4	16.4	0.0	4.8
Abdomen	2.4	3.5	2.1	2.0	0.2	0.0	0.0	4.7
Pelvis, hip	2.9	4.4	0.4	2.4	0.1	6.1	0.0	3.6
Thigh	2.6	4.5	0.8	2.2	0.3	3.6	0.0	0.2
Knee	12.0	16.5	8.6	20.2	0.1	3.9	0.0	7.0
Leg, lower	4.1	4.7	4.5	6.1	0.3	5.8	0.0	1.1
Ankle, foot	3.0	2.9	1.7	1.6	0.2	7.0	0.0	12.2
Lower limb*	1.6	1.8	1.2	4.0	0.2	0.2	0.0	0.2
Whole body	2.7	4.6	1.3	3.4	0.0	0.0	0.0	0.6
Unknown region	0.3	0.4	0.1	0.2	0.5	0.0	0.0	1.4

*Neck includes cervical spine. Back includes thoracolumbar spine. Upper and lower limbs include whole or unknown part only.

Source: National Safety Council analysis of National Highway Traffic Safety Administration, National Accident Sample System, Crashworthiness Data System, 1991.

WHO PAYS FOR THESE INJURIES?

The Insurance Research Council reports that 63% of claimants used their own automobile insurer, 55% used the auto insurer of another vehicle, 36% used health insurance, 20% relied on government programs, and 19% used workers' compensation benefits. Almost 60% report using two or more benefit sources.[12]

INJURY FACTS SOURCES

There are several sources for vehicle crash data in the United States.[5] Included are the Fatal Accident Reporting System (FARS); the Centers for Disease Control and Prevention (CDC); the National Accident Sampling System (NASS); and the National Safety Council (NSC), 444 North Michigan Avenue, Chicago. Also available are police accident-reporting systems such as the General Estimates System (GES), the National Health Interview Study (NHIS), the National Center for Health Statistics (NCHS), the NHTSA, and the National Crash Severity System (NCSS). Insurance and consumer surveys also are available. Other sources are medical records from hospitals, medical reports from ambulances, death certificates, and independent studies that may have federal funding or may be sponsored by the private sector such as automobile manufacturers.

When evaluating various accident studies, it is important to realize that many figures are estimates only, and may possibly be gross underestimates. When looking at the frequency of minor to moderate pain, it must be noted that many injuries are not reported because of the common delay in onset of pain. One 1990 US Department of Transportation study concluded that 42% of road accidents were not reported to the police, 15% of the injuries were not reported, 8% of all crashes were hit-and-runs, and 50% of all minor accidents were unreported.[13] A recent large insurance company study concludes that between 20% and 80% of all accidents are not reported to the police, depending upon the type of crash.[14]

HUMAN AND NONHUMAN FACTORS AFFECTING CRASHES

The average driver is confronted with 10 or more traffic situations per second, makes one to three decisions per second, and is confronted with at least one driver error every 2 minutes.[5] The average driver will cross over 1 million intersections in his or her lifetime.[5] Sivak showed that 93% of 420 accidents investigated were determined to be caused by human factors.[15] Nonhuman factors include road factors (in 10.9% of the cases),[16] age of the vehicle,[17] and vehicle defects.[1] The NHTSA reports that vehicle defects, including those of tires, braking systems, headlights, steering systems, and wheels, were reported by the police as contributing to 1.6% of all crashes.[1]

Human factors include risky driving, alcohol intoxication, drug use, improper lookout, inattention, failure to give way or stop, following too closely, loss of vehicle control, fatigue, physical handicap, decreased vision, driver history of accidents or violations, chronic illness, emotional stress, driving too fast, driver inexperience, vehicle/road unfamiliarity, sleep deprivation, urban driving, lack of vehicle inspections, too many hours driving, nutritional problems, and a driver too young or too old.[5,15–19] In addition, rubbernecking drivers create traffic congestion problems that result in many crashes. Table 14–2 shows the vehicle maneuvering and driving behavior involved in collisions; about 60% to 70% of drivers have some type of improper driving behavior.

Ferguson et al.[20] concluded that when age, educational level, and mental ability were evaluated individually, all affected injury rates; but when they were considered together, only educational level affected injury rates significantly. Drivers with lower intelligence were found to have 20% more accidents and receive larger numbers of speeding tick-

Table 14–2 Improper Driving Behavior in Accidents, 1993

Kind of Improper Driving	Fatal Accidents			Injury Accidents			All Accidents		
	Total	Urban	Rural	Total	Urban	Rural	Total	Urban	Rural
Total	100.0%	100.0%	100.0%	100.0%	100.0%	100.0%	100.0%	100.0%	100.0%
Improper Driving	57.7	54.7	59.4	72.7	74.3	69.6	68.6	69.8	66.1
Speed too fast or unsafe	16.5	14.4	17.7	13.5	11.8	17.6	12.2	11.1	15.4
Right of way	12.7	17.0	10.1	25.0	28.8	15.5	20.6	23.2	13.7
Failed to yield	7.8	9.4	6.8	17.3	19.3	12.3	15.1	16.6	11.3
Passed stop sign	2.7	2.7	2.7	2.7	3.0	1.9	2.0	2.1	1.4
Disregarded signal	2.2	4.9	0.6	5.0	6.5	1.3	3.5	4.5	1.0
Drove left of center	7.6	3.2	10.1	2.1	1.3	4.0	1.8	1.1	3.4
Improper overtaking	1.2	0.6	1.5	1.0	0.8	1.4	1.3	1.1	1.7
Made improper turn	2.9	2.7	3.0	3.4	3.3	3.7	4.5	4.6	4.2
Followed too closely	0.5	.4	0.6	6.2	7.2	3.7	5.5	6.2	3.6
Other improper driving	16.3	16.4	16.4	21.5	21.1	23.7	22.7	22.5	24.1
No improper driving stated	42.3	45.3	40.6	27.3	25.7	30.4	31.4	30.2	33.9

Source: Reprinted from Accident Facts, 1994 edition, National Safety Council, Itasca, Illinois.

ets.[21] People of lower economic status were reported to have higher rates of MVCIs and three times the occupant death rates of those in higher economic brackets, even though the latter drive almost twice as many miles.[22]

ALCOHOL AND DRUG USE

Many international conferences and articles discuss alcohol or drug use and traffic safety. It appears that alcohol-related injuries and deaths take a significant toll on most societies. Experiments on intoxicated volunteers have shown alcohol to be a fatiguing agent,[23] making subjects less able to execute avoidance maneuvers in response to unexpected obstacles.[24] Drivers' perceptions of their own car speed and distance are affected.[25] Decreased reaction times,[26,27] an overall increase in driving speed,[27] and diminished vehicle control[26] have all been associated with alcohol consumption. Intoxicated drivers have greater approach speeds on curves than normal[27] and have greater difficulty maneuvering out of potential crashes as well.[28]

There has been recent research into the combined use of alcohol and drugs, prescription and recreational, on its prevalence and causative effects in car crashes. Drug and alcohol combinations were found to be present in 22% of MVCI cases, according to Waller et al.[29] In a study by Terhune and Fell,[30] 497 MVCI drivers treated at a hospital were evaluated and 38% had alcohol or other drugs in their system. Alcohol was present in 25%, tetrahydrocannabinol in 9.5%, and tranquilizers in 7.5%; 10% of the drivers tested positive for two or more drugs. Terhune and Fell concluded their report by saying that tranquilizers did not pose a safety problem, but marijuana and hashish had high rates of MVCI involvement.[30]

Between 3% and 9% of all drivers on the road, at any given time, are intoxicated, according to an American Medical Association review of the literature.[31] There is one alcohol-related death every 30 minutes.[1] Thousands of lives are lost, young and old, as a result of driving under the influence of alcohol. Drunk driving involves many teenagers. DiBlasio found that 36% of all high school students report riding with a drinking driver on a regular basis.[32] Alcohol consumption is associated with increased likelihood of collision occurrence and collision outcome severity.[33] In 1981, 670,000 people were injured as a result of alcohol usage and driving.[34] Baker et al.[22] found that 50% or more MVCI deaths are due to intoxicated drivers in single car crashes or at fault in multi car crashes. Alcohol is a contributing factor in approximately 20% of all MVCI occupant injuries,[16] 41%[16] or 50%[35] of all fatal crashes (depending on the study), 60% of single-vehicle fatal crashes,[35] and 40% of pedestrian deaths.[36] The US Department of Transportation reports that about 7% of the driving population causes 66% of all fatal alcohol-related crashes, and alcohol is implicated in 50% of all fatalities.[5] A Texas study of 558 driver fatalities showed that 51% had a blood alcohol content (BAC) of 0.10% or greater and that accident reports on 34% of the cases showed alcohol as a contributing factor.[37] Alcohol involvement is most common at night and with drivers aged 20 to 49 years.[22] An unbelted driver having a BAC of 0.14% is 20 times more likely to cause an accident than a sober driver.[38] An unbelted driver is two times as likely to be intoxicated as a belted driver.[39]

A general guideline for per-hour decreases of BAC is 0.018%.[40] The person with a lower metabolism rate will require smaller alcohol doses to reach peak BAC and will require more time to eliminate it than people with higher metabolism.[41] Burns and Moskowitz showed that a given alcohol dose calculated for body weight will produce a significantly higher BAC in women than in men.[42]

There is an emerging trend for young women aged 21 to 24 to drink and drive.[43] In the past decade more women have entered the workplace, which may have something to do with this trend.

The 3-year study by Maull et al.[44] in Virginia concluded that injury appears to protect drivers from being convicted of driving under the influence of alcohol (DUI). None of the 56 injured alcohol-impaired drivers in this study were convicted.[44]

COLLISION TYPES

Figures 14–2 and 14–3 illustrate the frequencies of various types of collisions with resulting damage or injury, and the percentages and types of vehicles that were either the struck vehicle or the striking vehicle in the United States. Approximately 15% of all vehicle collisions involve multiple vehicles.[45,46] Figures 14–2 and 14–3 describe vectors of collision.

GENDER OF DRIVERS INVOLVED IN COLLISIONS

Collision involvement risk can vary depending on the gender of the driver. Female

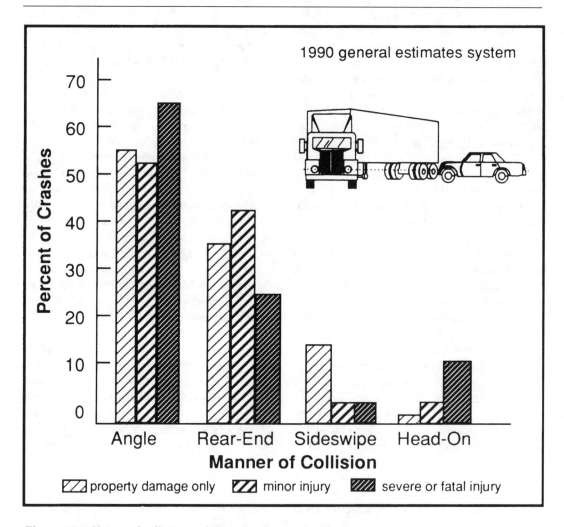

Figure 14–2 Vector of collision and property damage only, minor injury, and severe to fatal injury. *Source:* Reprinted from *A Review of Information of Police-Reported Traffic Crashes in the United States,* General Estimates System, National Highway Traffic Safety Administration, 1990.

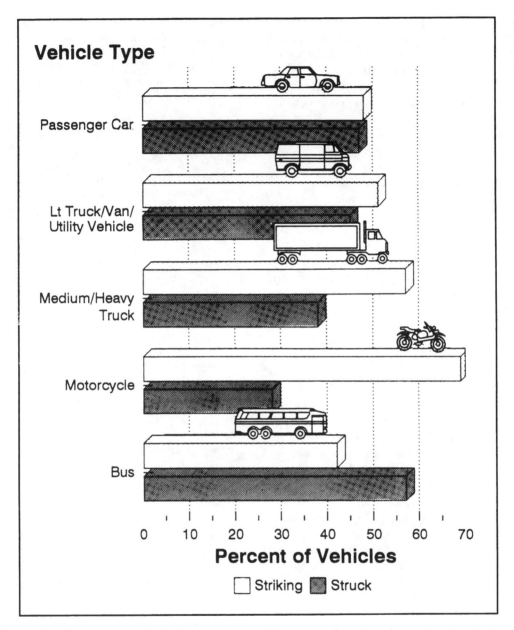

Figure 14–3 Vehicle type and whether it was the striking or struck vehicle. *Source:* Reprinted from *A Review of Information of Police-Reported Traffic Crashes in the United States,* General Estimates System, National Highway Traffic Safety Administration, 1990.

drivers represent 51% of the US population and account for approximately 55% of the number of collision claims receiving benefits.[45] Female drivers have been estimated to drive 50% fewer miles[47] and spend 35% less time driving than their male counterparts.[47] After age 34 females have higher rates of non-fatal accidents per million miles driven than their male counterparts.[48,49] The National Safety Council reports that in 1993 for all car crash accidents, females had higher involvement rates than their male counterparts.[1] About 12.9 million male drivers and 8.2 female drivers were involved in car crashes, with male and female drivers having rates of 87 and 101 crashes per 10 million miles driven, respectively.[1] Male drivers account for approximately 65% of the total miles driven in the United States.

RACE-CULTURE OF DRIVERS INVOLVED IN COLLISIONS

Several studies have attempted to determine whether certain races or cultures are overinvolved in automobile crashes. Racial comparison rates show that Native Americans had the highest crash rates per 100,000 miles (Native Americans had 51, whites 24, blacks 19, and Asians 9).[22] White occupant deaths in rural areas were three times higher, and blacks five times higher, than counterparts living in large cities.[22] A 1989 North Carolina study concluded that, except for individuals under 25, crash rates for nonwhites exceed those for whites in every age-sex category. Nonwhite males and white females were involved in more collisions per mile driven.[50] A 1991 study concludes that blacks and Hispanics have low rates of seat belt use.[51]

RURAL VERSUS URBAN COLLISIONS

MVCIs are mostly an urban phenomenon, with about 52% of 1987 injuries in the United States occurring in suburbs and central cities, 29% in medium-sized cities, and 19% in rural areas.[45] Urban accident patterns have been described as including rear-end collisions, drivers aged 35 to 44, minor head/face/neck injuries receiving primarily outpatient treatment, and crash speeds of 30 mph and below.[52] Rural crash characteristics include frontal collisions, skids or overturns, drivers aged 55 to 64, severe limb/abdominal/chest injuries that require hospitalization, and collision speeds of 50 to 60 mph.[52]

CONCLUSION

MVCIs are putting enormous strain on the United States in terms of quality of life, resource consumption, and economic costs. Most of the current focus on car safety, vehicle design, and laws that focus on lessening economic losses deal with the serious to fatal injuries, although most of the total costs in the real world relate to the minor injury.

Questions that the public needs to have answered include the following:

- Why do some comparable cars (size and weight) have two to nine times higher death and injury rates?

- Why are some cars allowed to be sold in the United States that do not meet the New Car Assessment Program's minimal 30 to 35 mph crash standards?

- Why is the current administrative focus on fuel economy pushing for small vehicle size instead of engine designs that will get 60 to 70+ miles per gallon in a 2000- or 3000-lb car? As long as there are large and small vehicles on the road that increase fatality and injury risks, small cars are dangerous.

- Why are children allowed to ride in the front seats of cars when studies show much less injury potential in the rear seats?

- Why are seats being manufactured with adjustable head restraints when higher fixed restraint–seat systems are cheaper to manufacture and are safer?

- Why are we manufacturing cars that travel over 80 mph?

- Why don't we require all vehicles to be certified for safety annually? This would include requiring an annual tune-up, brake check, and a check of other safety systems. Every year thousands of accidents are caused by rubberneckers when vehicles pull over because of mechanical or safety problems.

REFERENCES

1. National Safety Council. *Accident Facts.* Chicago: NSC; 1994.

2. Scott WE. *Epidemiology of Head and Neck Trauma in Victims of Motor Vehicle Accidents: Head and Neck Injury Criteria. A Consensus Workshop.* Washington, DC: US Government Printing Office; July 1983:1–6.

3. Rice D, MacKenzie E, et al. *Cost of Injury in the United States: A Report to Congress.* San Francisco: University of California; 1989.

4. National Highway Traffic Safety Administration. *General Estimates System 1990: A Review of Information on Police-Reported Traffic Crashes in the United States.* Washington, DC: DOT HS 807 781. US Dept of Transportation; 1991.

5. Holden JA, Cristoffel T. *A Course on Motor Vehicle Trauma: Instructors Guide—Final Users Manual.* DOT/OST/P-34/86-050. Washington, DC: Department of Transportation; September 1986.

6. Miller TR. Costs and functional consequences of U.S. roadway crashes. *Accid Anal Prev.* 1993; 25:593–607.

7. Committee on Trauma Research. *Injury in America: A Continuing Public Health Problem.* Commission on Life Sciences, National Research Council and the Institute of Medicine. Washington, DC: National Academy Press; 1985.

8. Luchter S. Traffic related disabilities and impairments and their economic consequences. In: *Crash Injury Impairment and Disability: Long Term Effects.* International Congress and Exposition; paper 860505. Detroit, Mich: Society of Automotive Engineers; 1986; SP-661:93–113.

9. Miller TR, Luchter S, Brinkman CP. Crash costs and safety investment. *Accid Anal Prev.* 1989; 21:303–315.

10. Luchter S. Multiple injuries in motor vehicle crashes. In: Proceedings of the 34th Annual Conference of the Association for the Advancement of Automotive Medicine; Scottsdale, Ariz; 1990:111–126.

11. National Highway Traffic Safety Administration. *The Economic Cost to Society of Motor Vehicle Accidents.* 1986 Addendum. Washington, DC: Office of Plans and Policy; 1987.

12. Insurance Research Council. *Paying for Auto Injuries: A Consumer Panel Survey of Auto Accident Victims.* Oak Brook, Ill: IRC; 1994.

13. Department of Transport, Scottish Development Departments. *Road Accidents, Great Britain, 1989: The Casualty Report.* London: Her Majesty's Stationery Office; October 1990.

14. Krafft M, Kullgren A, Lie A, et al. Car model safety rating based on real life accidents. In: Proceedings of the International Research Committee on the Biomechanics of Impacts, Berlin, September 11–13, 1991:25–39.

15. Sivak M. Human factors and highway-accident causation: some theoretical considerations. *Accid Anal Prev.* 1981;13:61–64.

16. Ministry of Transport, Motor Accidents in New Zealand. Statistical statement calendar year 1989, prepared by the Traffic Research and Statistics Section, Safety Standards Branch, Land Transport Division, ISSN 0550-5089; 1989.

17. Zlatoper TJ. Models explaining motor vehicle death rates in the United States. *Accid Anal Prev.* 1989;21:125–154.

18. Charlesworth KD, Cairney PT. *Development of Techniques for Studying Unsafe Driving Actions.* Australian Road Research Board, SR 39, Road Traffic Authority SR/87/4, Federal Office of Road Safety CR 58; 1988.

19. Evans L, Wasielewski P. Risky driving related to driver and vehicle characteristics. *Accid Anal Prev.* 1983;15:121–136.

20. Ferguson JC, McNally MS, Booth RF. Individual characteristics as predictors of accidental injuries in naval personnel. *Accid Anal Prev.* 1984;16:55–62.

21. Smith DI, Kirkham RW. Relationship between intelligence and driving record. *Accid Anal Prev.* 1982;14:439–442.

22. Baker SP, O'Neill B, Karpf RS. *The Injury Fact Book.* Lexington, Mass: DC Heath and Co; 1985.

23. Federal Office of Road Safety. *Driver Fatigue: Concepts, Measurement, and Crash Countermeasures (CR = 72).* Australia Transport and Communications; June 1988.

24. Ranney TA, Gawron VJ. Task demand and alcohol effects on simulated driving performance. In: Proceedings of the 30th Annual Meeting of Human Factors Society; Dayton, Ohio; 1986;1:265–269.

25. Stein AC, Allen RW. The effects of alcohol on driver decision making and risk taking. In: Proceedings of the 30th Annual Conference of the Association for the Advancement of Automotive Medicine; Montreal, Canada; 1986:59–74.

26. Stein AC, Allen RW. The combined effects of alcohol and marijuana on driving behavior. In: Proceedings of the 28th Annual Conference of the Association for the Advancement of Automotive Medicine; Denver, Colo; 1984:289–303.

27. Stein AC, Allen RW, Cook ML. The interaction of alcohol and fatigue of driver simulation performance. In: Proceedings of the 29th Annual Conference of the Association for the Advancement of Automotive Medicine; Washington, DC; 1985:91–104.

28. House EG, Waller PF, Stewart JR. Blood alcohol level and injury in traffic crashes. In: Proceedings of the 26th Annual Conference of the Association for the Advancement of Automotive Medicine; Ontario, Canada; 1982:349–359.

29. Waller PF, Stewart JR, Hansen AR, et al. Alcohol as a potentiating factor in motor vehicle crash injury. In: Noordzij PC, et al., eds. *Alcohol, Drugs, and Traffic Safety.* Proceedings the 10th International Conference on Alcohol, Drugs, and Traffic Safety. Amsterdam: Excerpta Medica; 1987:255.

30. Terhune KW, Fell JC. The role of alcohol, marijuana, and other drugs in the accidents of injured drivers. In: Proceedings of the 25th Annual Conference of the Association for the Advancement of Automotive Medicine; San Francisco; 1981:117–132.

31. American Medical Association Council on Scientific Affairs. Automobile-related injuries: components, trends, prevention. *JAMA.* 1983;249:3216–3222.

32. DiBlasio FA. Drinking adolescents on the roads. *J Youth Adolesc.* 1986;15:173–188.

33. Warren RA, Simpson HM, Buhlman MA, et al. Relationship of driver blood alcohol to injury severity. In: Proceedings of the 25th Annual Conference of the Association for the Advancement of Automotive Medicine; San Francisco; 1981:133–141.

34. Fell JC. Tracking the alcohol involvement problem in US highway crashes. In: Proceedings of the 27th Annual Conference of the Association for the Advancement of Automotive Medicine; San Antonio, Tex; 1983:23–42.

35. Haddon W Jr, Blumenthal M. *Determining the Drinking Driver: Legal Policy and Social Control* (Foreword). Lexington, Mass: DC Heath and Co; 1981.

36. Fell JC, Hazzard BG. The role of alcohol involvement in fatal pedestrian collisions. In: Proceedings of the 29th Annual Conference of the Association for the Advancement of Automotive Medicine; Washington, DC; 1985:105–126.

37. Pendleton OJ, Bremer R, Crowell S. Alcohol involvement in Texas driver fatalities: accident reports vs alcohol concentration. In: Proceedings of the 29th Annual Conference of the Association for

the Advancement of Automotive Medicine; Washington, DC; 1985:39–44.

38. Terhune KW. An evaluation of responsibility analysis for assessing alcohol and drug crash effects. *Accid Anal Prev.* 1983;15:237–246.

39. Stewart DE, Lawson JJ. Characteristics of Canadian impaired drivers: inferences from the 1981 nighttime surveys of drivers alcohol use. In: Proceedings of the 30th Annual conference of the Association for the Advancement of Automotive Medicine; Montreal, Canada; 1986:45–58.

40. Winek CL. Factors affecting predictions. *Trial.* 1983;19:39–46.

41. Stein AC. Factors affecting blood alcohol concentrations in humans: a review. In: Proceedings of the 30th Annual Conference of the Association for the Advancement of Automotive Medicine; Montreal, Canada; 1986:15–32.

42. Burns M, Moskowitz H. *Methods for Estimating Expected Blood Alcohol Concentration.* Los Angeles: Southern California Research Institute; NTIS, DOT HS-805-563; 1980.

43. Popkin CL. Drinking and driving by young females. In: Proceedings of the 33rd Annual Conference of the Association for the Advancement of Automotive Medicine; Baltimore; 1989:29–40.

44. Maull KI, Kinning LS, Hickman JK. Culpability and accountability of hospitalized injured alcohol-impaired drivers: a prospective study. *JAMA.* 1984;252:1880–1883.

45. All-Industry Research Advisory Council. *Compensation for Automobile Injuries in the United States.* Oak Brook, Ill: AIRAC; March 1989.

46. Otte D. Comparison and realism of crash simulation tests and real accident situations for the biomechanical movements in car collisions. In: Proceedings of the 34th Stapp Car Crash Conference; paper 902329. Orlando, Fla: Society of Automotive Engineers; 1990; SP-236:329–347.

47. Chipman ML, MacGregor CG. Time vs distance as a measure of exposure in driving surveys. In: Proceedings of the 34th Annual Conference of the Association for the Advancement of Automotive Medicine; Scottsdale, Ariz; 1990:421–432.

48. Chipman ML. Risk factors and automobile collisions: age, sex, and circumstances. In: Proceedings of the 24th Annual Conference of the Association for the Advancement of Automotive Medicine; 1980; Rochester, NY: 298.

49. Lee ME, Glover MF, Eavy PW. Differences in the Trip Attributes of Drivers with High and Low Ac-

cident Rates; paper 800384. Detroit, Mich: Society of Automotive Engineers; 1980.

50. Stutts JC, Waller PF, Martell C. Older driver population and crash involvement trends, 1974–1986. In: Proceedings of the 33rd Annual Conference of the Association for the Advancement of Automotive Medicine; Baltimore; 1989:137–152.

51. Kizer KW, Trent RB. Safety belts and public health: the role of the medical practitioners. *West J Med.* 1991;154:303–306.

52. Bourbeau RR, Laberge-Nadeau C, Latour R, et al. Road crashes and injuries in Quebec (1974): patterns among many variables. *Accid Anal Prev.* 1981;13:349–355.

Chapter 15

Collision Dynamics of Vehicles and Occupants

Lawrence S. Nordhoff, Jr. and Richard Emori

INTRODUCTION

This chapter addresses various collision types, crash dynamics, occupant motion at various stages in the collision, and the influence of interior vehicle structures, such as seat belts and head restraints, on injury production.

Vehicle and human crash data are obtained through several sources, including tests with human volunteers, animals, cadavers, dummies, computer simulations, and real-world accident reconstruction studies. Live human crash testing is presently less popular because of potential injuries or deaths. Larger animals, such as monkeys, pigs, and dogs, are very good in injury description, hierarchy of injury, and injury mechanisms, but results must be interpreted or extrapolated to humans. Human cadavers can be good in kinematic studies if adjusted for living occupants and can be good in determining various tolerance levels. Anthropomorphic crash dummies, which are used to re-create human frame sizes and anatomical accuracy and to apply data to real-world accidents, are commonly used. Several companies have emerged in the past decade

that run simulated crashes, using existing crash data and then feeding in accident-reconstruction information to predict human and vehicle kinematics and damage. All of the above methods provide useful information to vehicle safety engineers, physicians, and other professionals who deal with these injuries.

For the reader's benefit this chapter begins with crash statistics. Then the chapter is split into the precrash, crash, and postcrash phases. Phase 1 includes precrash variables such as mass ratio and use of seat belts. Phase 2 covers the specific crash dynamics for frontal, side, and rear-end collisions. Phase 3 includes postcrash injury variables such as head restraints and car interior impacts. Unless mentioned otherwise (e.g., low-speed, rear-end crash), this chapter primarily addresses the 30- to 35-mph passenger car crash.

When reviewing the following material, it is imperative to remember that there is no "typical" crash.[1] This is due to differences in vehicle crashworthiness, including factors such as injury or fatality risk for a specific car model; vehicle stiffness properties; safety design; curb weights; length of the vehicle; occupant space in which to move around during a crash; and a multitude of human factors, for which safety equipment may or may not be appropriate. "When style and safety clash, safety is a doubtful victor."[1]

CRASH STATISTICS

Frontal Collisions

The National Safety Council estimates that in 1993 there were 260,000 two-vehicle frontal crashes with 32,000 reported injury accidents.[2] Frontal collisions also account for 60% of all of the various vehicle collision types, including single- and multiple-car crashes.[3] A New Zealand study showed that 14% of passenger vehicles in frontal collisions have occupant-compartment damage and additionally 10% to 17% of frontal collisions have rear-passenger-area deformation.[4] In frontal collisions, 32.9% involve collision with another vehicle's side, 19.9% with another vehicle's rear end, 10.2% with a narrow rigid object, 6.8% with a rigid barrier, and 9.2% with the front of another vehicle.[5] The remaining 21% of collisions include rollovers, multiple collisions, side crashes, and undercarriage collisions.

Side Collisions

The National Safety Council estimates that in 1993 there were 3,010,000 two-vehicle side collisions with 242,000 injury accidents reported in the United States.[2] Approximately 30%[6] to 40%[7] of all two-vehicle crash types involve side collisions. Most side-collision impact points have been found to occur from 70° to 115°, with the usual point of collision just forward of the front occupant and the striking vehicle coming from the front at 65°.[8,9]

Rear Collisions

The National Safety Council estimates that in 1993 there were 2,750,000 two-vehicle rear-end collisions, resulting in 243,000 injury acci-

dents.[2] It is generally accepted that rear-enders produce the largest numbers of minor neck injuries.[10,11] Rear-end collisions account for approximately 2%[12] to 4%[13] of the total motor vehicle crash injury (MVCI) fatalities and 8% of the injury total.[3] Rear-end collisions of velocity change (delta V) of ≤10 mph were found in a National Crash Severity System report[10] to account for 45% of the injuries reported, whereas in frontal collisions only 2% had moderate or worse injuries. It has been reported by the National Highway Traffic Safety Administration (NHTSA) that 97% of all rear-enders produce no serious to fatal injuries.[10] The rear-end crash typically involves a stationary car being struck from the rear by another moving vehicle.

Rollovers

Approximately 10,000 people die and 30,000 serious injuries occur annually in rollovers in the United States.[14] Rollovers account for 17% of passenger car occupant deaths and for 41% of deaths in heavy truck rollovers.[12] They occur more frequently (60% to 80%) for pickups and utility vehicles and less commonly (30% to 50%) for passenger cars.[15] The best predictor for rollover tendency is the ratio of wheelbase to tread for cars and the ratio of truck width to the height of center of gravity for pickups and utility vehicles.[15] Digges et al.[14] suggest that the severity of injury to occupants in rollovers depends on the beginning velocity, number of quarter turns, vehicle damage, and environmental factors that may have initiated the rollover. Digges et al.[14] reviewed 1988–1989 National Accident Sampling System (NASS) data and concluded that around 60% of the economic costs for rollovers resulted from occupant ejection, and that the initial rollover speed was between 40 and 60 mph. Restrained occupants (48%), with a higher proportion of neck injuries than their unrestrained counterparts, account for about 22% of the total economic costs.[14]

Collisions into Poles and Trees

Approximately 1800 deaths occur annually in the United States from collisions into utility poles, and another 3600 from collisions into trees.[12] Utility pole collisions have 6.2 times more fatality risk than the average accident and three times more injury risk, accounting for 3.3% of all reported accidents. Studies show that 43.3% of pole collisions result in injuries.[16] Of pole collisions, 72.9% are full frontal contacts, with either right- or left-front sides having almost equal frequency of 25%.[16] Approximately 55% occur at the 12-o'clock position. In frontal pole collisions, crush distances of 21 to 50 inches resulted in 15% severe to fatal injury, while 20 inches or less resulted in 3% severe to fatal injury. In side pole collisions with more than 10 inches, dramatic increases in severe/fatal injury occurred.[16] Severe to fatal injuries from pole collisions occurred at delta V of 22.5 mph for small cars and 30.7 mph for large cars.[16] Smaller car-to-pole collisions were found to have higher delta V of 18.1 mph versus larger car-to-pole collisions having a delta V of 15.5 mph. In addition, since side structures of motor vehicles are weaker, the side of the vehicle may wrap around the pole if the collision speed is high.

Multiple-Vehicle Collisions

Multiple collisions, in which the vehicle is submitted to several successive collisions during the whole accident phase, are of special significance, as far as the injury severity is concerned. It appears that in this case injuries may be caused by almost all parts of the interior, due to the actual impact situation and the consequent relative motion of the occupants.[17]

Multiple-vehicle collisions occur in about 15% of total crashes, and the second-collision speed has been found to be just as high as or higher than the first crash 43.2% of the time.[9]

An example is the rear-end collision in which one car is pushed into a vehicle ahead, starting a chain reaction. Reckless driving behavior such as tailgating and continuing high speeds in fog and rainy conditions create the potential for these multiple-car collisions.

PHASE 1: PRECRASH VARIABLES

Precrash variables include factors that exist within the vehicle, the vehicle design, pre-existing human factors, road conditions, and others. For example, the size, weight, and safety design of the vehicle exist before the crash and may influence crash dynamics and injury production.

Collision Velocity and Injury Risk

We cannot assume that the crash velocity always correlates with individual occupant injury. The crash delta V (instantaneous change in velocity) is the best predictor of occupant injury severity or fatality; however, "the relationship between instantaneous change of velocity and injury severity (from the point of view of threat-to-life) is neither linear nor necessarily applicable to any one individual in any one crash. It is the probability of car occupant injury or death that increases with increasing delta V of the vehicle."[1] Humans have different tolerances; therefore there are many factors to consider when dealing with risk, such as variations in human tolerances, precrash variables, and crash variables. There are varying thresholds at which people suffer substantial risk of critical injury to fatality. There are crash victims having injury at 5-mph crashes while others do not have significant injury at 45- to 55-mph crashes. Ryan et al.[18] found in their 6-month study of neck injuries that the crash velocity correlated statistically with initial neck injury severity.

Positive correlation between high-speed collision velocity and crash injury have been reported, especially for side and frontal collisions.[19] However, in the lower-speed crashes, the correlation between crash velocity and injury occurrence is less predictable. For example, Foret-Bruno et al.[20] found that in rear-end impacts at speeds under 9.3 mph the risk for cervical injury frequency was 36%, and those occupants involved in speeds in excess of 9.3 mph had 20% neck injury frequency. The authors attributed the lesser neck injury frequency at higher-speed crashes to seat breakage. A recent NHTSA study concluded that there is significant risk for soft tissue injuries with delta V above 12 mph with the exceptions of lower-extremity injuries and lap belt hematomas, which may already occur at 6 mph.[17] Malliaris et al.[21] found in head injuries that minor (AIS-1) injuries occurred at 10 mph and that one-severity-ranking level worse injuries occurred for every 5 mph increase in crash velocity. Figure 15–1 illustrates a general graph showing a more linear gradual increase in neck injuries as crash velocities rise. The rear-end crash is unusual in that significantly more injuries occur at low speeds with a much sharper incline in the injuries seen.

Other injuries in rear-end crashes would probably follow trends similar to those seen in the frontal and side crashes.

Several studies have concluded that collision speed (delta V) and occupant age are the most important variables in injury prediction.[22-24] The kinetic energy (KE) that a vehicle possesses in a crash is proportional to the square of its velocity. In the frontal crash, when two vehicles are going in opposite directions, the delta V (collision speed) is equal to the sum of the speeds of both vehicles. In rear-enders, the delta V is the difference between the two vehicle speeds. Recently, White and Panjabi described a car that weighs 3,290 lbs traveling at 30 mph as having a KE of approximately 167,000 ft-lb of force.[25] If the vehicle speed is doubled to 60 mph, the KE is four times greater, which means that four times as much force is necessary to absorb the energy in the crash.[25] Of course, the crush design characteristics of the vehicle, time of exposure, and vector of collision play a significant role in whether the increased KE will create injuries.

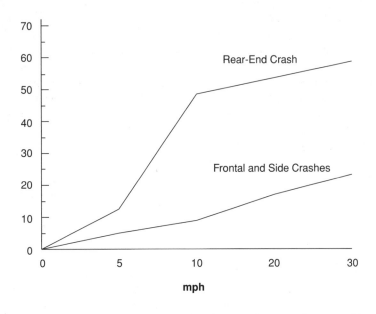

Figure 15–1 Neck injury frequency increases with collision velocity and vector of impact.

At What Crash Velocities Do Fatalities Occur?

A comparative study of the United States and Germany concluded that a crash having a delta V of 20 mph was the threshold for critical to fatal neck injuries.[11] A 1991 Washington Traffic Safety Commission study of 337 crashes concluded that a delta V of 40 mph or more is considered to be nonsurvivable.[26] The risk of being fatally involved in a collision per vehicle mile of travel is eight times higher at 55-mph speeds than at 25 mph.[27] Four occupant deaths occur per 1000 injuries when the speed limit is 30 mph or less. This rate goes up to 25 for 55-mph speed limit areas.[12] The probability of death doubles at 45 to 60 mph and then doubles again at 60 to 70 mph.[25]

Vehicle Size and Mass Ratio Factors

The majority of automotive crash studies show that the weight or mass of the striking and struck vehicle have significant influence on injury occurrence and trauma extent.[28,29] Figure 15–2 illustrates a mass ratio graph and the velocity changes that one might see in a collision of two vehicles of dissimilar masses. One 1987 English study reported that in frontal collisions, mass ratios were the most important factor for injury production.[30] A vehicle's "aggressiveness" results from its weight advantage, stiffness, size, and structural characteristics. The aggressiveness resulting from large mass ratio differences greatly influences the injury risk and severity to the smaller-vehicle occupant.[31,32] Increased risks for smaller vehicles include collisions from any vector, and relate to the occupant compartment space for the occupant and structural stiffness design. In the past two decades all car sizes and weights have been reduced dramatically as a result of federal requirements to improve vehicle emissions and gas mileage. Newer vehicles are easily 1000 lbs lighter today than comparable cars made 20 years ago. Newer technology has allowed smaller engines, lighter car-frame structural

materials, and better design. Although newer cars have better safety design overall, the safety value of being in a larger car in a crash is still significant. One large insurance study concluded that for every added 45 lbs of car weight, injury frequency was reduced by an average of 7.7% to 11.8%.[33] This study also concluded that there were 47.7% fewer head injuries and 40.9% fewer neck injuries in occupants of large cars as compared with small cars.[33]

Every vehicle could be considered crashworthy if it had a deformation (ability to absorb energy) capacity proportional to its own mass.[34] For example, in order for a 3000-lb car to have nonaggressivity with a similar size car, it should crush 38 inches. A 4000-lb car should therefore be able to crush 47½ inches.[35] Light trucks have been found to be more aggressive than passenger cars.[4]

The delta V of two vehicles is inversely proportional to their weight ratio[36,37] and has similar effects in side and frontal collisions. Consider a large car of 4000 lbs and a small car of 2000 lbs hitting head on and having mass ratios of 2:1, with both vehicles traveling at 30 mph. At the time of collision, the larger car will slow to 10 mph, whereas the smaller car will instantaneously be propelled backward at 10 mph.[25] The larger vehicle has a 20-mph total velocity change and the smaller car has a 40-mph velocity change, which raises the risk of injury or death for the smaller vehicle. Figure 15–3 illustrates the advantages that a larger car has in changes in velocity (delta V) and fatality risk. If a 3000-lb car hits an empty tractor-semitrailer weighing 30,000 lbs head-on, with both vehicles going 25 mph, with a mass ratio of 10:1, the smaller car will undergo a 90% velocity change, immediately going backward at 20 mph, having a delta V of 45 mph.[38] The truck will have less than a 5-mph velocity change. A streetcar colliding with a small car at 3 mph is estimated to be equal to a small car hitting another small car at 40 mph.[39] A large truck can weigh up to 80,000 lbs if fully loaded.

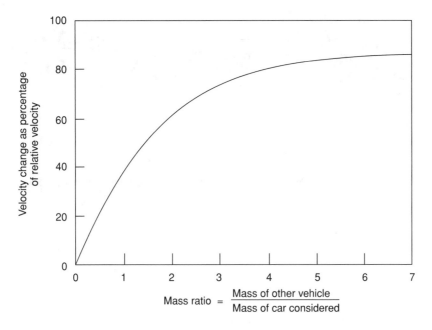

Figure 15–2 Mass ratio and velocity changes. *Source:* Reprinted from *Handbook of Road Safety Research* by G. Grime, pp. 86–92, with permission of Butterworth-Heinemann, © 1987.

Car Size Determined by Weight

- Minicompact—up through 1,949 lbs
- Subcompact—1,950 through 2,449 lbs
- Compact—2,450 through 2,949 lbs
- Intermediate—2,950 through 3,449 lbs
- Full size—3,450 through 3,949 lbs
- Large size—3,950 lbs and over

The velocity change for the occupant depends mainly on the mass ratios of the vehicles involved.[32] Vehicle size is the primary factor in injury severity: full-sized cars have 5 deaths per 1,000 accidents, whereas smaller cars have 15 deaths per 1,000 collisions.[40] Smaller cars (around 2,000 lbs) have 2 to 20 times more frequent injuries and fatalities than larger (around 4,000 lbs) passenger cars (2:1 ratio) in two-vehicle collisions.[27,28,36,41,42] Figure 15–4 shows the fatality risk by the size of the vehicle. An NHTSA study classifies two-vehicle crash driver fatality risk by the size of car, with the risk going up four times

for cases where skips in two size classifications (minicompact to large car) are seen.[41]

Smaller cars have more severe crash injuries and fatalities because they have less mass and less front-end crush distance and shorter stopping distances. Small cars may have less than 6 inches of side-impact crush space, making small cars prone to more occupant thoracic injury or fatality.[43] If a small vehicle collides with a car twice its weight, the smaller car must absorb about 33% more deformation and 20% more dynamic crush.[44] Figure 15–5 illustrates the design issues confronting the car safety engineer. When comparing the small vehicle with the large vehicle there is a large difference in crush distance available to the occupant and the velocity profile of the occupant.

In head-on crashes, unrestrained occupants in large-car to large-car collisions will strike their car interiors at lower relative velocities than will those in small-car to small-car crashes. Large-car occupants are safer.[19,45]

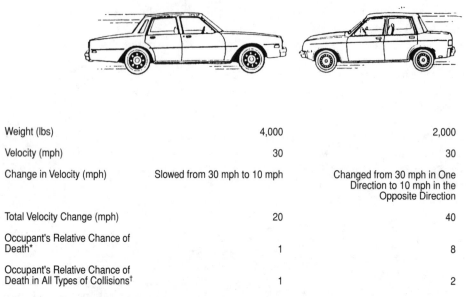

Weight (lbs)	4,000	2,000
Velocity (mph)	30	30
Change in Velocity (mph)	Slowed from 30 mph to 10 mph	Changed from 30 mph in One Direction to 10 mph in the Opposite Direction
Total Velocity Change (mph)	20	40
Occupant's Relative Chance of Death*	1	8
Occupant's Relative Chance of Death in All Types of Collisions†	1	2

*Based on 1979 FARS accident data in two-car collisions.
†Nearly half of all fatal collisions involve only one vehicle, e.g., car into a telephone pole.

Figure 15–3 Effects of a large car and a small car in a frontal crash. *Source:* Reprinted from *Small Car Safety in the 1980s*, National Highway Traffic Safety Administration, 1980.

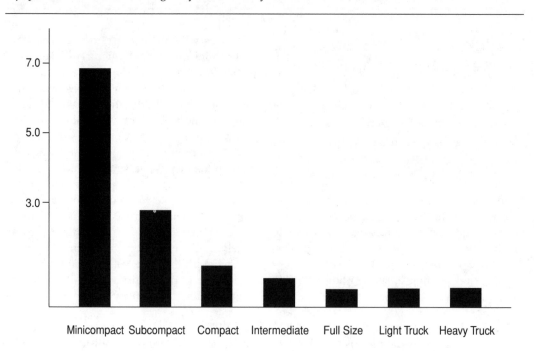

Figure 15–4 Fatality risk for the size of vehicle. *Source:* Data from Cerelli, E.C., Relative Risk of Fatal Injury in Vehicle to Vehicle Impacts Involving Cars of Different Sizes, in 29th Proceedings, Washington, DC, Association for the Advancement of Automotive Medicine, 1985.

Generally speaking, one study concluded that size is more protective than weight to the occupants,[45] but both have a role in injury. Another study concludes that the heavier the car, the more the occupant protection.[42]

Large Vehicles (Trucks and Commercial Vehicles)

Large trucks frequently are not compatible with passenger cars in collisions because of large mass ratio differences; stiffer front ends; and the height differences of the front, side, and rear truck structures that overrun the passenger car. The overrun allows the car to go underneath the truck structures. For example, the bumper of a truck may not even hit the passen-

ger car structures designed for collision and, instead, may even make direct contact with the occupants. A Berlin study of truck-car crashes concluded that 100% of the cars involved had interior compartment intrusion. Truck occupants had a 12% injury rate whereas car occupants had an 83% injury rate. The primary factor affecting injury severity was mass ratio.[46] If a car strikes a medium to heavy truck, the occupants of the car have a seven times higher risk of death than the truck driver.[38] Fortunately, newer trucks have bumpers and rear structures that are more compatible with passenger cars. It will take years before most of the older trucks are phased out.

An unloaded truck will roll over at 0.7g and a loaded truck at 0.3g, whereas passenger cars

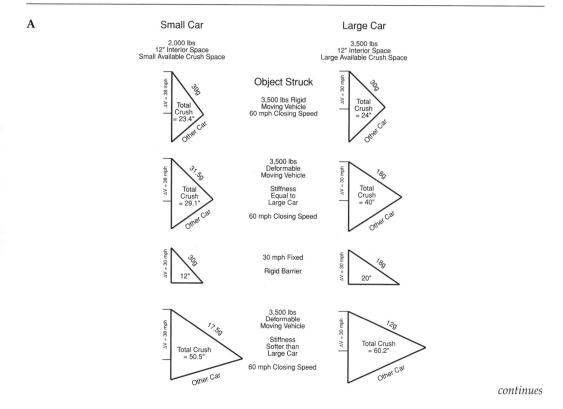

A

continues

Figure 15–5 A, simplified diagrams for large and small cars for various collisions. B, air cushion design constraints for large and small cars. *Source:* Reprinted with permission from Mertz, H.J., and Marquardt, J.F., Small Car Air Cushion Performance Considerations, Society of Automotive Engineers, Inc., paper 851199, 1985.

Figure 15–5 continued

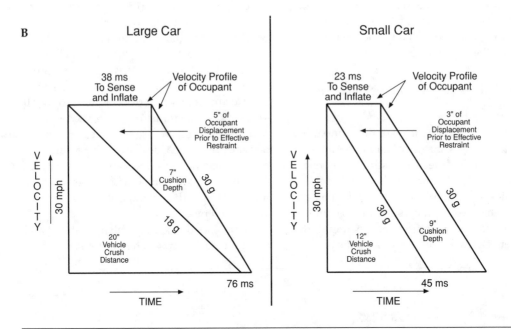

do not roll over until going over 1.1g in side acceleration,[38] which means that these larger vehicles are less stable when making lane changes and going around corners. Utility vehicles are involved in more single-vehicle crashes, nighttime crashes, rollovers, occupant compartment intrusion, driver ejection, and driver deaths than pickups and vans.[47] Light-truck (van, pickup, and utility vehicle) occupants have higher injury risk than passenger car occupants[48] and, in addition, their vehicles are more aggressive than cars and have higher rollover rates in single-vehicle crashes.[4]

Until about age 27, drivers of large/heavy trucks are overinvolved by three times[49] in fatal crashes. Drivers under age 21 are overinvolved in fatal crashes by a factor of 6.[50] Commercial-vehicle crash-occupant fatality risk is 0.4% when compared with noncommercial-vehicle occupant fatality risk of 4.5%.[51] It has been estimated that 68% of commercial vehicle crashes involve two vehicles; 25% are three-axle trailer/two-axle semitrailer combi-

nations; 3.4% of these vehicles jackknife before collision, 3.9% jackknife after, and 6.2% involve cars underriding the commercial vehicle. In addition, 24% are two-axle trucks, tractors, or buses; 17% are two-axle tractor/one-axle semitrailer/two-axle full-trailer combinations. Also, 45% of these collisions are deemed to be driver fault and 10.8% equipment fault; 60% of the time these vehicles are laden.[51] A 1987 Finland study on large tractor combinations found that 22% of the single collisions were due to avoidance of rear-ending, 44% of the rear-enders were due to following too closely, and the tractor driver was guilty in 39% of the cases.[52] Tractor-trailer drivers were found to be driving beyond the US Department of Transportation time guidelines in 58% to 90% of the cases in another study.[53]

Occupant Ejections

Around 36,000 occupant ejections from vehicles occur annually, with 42% of these ejections occurring at vehicle speeds of less than

30 mph.[54] These ejections happen mostly to unrestrained occupants in frontal collisions and rollovers, but also occur in side crashes. It is estimated that 11% of unbelted front-seat occupants are ejected in side crashes.[55] Most cervical injuries occur before or in the process of ejection as the occupant hits vehicle parts.[56] Seat belt use prevents this from happening.

Effect of Seat Belt Use on Reducing Serious Injury and Fatalities

The use of seat belts for drivers and occupants has gradually increased over the past two decades as a result of public education and federal and state laws. As of early 1990, 33 states have enacted mandatory seat belt laws. Recent overall seat belt use in the United States is between 46% and 50%.[57,58] The three-point lap and shoulder harness system is referred to in this text as a seat belt; single entities will be specified as shoulder harnesses or lap belts. The evidence is overwhelming that seat belts lessen fatalities if used properly,[37] primarily by eliminating ejections. It is estimated that if all front-seat occupants had used seat belts in 1989, 15,000 lives would have been saved.[57] A 2-year Virginia pre- and postbelt law study found that injuries resulting from windshield contact decreased from 11% to 6% and head-hitting steering-wheel contact injuries went from 14% to 10%.[59]

Air Bags

In a typical motor vehicle collision, an air bag will be fully deployed and inflated within 40 milliseconds.[60] When air bags are used in combination with the seat belt system, an 8% additional protection from air bags is observed.[24] Other studies show that air bag effectiveness is 21% for two-car collisions and 16% for single-car collisions.[61] Recently air bags have been compared to seat belt systems, using Fatal Accident Reporting System data finding that air bags reduce fatalities in large cars by 50%, midsize cars by 19%, and small cars by 14%.[62] The additional protection from the air bag assumes that the occupant is properly seated in the vehicle.

Improperly seated occupants, frequently children, who are sitting on passengers' laps, or the unbelted driver or occupant who prebrakes or is reaching for something and now has the upper body close to the air bag ejection port, can suffer high air bag loading.[63] There is nearly a 100% risk of having a serious injury if the bag is restricted by the person's body when the air bag is deployed.[63] The normal pressure is 170 kPa for an unrestricted path, whereas in a blocked path pressures exceed 550 kPa.[63] An air bag that is being deployed in a crash can propel a 29- to 34-lb child rearward over the front seat back if the child is improperly positioned at the time of bag deployment.[64]

Bumpers

Bumpers can either increase or decrease occupant or pedestrian injury, depending on design, bumper height, collision vector and speed, and collapsibility characteristics. Mismatching of bumper heights and braking can result in one vehicle's diving and the other vehicle's bumper underriding.[65] Underruns are a safety problem for drivers of cars that either hit or get hit by a vehicle having mismatched bumper heights. Bumper height can affect how much door crush intrusion will occur in a side collision. If the higher bumper overrides the stiffer lower frame, hitting the weaker door panels, more deformation will occur. One English study concluded that if underrun guards were put on large vehicles, there would be an estimated decrease of 3% in fatalities.[66] Fatal underrun collisions result in 85% having occupant compartment intrusion in frontal crashes and 17% in rear-end crashes,[66] which is higher than that for the normal crash population. Bumper heights also play significant roles in the pedestrian injury. (For more information about bumper role in frontal and rear collisions see section on vehicle damage relating to injury.)

Braking

Road-tire friction may possibly play a minor role in reducing vehicle velocity[67] and mitigating injury occurrence in low-speed collisions. However, in higher-speed collisions, friction from braking will have no significant injury-reducing effect. Braking converts kinetic energy to thermal energy by removing tire rubber.[68] Friction is the force that exists between the road and the tire interface, which acts to resist or retard relative sliding motion between the two surfaces.[69] Kinetic energy (KE) is expressed as follows: $KE = (W/2g)V^2$ lb-ft, where W is vehicle weight in pounds, g is gravitational acceleration at 32.16 ft/s^2, and V is vehicle speed in feet per second. Although most drivers are aware of the impending frontal crash, many do not have time to prebrake. In frontal crashes it has been found that in 57% of these crashes no prebraking was involved, and of those who braked, the average time of prebraking was 0.78 second.[5] Prebraking, however, will usually result in the occupant's head being closer to the windshield or dashboard.[70] Most car brakes can decelerate a car at 15 ft/s^2. A car going 100 mph needs 717 ft to stop. At 50 mph it needs 170 ft to stop.[45] Speeds of 60 mph on a dry road surface require a braking distance comparable to that for 45 mph in wet conditions.[71] Dry road-tire friction is 0.72g, and wet road-tire friction is 0.61g.[68]

Seating Orientation and Out-of-Position Occupants

In general, the seating position of an occupant and whether the occupant is out of position can have significant factors for injury production. Jakobsson et al.[72] conclude that the risk of sustaining neck injury can be related to occupant seating orientation, such as having one's neck turned at the time of impact. Figure 15–6 illustrates injury production by occupant seating position, with the driver having higher frequency because of the steering wheel (more hostile environment). Any occupant who is outside the normal upright seating position or is nonrestrained is out of position for a typical crash. This includes passengers who are sitting on laps, leaning or bending over at the time of the crash, or standing, or passengers seated unrestrained in the rear of a truck. Any of these situations put the occupant at risk for more injury. For example, in a frontal crash, the unrestrained occupant may have the chest near the air bag deployment device, causing high chest loading and injury. Unrestrained occupants may fly around the vehicle, hitting other occupants. If the occupant is seated forward at the time of a rear-end crash, a longer time will elapse before the seat forces will build up, which increases the relative occupant velocity between the vehicle and the occupant.[13] Romilly et al.[73] report that the forward-leaning driver or front passenger in a rear-end collision will have a higher level of injuries due to further seat and occupant head displacements. In rear-end collisions of 8.1 km/h, where the occupant has a 20° forward head-leaning position, the head deflection relative to the shoulder produces effects comparable to responses at twice the crash speeds, when compared with the normally seated occupant.

Vehicle Damage Correlation to Injury Severity

Historically, insurance company claims adjusters have assumed that collision injuries correlate to the vehicle external structural damage and costs of repair. A claims adjuster might state that since there was only $100 worth of damage to the car's bumper, the person could not possibly be hurt. On the other hand, the same adjuster might assume that since the car was totaled, the damage to the occupant must be great. The assumption that injuries relate to the amount of external vehicle damage in all types of crashes has no scientific basis. Three fundamental concepts of exterior front-end and rear-end vehicle design

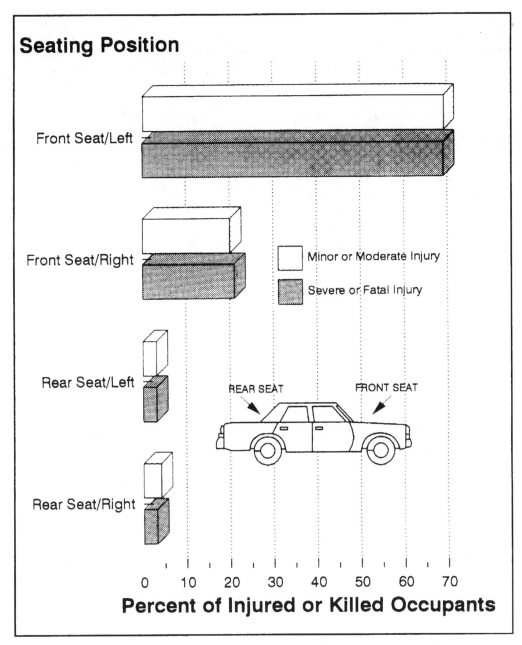

Figure 15–6 Percentage of occupants injured or killed by seating position. *Source:* Data from General Estimates System, National Highway Traffic Safety Administration, 1990.

currently are employed by automobile manufacturers: (1) to reduce the aggressive nature of the striking vehicle, (2) to protect the occupant from injury, and (3) to reduce repair costs

in low-speed collisions. The vehicle's front end and rear end must possess a suitable level of stiffness and still protect the occupant, and at the same time keep repair costs manageable. There is a conflict between the bumper stiffness requirements and vehicle compliance for occupant protection.[73] Much of the current crash performance standards address the higher-speed collisions as well.

A recent NHTSA report shows that crash characteristics become more favorable for the occupant as the amount of residual deformation increases.[74] There can be a very strong *inverse correlation* between residual deformation and injury levels in some instances. Injury levels decrease as residual deformation increases (car crush is good for occupant). There are several important factors that influence vehicle damage correlation to injury that must be considered: speed of collision, vector of crash, model year of vehicle, mass ratios, and vehicle crashworthiness. In addition there are two aspects to vehicle damage that warrant attention: the exterior residual crush and internal occupant cage crush. Collisions that are off-center result in more extensive crush distance and repair bills. The amount of crush that happens in the last half of the crash, and is still visible and measurable after the collision, is termed *residual deformation*. Dynamic deformation is what happens in the first half of the crash, and is the amount of total crush that occurred minus the elastic properties of the structure hit. For example, a bumper might have mostly elastic deformation; that is, the car is struck and moves forward rapidly with little or no measurable crush. The front and rear bumper characteristics include rebound at lower-speed collisions. In a side crash, there is mostly residual deformation. Hyde[1] reports that about 1 inch of crush occurs for every 1.5 mph of delta V.

There is little correlation between neck injury and vehicle damage in the low-speed rear-end collision. Ryan et al.[18] found that neck strains can occur from very minor crashes, even where there was almost no vehicle damage. Other evidence that supports neck injuries occurring at low velocities includes the consistent data showing that most nonfatal neck injuries occur in the low-speed

rear-end crash. In rear-enders, only slight increases in injury-producing forces are seen from 10 to 30 mph.[75] These same data show that higher crash speeds are usually required to cause neck injuries in side and frontal collisions. Another factor to consider is that cervical soft tissue and joint anatomy, combined with poor head restraint positioning and lack of awareness of the impending rear-end collision, make this injury more frequent and severe for all collision speeds. One cannot assume that all collisions are equal in producing injury in attempting to correlate.

In a recent NHTSA report, Romilly et al. state:

> The mechanics of a high speed collision are relatively well documented. The vehicle structure deforms, converting the system's kinetic energy into sound, thermal, and strain energies. The rate of deformation is a result of the vehicle's stiffness characteristics while the amount of recoverable deformation is a function of its elastic properties. At high impact speeds, very little elastic recovery occurs and the vehicle generally behaves as a plastic body. At low impact speeds, however, plastic behavior may be absent allowing most of the total impact energy to be recovered in elastic rebound. For the occupant, the best ride down profile occurs when the vehicle behaves as a plastic body with large deformations to reduce the overall acceleration. This creates a major dilemma for the manufacturer, occupant, and insurer. Each would like the vehicle to provide the maximum protection for the occupant with the minimum material damage to the vehicle during a collision. As the vehicle becomes stiffer, the vehicle damage costs are reduced as less permanent deformation takes place. However,

the occupant experiences a more violent ride down which increases the potential for injury. This implies that vehicles that do not sustain permanent damage in low speed impacts produce correspondingly higher dynamic loadings on their occupants than those that deform plastically under the same or possibly more severe impact conditions.[73]

In the side and frontal collision the best indicators of occupant injury are findings consistent with high direct loading within the occupant cage (thus transmitting forces to occupant). Intrusion of a vehicle into the occupant's protective space is often correlated with injury severity and collision dynamics. Indicators of interior intrusion may include the side door collapsing inward; side door being unable to open; or floor pan, knee bolster, dash, or steering wheel intrusion. If side or passenger compartment intrusion occurs, there is a 1 to 10 times greater risk of having a serious to fatal injury.[7] In the frontal crash this includes side door jamming and intrusion or damage to the interior of the car. In the side collision, inward bulging speed of the crushing door against the body of the occupant, "occupant-wall velocity,"[55] is the best indicator of high occupant loading and injury for the torso and abdomen. Head and neck injuries have been attributed to side wall penetration also.

Vehicle damage and occupant injury do not necessarily correlate with the collision delta V[76,77]; however, one study concluded that there is a significant relationship between the probability of a severe injury and the magnitude of lateral delta V in side and total delta V in frontal collisions.[23] High-speed collision damage may indicate severe crash dynamics or substantial crash energy deformation.[19] In a study by Jones and Champion,[78] velocity changes of 20 mph or more in direct frontal collisions, 22 mph or more in offset frontal collisions, and 15 mph or more in side collisions

were experienced by 90% of the patients having serious to fatal injuries. Vehicle crush damage in direct frontal collisions was measured at 20 inches, 28 inches in offset frontal collisions, and 15 inches in side collisions. There are normally 12 inches of precrash distance between a driver's chest and the steering wheel and 18 inches to the instrument panel.[79] In a typical frontal collision of 30 mph, the front of the car is pushed in 36 inches.[80]

Rigid and Soft Collisions

Most collision durations average around 100 milliseconds with a range of 0.1 to 0.2 seconds.[44,81,82] Short-duration crashes include front-to-front crashes, front-to-barrier crashes, and front-to-narrow fixed-object crashes. Rigid barrier collisions have shorter impulses[83] and have higher crash intensities when compared with long-duration collisions (Figure 15–7). Long-duration collisions involving less-stiff material are typically seen in crashes such as offset frontal crashes, front-to-rear collisions, and heavier-mass collisions.[5] Vehicle damage is greater in these situations, which makes the duration longer. The crash duration will increase as vehicle weight increases for a given delta V.[5] One study concluded that passenger car collisions into a fixed object would increase likelihood of serious injury by three times and death by five times.[7]

PHASE 2: PASSENGER CAR COLLISION DYNAMICS

Vehicle and Occupant Dyamics in Frontal Collisions

Frontal collisions take an average duration of 100 milliseconds, or the time it takes to blink an eye.[30] In a 30-mph frontal crash, the passenger compartment goes from 30 mph to zero in 91 milliseconds, with an average deceleration of 15g.[3] Frontal crashes at 30 mph will result in about 2 ft of permanent crush.[30] This

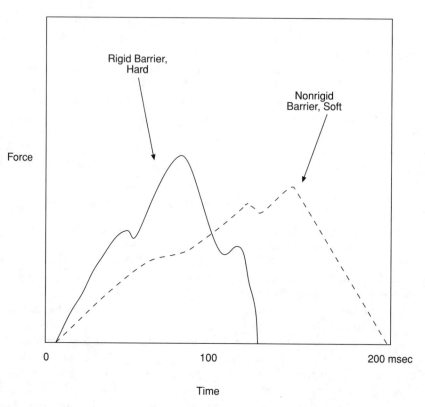

Figure 15–7 Typical forces and duration for collision seen for rigid barrier and nonrigid (soft) barrier collisions.

crash will have net effects similar to those produced by two vehicles, of equal weight, both traveling at 30 mph, having a closing speed of 60 mph. A recent study by Viano and Arepally showed that for a 30-mph frontal crash, a 165-lb occupant may develop 0 to 6733 J of kinetic energy with respect to the occupant compartment.[84] For frontal collisions of moderate to high speeds, some accident reconstructionists use a rule of thumb that crush distance in inches approximately equals velocity change in miles per hour.[83] This rule becomes less valid in offset collisions due to the fact that the central front end of the car is the stiffest, and as you proceed laterally, the stiffness lessens; thus crush distance will vary depending on the stiffness, and unless it is known how stiff, calculations can become more obscure.

Restrained Occupants in a Central Frontal Crash

Stage I. Typically, in a frontal crash, the vehicle will crash into another moving or stationary vehicle or lose control, hitting some object. The striking vehicle's front end will be pushed inward, directing forces into the structural members of the struck vehicle's body frame, usually off-center to some degree. If prebraking occurs in the frontal crash, the nose of the striking car will dive downward as well. In many frontal crashes the occupants know of the impending crash and try to prebrake and brace themselves. Unfortunately, only in about one half of these crashes do the drivers have time to prebrake. The braking deceleration may cause the occupant's body to move forward, or the driver may brace himself or herself against the steering wheel with the back forced into the seat back, or the front passenger may brace against the dash or windshield. As the crush proceeds into the engine compartment, in a central frontal crash, the supports of the engine are designed to minimize the risk of engine and firewall from protruding into the occupant compartment. As these forces continue to be transmitted from the firewall into the frame under the seat, dash, floorboard, and steering wheel, rapid deceleration forces occur within the occupant cage. The front of the car typically will crush in 2 ft, allowing the vehicle to move forward about 2 ft before stopping abruptly. As the vehicle stops before the occupant does, the occupant literally runs into the slowing or stopped car interior, such as the seat belt system or other interior structures. The occupant's compartment space is critical for ride down and can lessen the occupant's risk of striking the car interior. Seat positioning, occupant size and posture, vehicle interior design (front window angle and steering wheel shape and size), and size of car (less space for small cars) may leave the head or chest having a range of 4 to 18 inches from the front windshield, header, or steering wheel. Some drivers have their seats positioned forward to the point where their torsos are nearly touching the steering assembly.

Stage II. The vehicle is now reaching maximal deceleration. The 2 ft of front crush has ended with the driver's and front passenger's head, neck, torso, hips, and knees moving forward much faster than the now stationary seat under them. During this rapid deceleration, the restrained driver's left shoulder will move forward until the shoulder harness reaches its limits, holding back the left shoulder as the right shoulder continues forward. The driver, for example, can have the right shoulder and torso continue to move forward, causing head rotation and increasing the probability of sustaining concussion, intercostal sprains, and other soft tissue injuries. If the seat belt is

loose, the occupant's body can stop abruptly at the belt's tension point.

Once the seat belt slack has ended, the upper body will pivot around the shoulder harness, which acts like a fulcrum, allowing the unrestrained right shoulder to rotate forward and allowing the head, neck, and shoulder to rotate as they continue their forward trajectory.

Stage III. The driver's and front passenger's head, neck, and torso are now reaching peak deceleration levels. The vehicle has stopped all forward motion at this point. Shoulder belts may be loading up to 2000 lbs of force, depending on the collision speed. The pelvis has now moved forward and upward approximately 4 to 6 inches, depending on belt slack present before the crash, which can be reduced if a pre-tensioner is employed in the automatic safety system. The belted occupant's chin will usually not hit the chest with head flexion motion, as frequently believed, because of the forward inertial effects of the head, neck, and thorax pulling the entire neck forward as it flexes, while the torso is restrained, causing an axial stretch to occur.

During a frontal collision, the colliding forces first will be transmitted to the driver's feet, which act as a fulcrum, allowing the body to angulate around the feet until the knees contact the knee bolster at 72g and 23 mph, resulting in 3 inches of panel crush. The body will then angulate around the knees at around 62 milliseconds. At 76 milliseconds the chest hits the steering wheel at 78g and 28 mph, crushing the steering wheel 4 inches. Belted passengers' heads may strike their knees in situations with loose shoulder harnesses or older-model cars having only lap belts, if there is enough room in the car available. By 91 milliseconds the car has stopped, moved forward 2 ft by way of crush, and the driver's head has moved 2 ft forward for a net head movement of 4 ft, if crush distance is included. For taller occupants, the steering wheel now acts as a fulcrum. The driver's head rapidly decelerates in the now-stopped car, hitting the windshield and bulging it outward 5 inches at a contact velocity of 30 mph and 72g. If the head hits the header above the windshield, the 30-mph contact velocity and 0.5 inches of crush at 721g will occur. These experimental crash figures are averages; real crashes can have higher accelerations.[3,85] (See Figure 15–2 for illustration.)

A recent study by Viano and Arepally showed that for a 30-mph frontal crash, a 165-lb occupant may develop 0 to 6733 J of kinetic energy with respect to the occupant compartment.[84] The driver's chest and head will hit the steering wheel or windshield less frequently while he or she is belted. In frontal collisions more than 80% of all head impacts with the vehicle interior are contacts with windshield, rearview mirror, steering wheel, instrument panel, structural pillars, or windshield header.[86]

The front passenger will have different kinematics than the driver, due to the absence of the steering wheel in front. The unrestrained passenger's head frequently hits the windshield at the original collision velocity, with knees hitting the dashboard in early stages and torso contacting the dash later.[87] See Figure 15–8 for a comparison of driver and passenger in a 30-mph frontal crash.

Stage IV. The once-stationary vehicle is now going through a rearward recoil mechanism in this stage, especially if the striking vehicle hits another bumper at lower speeds. Most full frontal crashes will have about 10% recoil velocity or rebound. The driver's and front passenger's head, neck, and torso are now rebounding backward into a seat that will move rearward and then rebound the occupants forward. Sometimes the occupant's head may fully flex forward and backward twice before hitting the seat back. This rebound motion comes at a bad time for the occupant.

Unrestrained Occupants in a Central Frontal Crash

In a 30-mph frontal collision the body of an unrestrained occupant will immediately move forward within the occupant compartment.[3] The occupant's body will continue to move at 30 mph until contacting the vehicle interior just after the car stops. At about 60 milliseconds the occupant's knees will strike the dashboard. The lower body stops at this point, and now the occupant's torso pivots and flexes forward with the torso impacting the steering wheel at about 75 milliseconds. By about 90 milliseconds the front of the vehicle has crushed around 2 ft and the vehicle essentially has stopped. The occupant's head continues to move forward, pivoting over the steering wheel striking the windshield at 30 mph. When the passenger compartment has come to rest prior to head contact, the most severe injury conditions can occur.[3] In frontal crashes, the unrestrained occupant will either go down and under or up and over, with the knee acting as the fulcrum.[88] Unbelted occupants have about 10 milliseconds to stop, compared with 100 milliseconds for a belted occupant.[58] See Figure 15–9 for dynamic comparison.

For unrestrained occupants, the likelihood of benefiting from car ride down can increase in two situations: first, when there is only a small gap between the occupant's body and the vehicle structure; second, if the collision duration lasts more than 0.1 second.[89] Ride down occurs if an occupant slows down as the vehicle decelerates, e.g., a situation created by a seat belt. The unbelted driver definitely gets benefits from the steering wheel that the unbelted passenger does not, deriving additional ride down and less space to build up acceleration. Figure 15–10 shows major areas of impact injury in an unrestrained occupant.

Offset Frontal Collisions

About 60% to 80% of all frontal collisions are offset[9,30] to some degree, often due to the driver's attempt to avoid collision. A 12-o'clock-position frontal crash at 31 mph has an impact duration of 100 milliseconds with 41g of deceleration. The problem with asymmetric collision loads is that car structures in the center front are stronger, and as one moves away from the center toward the headlights, these

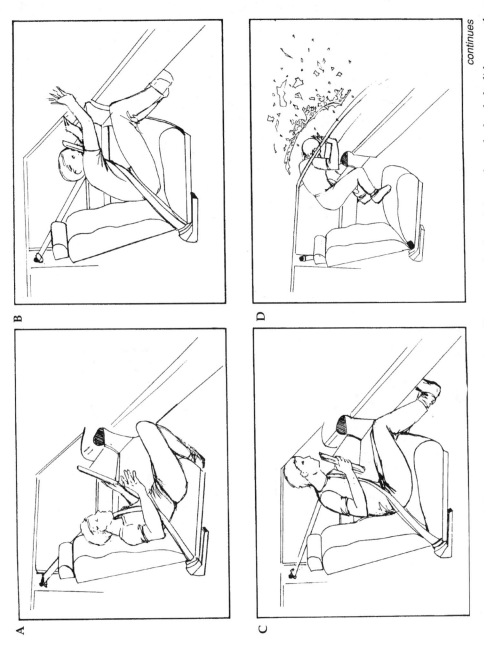

continues

Figure 15-8 Variations in frontal collision dynamics in a 30-mph crash. A, Illustration of submarining, where the lap belt slides over the anterior iliac spine into soft abdominal structures. B, A short driver may hit face in the steering wheel. C, A tall occupant may hit header. D, Unrestrained occupant may eject from vehicle. Restrained driver hitting head on steering wheel, caving it inward. F, Passenger in older vehicle with only lap belt, his head hitting his knee.

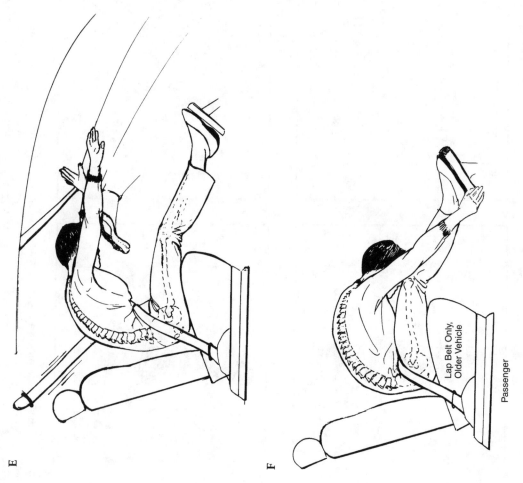

Figure 15–8 continued

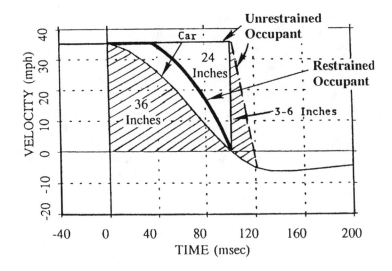

Figure 15–9 Comparison of car, restrained, and unrestrained occupant velocity changes in a 35-mph barrier frontal crash. *Source:* Adapted from Hofferberth, J.E., Restraint System Design and Crash Response, *Bulletin—New York Academy of Medicine*, Vol. 64, No. 7, pp. 706–707, with permission of the New York Academy of Medicine, © 1988.

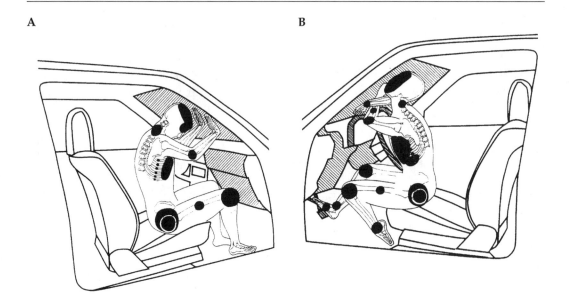

Figure 15–10 Major areas of impact injury (black) in unrestrained front seat passenger (A) and driver (B). The "hostile" contact areas (windshield, steering column, dashboard, and foot pedals) are striped. Note the involvement of forearm, hand and wrist, and foot and ankle. *Source:* Reprinted from Daffner, R.H., et al., Patterns of High-Speed Impact Injuries in Motor Vehicle Occupants, *Journal of Trauma*, Vol. 28, No. 4, pp. 498–501, with permission of Williams & Wilkins, © 1988.

structures have about one half of the energy-absorbing capability.[36,90] Off-center crashes always cause some rotation of the vehicle during and after collision, increasing the crash time and amount of deformation. A 30°-offset frontal collision will have a 180-millisecond duration impulse and 18g of deceleration. In addition, cars in 30°-offset collisions undergo rear spin of 13°.[36] Offset frontal crashes have 1.6 to 1.8 times more crush than full frontal collisions.[30,36]

Do offset frontal collisions have any role in the vehicle dynamics or any harmful or benefiting effects for the occupants? The car rotation in an offset frontal crash does not reduce the collision velocity, but it will increase the duration of the crash.[30] This can reduce belt loading to the occupant by 30%.[30] Unrestrained occupants will have about 10% to 15% less collision velocity because of the increased vehicle deformation,[36] and restrained occupants will have about 30% less loading in these offset collisions. Approximately 10% of the kinetic energy from the crash is used in the rotation of the car.[30,36]

Vehicle and Occupant Dynamics in Side Collisions

Most side collisions have the same crash time as frontal collisions, being about 100 milliseconds in duration.[6] Figure 15–11 illustrates common occupant dynamics in a side crash.

What Makes the Side Collision Complicated?

Side collisions are more complicated than either frontal or rear collisions. Many of the collision elements that apply to side crashes do not have any significance in other vectors of collision. Although most side collisions do not end with the occupant's head going through the side window, it is common for the head to hit the side window and bounce off. A 1990 German study found that in side collisions, 60% of the time, occupant compartment deformation was observed.[9] Following are important elements that must be understood by the doctor diagnosing and treating patients injured in side collisions[6,30,91,92]:

- There are no large mass elements in the side of the vehicle involved, such as the engine, wheels, bumper, and transmission, to lessen or disperse the incoming collision. Added protection may be given to the front occupant if energy-absorbing support structures are put between the driver's and the passenger's seats.

- The crush pattern from the striking vehicle's geometry plays a significant role in whether impact is narrow or wide, shallow or deep. The angle of the impacting bumper plays a significant role. The extent of dynamic crush of the doors is often hidden to the investigators, because of changes in door shape after the crash.

- Impact points of 6-inch distance from one point to another may make a significant difference in the stiffness of the target vehicle and therefore may have significant effects on injury.

- Side structural members of the target vehicle are usually of lighter-weight construction than other areas. The stiffness ratio of the side structures that are hit plays a more significant role than mass differences.[6] Figure 15–12 compares stiff and soft vehicles and effect on door velocity.

- Side collisions usually involve more vehicle rotation than most frontal or rear collisions. Unless the struck vehicle is stationary and hit at 90°, both vehicles will rotate. Vehicle rotation is dramatically influenced by mass ratios. Figure 15–13 shows the difference on the striking and struck vehicle when difference of mass is doubled for the striking vehicle.

- Side-vehicle structures have less depth, sometimes leaving only 7.9 to 11.8 inches of crush distance between the occupant's body and the striking vehicle's bumper.[93,94] At least in a frontal collision the

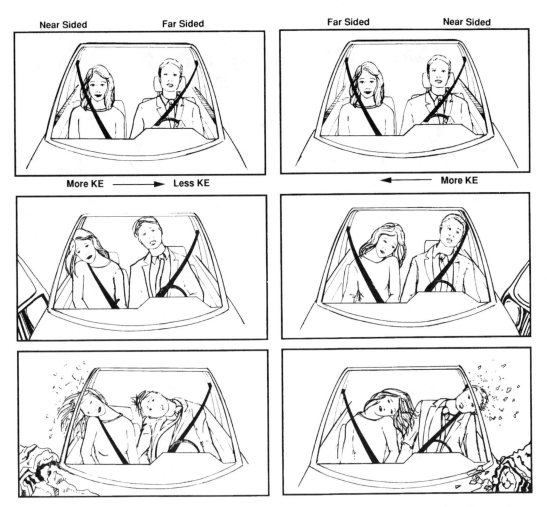

Figure 15–11 Illustration of driver and front passenger occupant dynamics in a side collision. Comparisons for near- and far-sided occupants are observed.

space is 39 to 47 inches, and includes the engine, firewall, and wheels, all of which act to absorb energy and protect the occupant. Larger spacing between the occupant and the side door is associated with increased injury.[82]

- Side structures provide less energy absorption than frontal structures, so the door often may hit the occupant near the striking vehicle's speed. The side doors' locking mechanisms and design characteristics may have a role in injury prevention or causation. For example, if the side

door is designed to lock into the door sills during a crash and thus stiffen the door, the occupant will have added protection. Side-door padding may decrease the spine and rib accelerations in side crashes.[82] Adding energy-absorbing door materials can reduce injury-related costs by 10 times and is effective in reducing injury by 10% to 20% in low-speed crashes with delta V of 4 to 8 m/s.[95] Side-door surface gaps or irregularities also may be associated with increased injury[96] due to tissue filling in the gaps.

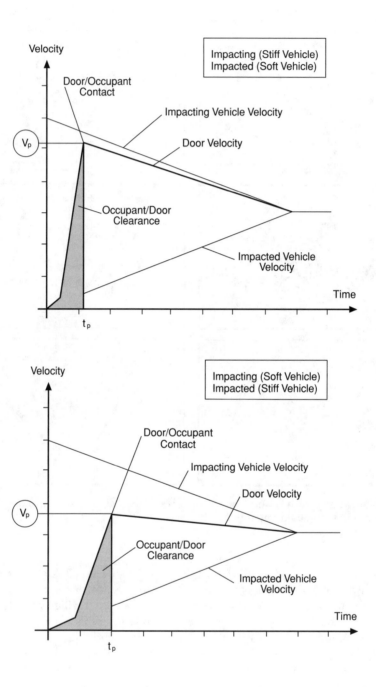

Figure 15–12 Door velocity (V_p) at the instant (t_p) of door contact in two configurations of relative rigidities of the vehicles involved. *Source:* Reprinted with permission from Foret-Bruno, J.Y., Occupant Velocity Change in Side Impact Method of Calculation-Application to a Sample of Real-World Crashes, Society of Automotive Engineers, Inc., paper 801308, 1980.

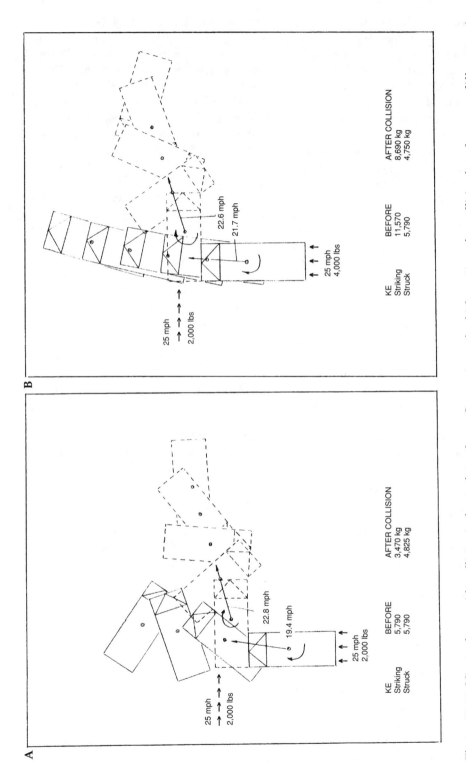

Figure 15–13 Ninety-degree side collision in front of struck car. Comparison of vehicle motion after collision based on mass differences. A, Two cars having equal masses. B, Striking vehicle has double the mass of the struck car.

- The presence of an occupant next to the door of the target vehicle will have considerable influence on the vehicle structural response during impact. The door may, in fact, wrap around the occupant, whereas in frontal and rear collisions, occupant presence plays no role in crush pattern.
- Normally, the occupant's movement is in relationship to the movement of the struck vehicle. When side intrusion occurs, this relationship to the vehicle changes. Deformation will alter the occupant's response to acceleration. Figure 15–14 illustrates struck car door and the driver's spine velocity levels in a side impact.

One study concludes that side collisions produce more severe injuries than either frontal[31] or rear crashes. This is primarily due to less structural mass and strength, less distance between the striking vehicle and the occupant, and higher overall delta Vs for the occupant. Studies show that the velocity of side doors in lateral crashes can be very close to the closing delta V of the striking vehicle.[3] In fact, in side collisions, the occupant's head has been documented going through the side window and actually hitting the striking vehicle.[3] See Figure 15–14 for an illustration of the effects on an occupant in a side collision. An occupant's body may fully eject in side crashes as well.

In side collisions, as in frontal and rear collisions, occupant injuries become more dangerous as the crash angle becomes less oblique and becomes more lateral or near 90°.[97,98]

In side collisions, crushing force from the striking vehicle is the primary mechanism of death. Crush is seen more often in lateral collisions than in those from any other direction.[99] More than 80% of head contacts with the vehicle interior are side-window car frame, A and B pillars, and side doors.[100]

A study in England concluded that the delta V was not the best measure of injury severity but that the collision speed of the striking vehicle was more significant.[101] In side collisions,

mild injuries dominated the 50th percentile occupant, with delta V being around 9 mph. For serious injuries, delta V was about 17 mph; for fatalities, it was near 31 mph.[7] In side crashes of 25 to 37 mph, the C-5 to C-6 area is the primary neck area injured, with strains at C-6 in 16% of patients. Disc injuries were found to be primary, with joint injury being secondary and muscle injury being tertiary.[102]

Near-Sided Dynamics in Side Collisions

A near-sided frontal occupant is the person seated on the side closest the striking vehicle in a side collision. In the United States, if the crash happens at the 9-o'clock position the near-sided occupant is the driver. Studies show that near-sided occupants in lateral crashes have two to three times higher risk of sustaining injury and fatality,[7,31] more compressive spinal column forces,[102] and significantly higher head and neck velocities and angular acceleration levels than the levels for far-sided occupants.[103] The four stages of a 9-o'clock-position side collision when both cars are moving through an intersection and collide, and the driver's door is struck squarely are described below.

Stage I. The struck vehicle, usually traveling straight ahead, is usually hit by an incoming vehicle in an intersection. The bumper of the striking vehicle hits the driver's door, door sill, and frame structures from the side, with the striking bumper being 7 to 10 inches away from the driver's body. The inside of the door frame, including armrest, is 4 to 7 inches away from the driver's torso and hip. The side window, which is usually inclined inward at the top, is about 4 inches away from the driver's head. The left arm is usually holding onto the steering wheel. The driver's head is turned toward the striking vehicle, as the driver realizes that he or she is going to be hit. The interior of the side door strikes the driver's body at the same striking collision velocity. The lower vehicle sill and side door are crushing inward, pushing the driver's seat toward the passenger's seat. The driver is also restrained. The near-sided occupant will interact with the

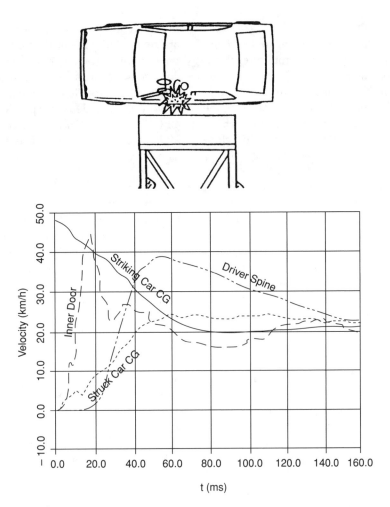

Figure 15–14 A side crash where a stationary occupant is struck by the encroaching door at high speeds with a self-limiting stroke. The door velocity-time history during occupant contact defines the severity of the side-impact punch. *CG* = center of gravity. *Source:* Reprinted with permission from Lau, I.V. et al., A comparison of Frontal and Side Impact: Crash Dynamics, Countermeasures, and Subsystem Tests, Society of Automotive Engineers, Inc., paper 912896, 1991.

intruding car structure well before the overall vehicle structures show impact forces.[104]

Stage II. The struck vehicle's side door, driver's seat, and driver's body reach maximal velocity at nearly the same time. The driver's head and neck remain stationary as the side of the door slams into the torso and lower body. The side window may be pushed directly into the side of the driver's head as it starts to move. The head and neck laterally accelerate rapidly toward the striking vehicle as the torso and lower body are being pushed and stretched in the opposite direction. Depending on the driver's height, the design of the vehicle, and the size and design of the striking vehicle, the top to the door and shoulder may act as a fulcrum to allow the driver's head to smash through the side window, even as much as ejecting partially or fully. The driver's head may hit the hood of the striking vehicle, especially if the vehicle has been modified (postfactory) to lift it up, as seen in some pickup trucks. The lap belt does limit the occupant's lower body motion. In side collisions, the head may initially rotate rearward 15°. In neutral head position in a side crash, lateral flexion predominates over torsion, and if the head is initially forward-flexed 7° at the crash time, the torsion predominates over lateral flexion.[105] At a 90°, 18.6-mph side collision, the near-sided occupant has 82g to 120g on the thorax and 64g to 98g on the pelvis. At 28 mph, there are increases to 149g to 158g on the thorax and 150g to 166g on the pelvis. At some 18.6-mph collisions and all 28-mph side collisions, pelvis tolerance levels are exceeded.[106]

Stage III. The velocity of the vehicle and the driver are still near striking velocity. The inertial effects of the driver's body on the struck body, which will tend to go in the same forward direction as it was precrash, now gets side forces of nearly striking velocity. To complicate matters, the struck vehicle spins, adding a rotational component to this already dynamic and very complex type of crash. The front passenger's entire body (unrestrained) or arm (restrained) may now hit the driver.

Stage IV. The vehicle has stopped and it may have struck another moving or fixed object while it spun around. The head, neck, and torso are now moving sideways away from the striking vehicle, with body rotation into the center of the vehicle. The occupant's head may hit the steering wheel or other occupants.

Far-Sided Occupant Collision Dynamics

The far-sided occupant is the person seated away, or opposite, from the collision of the striking vehicle. If a lateral collision occurs at the 9-o'clock position, the far-sided occupant is the front right passenger. Many side collisions involve secondary rotatory and forward velocities large enough to cause the far-sided occupant to hit the car interior in the front and side.[107] One study showed that almost 75% of all real-world side collisions had forward velocities significant enough to cause the far-sided occupant to hit the car interior in front of

the occupant.[108] A 1991 report concluded that approximately 39% of far-sided belted occupants get mild to moderate head injuries from contacts with the side window or roof, other occupants, near-sided door, steering wheel, or header.[109] Far-sided occupants also sustain 42% of torso and 23% of mild to moderate and abdominal injuries[109] and sustain harmful tension forces on the spinal column.[102]

Seat Belt Use in Side Collisions

In side collisions, forces produce lateral angular head and body motion toward the upper-side car structures, resulting in the unrestrained occupant's being lifted and sometimes ejected through the side window.[110] Seat belt use may reduce the risk of the occupant's hitting side interior structures by almost one third, but will have little effect on incidence of the head hitting the side window.[111] Seat belts provide an anchor for the far-sided occupant, limiting motion and reducing the likelihood of his or her body striking the near-sided occupant.

Rollovers

Rollovers are usually caused by the vehicle's hitting curbs or obstacles, dropping off embankments, or sliding through sod or soil.[112] Some rollovers are caused by sharp overswings of the steering wheel in reaction to potential danger. In a 32-mph rollover study, it was found that the car would roll around one revolution per second. The dummies in the car were pinned to the sides of the car by centrifugal acceleration forces of around 3g to 4g.[113]

Roof strength is not an important factor in injury production in rollovers as long as enough space is maintained for the occupant during the particular rollover.[113] In rollovers, 20% of the head-impact injuries incurred are probably from the occupant's colliding with the ground through the side window.[113] Bracing and muscular reactions have no significant effect on mitigating the rollover injury.[114]

Especially for the unrestrained occupant, there is violent and complicated motion in rollovers, with the most violent motion occurring 1 to 2 seconds after the roll starts, when the car is upside down for the first time. The occupant's head is close to the roof, especially so with a tall person, so most neck loading does not come from the roof, but rather through the occupant's torso and lower body pushing against the head. Studies with human volunteers indicate that three-point-belted occupants in a slowly inverted vehicle typically experience 4 inches of vertical head displacement when the vehicle is turned upside down.[113] Lateral head impacts and limb flailing are the primary sources of trauma for these people.[115] Lap belt forces in a rollover can give a few peaks at almost 2000 lb, and upper arm and window forces can reach 800 lbs.[115]

Vehicle and Occupant Dynamics in Rear-End Collisions

Most automotive crash research traditionally has focused on the frontal and side collisions because of their higher fatality risk. Recently more research has focused on the low-speed rear-end crash, primarily because of the frequent neck injury incidence and associated substantial economic costs. Typically, in a rear-end collision, a stationary vehicle is hit from behind by another vehicle whose driver is either tailgating or misjudging distance, or who does not see the car in front until too late. Unless the struck occupant hears the squealing brakes of the striking car or sees the vehicle coming in the rearview mirror, the occupant seldom knows about the impending crash and is not braced. This is usually opposite for the frontal and side collisions. We focus on the lower-speed crash dynamics, since most of the controversy does not focus on the higher speeds (Figure 15–15). The reader needs to be aware that there are still limited data on the lower-speed rear-end crashes and that there are some gray areas. There are four stages of collision dynamics for the rear-end collision.

Occupant Dynamics in Low-Speed Rear-End Collisions

Stage I: Vehicle Impact. Typically the bumper of the striking vehicle hits the rear bumper of a stationary vehicle, frequently stopped at a light or stop sign for slowed traffic on a main street at a low velocity, often under 10 mph. The striking vehicle's bumper and front end will usually collide with the struck vehicle's bumper and trunk, transmitting energy and forward motion forces into the underframe, which are then transmitted into the seat frames of the struck car. At these low velocities there is often negligible permanent deformation, depending on the age of the vehicle, angle of collision, and structural characteristics of the bumper. If the striking vehicles bumper (center of gravity[116]) is higher or is braking with the nose of the vehicle diving downward, the car frame and seats of the struck car will be accelerated rapidly forward and downward several inches. Downward motion occurs when the suspension system and tires are loaded. By 50 milliseconds the front occupants have not moved and the vehicles front seats will move forward about 2 to 3 inches in a 5-mph rear impact.[117]

Stage II: Peak Vehicle and Seat Loading. In the lower-collision velocities, peak vehicle and seat loading occurs from 50 to 100 milliseconds. Thomson et al.,[116] in a 5-mph rear-end crash study, found that at 50 milliseconds the struck vehicle has reached about 60% of its maximum speed. At about 60 milliseconds the seat back cushion is compressed enough to move the subject's hips and low back forward and upward. At the same time the seat back is flexing rearward in respect to the vehicle's motion.[117] The struck vehicle is now reaching peak acceleration. As the rapidly accelerating forces of the seat build up, the occupant's torso starts to slide up and backward, against the seat that is also deflecting backward, leaving a gap under the occupant. This ramping

Proper Headrest

Low Headrest

Absent Headrest

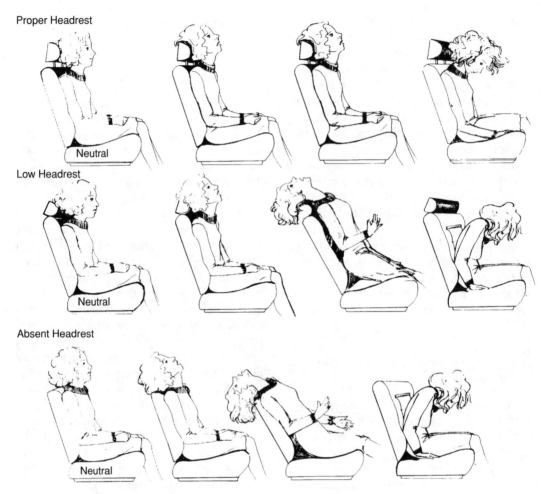

Figure 15–15 Rear-end collision dynamics for a typical occupant with proper, low, and absent head restraints.

effect can occur even at 5 mph[73] and is dependent on the seat angulation before and during impact, collision forces, friction between occupant and seat (seat material and clothing effect), and occupant's body shape and size. As the occupant's torso is pushed forward with the accelerating seat motion, the head and neck movement initially will rapidly flex or extend, depending on the occupant's preimpact orientation to the seat and head restraint position and shape. If the seat back and head restraint are close to the occupant, rapid extension occurs first. If the occupant is sitting forward, or the seat back is oriented at an angle that leaves a large gap, or the occupant is very kyphotic, then neck flexion can occur first.[118,119] The neck will flatten and possibly reverse—if the head restraint design permits—to fill in the gap, thus causing an initial forward head motion.

Stage III: Peak Occupant Loading. The driver's and passenger's shoulders reach peak acceleration levels at about 100 milliseconds, with the occupants' heads reaching peak acceleration levels at about 120 milliseconds. The struck vehicle's acceleration levels are now slowing down. Significant occupant motion has been demonstrated in the low-speed rear-end collision because of the elastic rebound properties of the seat back,[116] head restraint,[120] and bumper system.[74] At about 100 milliseconds the seat back has reached its maximum rearward rotation of about 10°.[121] High-speed film analysis shows that there is a seat back acceleration-related straightening of the normal cervical, dorsal, and lumbar spinal curvatures against the forward-moving seat back, causing an axial lengthening of the spine. The initial upward motion is immediately followed by a sudden and surprisingly vigorous descent of the torso, much like a rubber band, as the stretched and straightened spine structures are restrained and limited by the seat belt, with the spine forcefully returning to its normal curvature state.[117] One study showed that in rear-end collisions the head may have two impacts onto the head restraint, with the second impact having a higher magnitude than the first.[122] The seat back and usually more elastic head restraint are now rebounding forward, unless the hinge or frame structures fail, pitching the occupants' torsos forward at the worst possible time, as their heads are extended and the jaws open. The head will have higher acceleration levels when rebounding forward due to the elastic spring effect of the head restraint.[73] The forward torso and shoulder motion is occurring at the same time the head and mobile neck structures are reaching peak rearward acceleration levels at about 108 milliseconds. The shoulder has been found to rebound forward of the head in all low-speed tests. Photographic analyses show that the elastic properties of the seat allow the vehicle almost to reach its maximal forward velocity as the occupant's head reaches its maximal rearward velocity.[73] These rapidly opposing, and almost instantaneous, simultaneously accelerating forces cause the commonly termed whiplash injury. When the head is accelerated backward in a whipping motion, McKenzie and Williams[123] found that the head and shoulders may accelerate at levels 2 to 2½ times greater than the striking vehicle. Thomson et al.,[116] in Figure 15–16, verify earlier studies finding that head acceleration

levels can exceed those of the vehicle in low-speed rear-end impacts. Other authors have found that the rebound effect of the seat back, in conjunction with the ramping tendency, acts to increase the effective occupant change of velocity during collision (delta V) and thereby increases the potential for injury.[124] Romilly et al. found that in some cases the passenger seats had a rebound velocity 150% higher than the initial impact velocity.[73]

Stage IV: Occupant Dynamics after Vehicle Motion Stops. Both vehicles are stopped by this time. Occupant motion will continue to occur for up to about 200 to 400 milliseconds after impact, with the occupant's having the second peak acceleration level (about 6g) at about 220 milliseconds.[116] Rebound is an important factor in low-severity neck injuries.[125] The occupant's seat back has moved forward and the head and neck are now rebounding forward due to the elastic recoil of the seat back and the head restraint. The elastic seat back rebound, along with ramping, can increase the risk and violence of neck injury.[120,124–126] The risk is higher for taller occupants. The seat back will continue to load the occupant even after the external crash forces have subsided.[116] At about 250 milliseconds the seat back has returned to precrash angulation, or at the modified rearward angulation in many cases where structures have failed.

This is where the opened jaw can snap shut, damaging the meniscus. The occupant's chin will usually not hit the chest, due to the forward head inertia pulling the head forward to the shoulder harness and now backward as seat back rebound occurs, both holding the torso back. The occupant's head may whip forward and backward several times. Secondary injuries typical for a frontal crash may occur in this stage if the occupant hits the car interior; if the seat frame bolts break, allowing the seat structure to move; or if the struck vehicle strikes a car or another object in front, complicating and magnifying the already existing injuries. It is not uncommon in higher crash velocities to see cases where the entire seat frame has broken away from the car

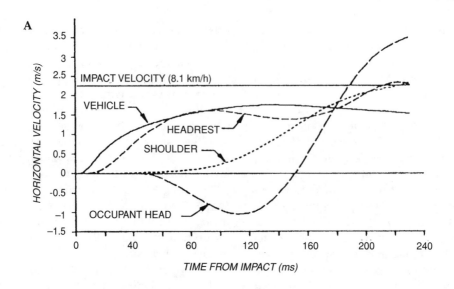

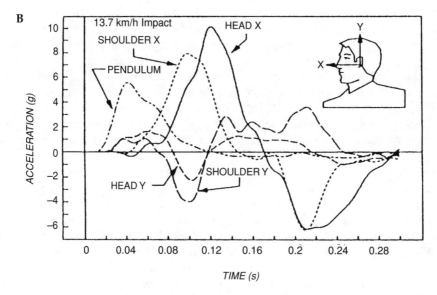

Figure 15–16 Occupant responses (A) and acceleration levels (B) in a rear-end impact of 8.5 mph (13.7 km/h). *Source:* Reprinted with permission from Thomson, R.W., Romilly, D.P., Navin, F.P.D. et al., Dynamic Requirements of Automobile Seatbacks, Society of Automotive Engineers, Inc., paper 930349, 1993.

frame or where the seat back has been broken as well.

Unrestrained occupants in rear-end collisions endure forward motion for about one third of the crash duration. During the second two thirds of the crash, usually about 25 milliseconds, the car continues to accelerate at 10*g*

to 15*g*. The seat will produce a rebound occupant acceleration of about 6*g* to 9*g*.[13] Rebound injuries involving contact with front occupant cage structures such as the steering wheel account for about 28% of all reported injuries, making them nearly as common as the hyperextension injury.[10]

Injury Mechanisms in Low-Velocity Rear-End Collisions

A low-velocity rear-end crash is defined for this text as 8 mph or less. There are many variables in the rear-end crash, explaining the complex but common injury mechanisms at low velocities. (See Chapter 1 for further details.) Figure 15–16 illustrates how complex the rear-end collision can be with elastic bumpers, elastic seat backs, and the cantilever seat system, and how these can all work to create a situation in which there is magnification of striking vehicle acceleration forces, creating injury potential at low velocities.

First of all, an occupant may sustain neck injury in cases having no cervical hyperextension or hyperflexion.[117,119] Several studies have analyzed human test subjects in low-velocity rear-end crashes (under 8 mph); they found that as the occupant's body was pushed against and flattened against the forward accelerating seat back, the lumbar lordosis, thoracic kyphosis, and cervical lordosis curvatures became flattened and elongated. The effect was similar to an accordion opening and closing. They concluded that the principal mechanical stress was rapid "compression-tension" cycle.[117,121]

It is also evident in a recent NHTSA report on low-speed rear-end collisions[73] that there is a differential motion between the occupant's head and shoulders in a rear-end collision. The subsequent rebound of the seat and head restraint tends to pitch the shoulder ahead of the occupant's head. This is due to different rebound speeds off the seat and head restraint. The elastic behavior of the seat catapults the occupant forward in the order of 150% of the original collision velocity. This elastic rebound of the seat allows the vehicle almost to reach its maximum forward speed as the occupant's head reaches its maximum rearward speed. This differential speed and displacement among the head, neck, and shoulder/upper torso cause the whiplash injury potential to occur. Significant occupant motion can be encountered in low-speed impacts because of the elastic rebound of the seat back.[116]

If the head restraint is low or absent and the occupant's head is able to extend backward beyond anatomic limits, the soft tissues may fail to tolerate the rate of loading. The neck may extend up to 120° if the occupant is tall enough in relation to the seat back and head restraint height. Ono and Kanno found that the neck bending moment of the low head restraint test was 50% higher than that seen in the standard height.[127] Emori and Horiguchi[128] found when using human volunteers in vehicles with no head restraints that neck extension in rear-end collisions with a standing similar mass vehicle was almost 60° at collision speeds as low as 1.6 mph. This range is near human limits of normal extension, so a low head restraint or the lack of a head restraint may be potentially dangerous for the occupant.[128]

The head restraint is the only passive safety measure for cars involved in rear-end collisions.[129] Fixed head restraints are cheaper to manufacture and safer for occupants, but the industry continues to make mostly adjustable types. In one study of over 300,000 crashes, it was concluded that fixed head restraints reduce neck injury by 24.5%, whereas adjustable head restraints reduce neck injury by 14.8%.[33] There are three primary designs for head restraints in today's vehicles: (1) the head restraint is absent, as is often the case in pickup trucks, vans, or older passenger cars; (2) a vertically adjustable head restraint is present, usually in the downward position; and (3) there is a rigidly fixed, permanent head restraint. When most people drive or ride as a passenger, they do not know which position is correct on the adjustable head restraint, so the majority of people leave it down all of the time for the sake of appearance and visibility.

The proper head restraint system should be designed to protect the front occupants in rear collisions and the rear occupants in frontal collisions. Head restraints should be positioned so that they contact the back of the occupant's head,[20] and should be elevated to the top of the occupant's head. The primary benefit of having a head restraint in a rear-end crash is that it will limit the amount of head extension, thus lowering the overall head angular acceleration by limiting the distance the head travels, and dampen (plastic behavior) the head rebound velocity. This frequently is not the case, because in the real world many head restraints have elastic effects on the head, causing high rebound velocities, and are not positioned properly. See Figure 15–17 for illustration.

Hyperextension neck injuries from rear-enders have been found to produce more damage to the occupant's neck than either frontal or side collisions.[10,130] It appears that only 25% of adjustable head restraints have been found to be positioned properly.[10] There is mounting evidence that properly adjusted head restraints will reduce injury frequency and severity for front-seat occupants in rear-end collisions[36] and rear-seat occupants in frontal collisions as long as the head restraint is high enough and positioned close to the back of the occupant's head. Several studies conclude that for front occupants a proper head restraint system will reduce rear-end collision neck injuries by approximately 13% to 50%.[10,20,33,129,131,132]

Low or absent head restraints may act to increase the amount of hyperextension and degree of angulation of the head backward when the vehicle is rear-ended. A low head restraint may act as a fulcrum.[133] A low head restraint or absent head restraint can magnify the occupant's head acceleration levels and increase the injury risk. The top of the seat or a low head rest can act as a fulcrum as the high acceleration forces push the chest forward while the head stays stationary, resulting in an upward, backward stretch of the neck over the low head restraint or seat back.[134]

Olsson et al.[126] report that the duration of neck symptoms may relate to the horizontal distance of the back of the occupant's head and the front of the head restraint. In a typical rear-ender, McKenzie and Williams[123] found

that the head and shoulders sustain two to three times the acceleration of the torso. If the fulcrum effect of a low head restraint is added, this process of magnification is further increased, even to the point where in some cases the occupant's face is fully facing the rear window! Head restraints that are low or are positioned backward from the occupant's head allow for more horizontal head and neck displacement.

If the head restraint is absent, the occupant's seat will maintain the car's forward accelerating velocity on his or her body mass below the neck, pushing the chest forward. The head will lag behind, staying in its initial position, resulting in the neck being extended or stretched over the top of the seat, creating increased neck tension. Next, the seat will bend backward due to the increased loading to the point where the seat will bottom out and rebound, projecting the occupant forward, sometimes into the front interior car structures.[3] Belt usage has value here.

Ryan et al. found that occupants who were aware of the impending rear-end crash had less severe injuries and at 6 months those who were unaware had 15 times more risk for persisting neck symptoms.[18] At low-collision velocities bracing can mitigate injury by lessening neck motion and thus focusing forces within myofascial tissues, which are preferred over ligament or disc injuries more typical for motion extremes. Jakobsson et al. found that the distance between the occupant's head and the head restraint was an important factor for injury risk.[72]

Depending on the occupant's seating orientation in relationship to the seat and head restraint, the neck will go into immediate extension or flexion. Recent rear-end crash studies have found that in some cases neck flexion occurred first.[118,119] This motion pattern is seen primarily in cases where the occupant is sitting forward of the seat. Some seat back designs promote large distances between the occupant and the seat, and in some instances the occupant may slouch or be ex-

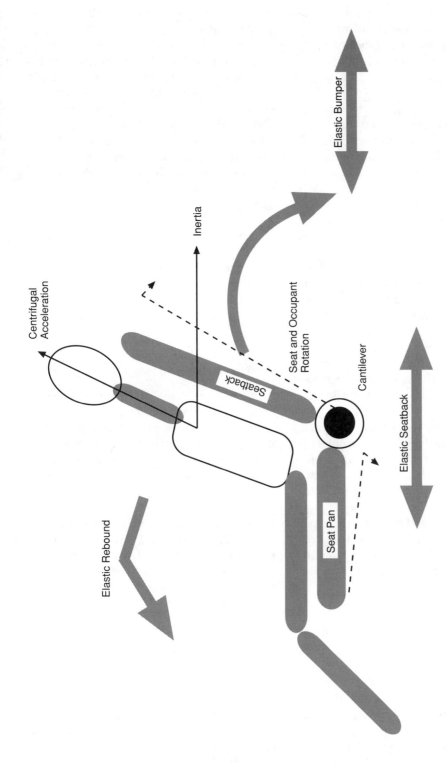

Elastic Bumper

Inertia

Centrifugal
Acceleration

Seat and Occupant
Rotation

Cantilever

Seatback

Elastic Seatback

Seat Pan

Elastic Rebound

Figure 15-17 How elastic rebound can occur to occupants in low-velocity rear-end crashes with negligible damage to either vehicle.

tremely kyphotic, leading to the same problem. Neck flexion may also occur initially if there is a large enough space between the head restraint and the seat back, allowing the neck literally to fill in the gap as the seat is loaded.

A low-velocity (1.6 to 3.6 mph) rear-end crash (sled-pendulum) simulation study of 26 human test subjects was performed using X-ray, cineradiography, accelerometers, and electromyography.[119] These tests compared 19 rear-end, 4 frontal, and 3 side crashes in seats having properly positioned head restraints. This study concluded that normally sitting occupants had their cervical and dorsal spines straighten and lengthen, whereas in stooped-shoulder and forward-sitting occupants the thoracic spine lengthened while the cervical spine shortened. Other observations made in this study include the following: the cervical spine goes into flexion before extension; higher head acceleration levels were found in belted occupants than in the unbelted occupants; and six subjects reported mild neck pain the day after the test that lasted for 2 to 4 days.

Head restraints for rear-seated occupants serve a different role than those for frontal occupants. The head restraints act as a face shield for them, and should be built to serve that purpose, because approximately 25% of all occupants sit in the rear seats.[3]

According to an NHTSA report, head restraints may be less effective for tall occupants, those in rear collisions having significant ramping, or occupants positioned forward from the seat.[10]

Unrestrained occupants are at higher risk of hitting vehicle interior structures, such as the steering wheel and windshield, when rebounding from the initial rearward motion. Unrestrained occupants may have injuries similar to those of the frontal crash victim if they hit the vehicle interior. One study concludes that seat belts may prevent thoracic and abdominal injuries in rear-enders, but may increase neck injuries by restricting pelvis movement.[134]

PHASE 3: POSTCRASH INJURY FACTORS

Several postcrash factors influence the frequency and severity of injury to the occupant. If the occupant's body hits or interacts with some part of the vehicle after the initial crash and sustains injury from tension or compressive forces, this is termed a postcrash injury. These include injuries sustained from hitting steering wheels, dashboards, windows, other occupants, or structural pillars, or from interacting with restraint systems. Some of the postcollision injuries can be reduced by proper car equipment placement, as in proper use an adjustable head restraint or wearing the seat belt properly. Other factors are influenced by the vehicle design and size. For example, larger cars may afford more distance between the occupant's body and the interior of the car.

Passenger Seats

Passenger vehicle seats have a very important backup role to the single or combination seat belt and air bag systems, especially in multiple collisions. The front seat may break from its floor mountings or the seat back may be distorted backward in rear-end collisions.[100] Federal standards now call for seat strength requirement of 20 times the weight of the seat back. Considering the weight of a seat back at 40 lbs (times 20), equaling 800 lbs of retention, this is woefully inadequate, especially if there are unrestrained passengers or materials behind the front seat.[100] Sharp and Stapp further add that "there is a second problem with this minimal standard of a 20 G retention for seat backs. In a rear end collision, the front seat occupants are thrust rearward. With a failure of the seat back, the occupants have now lost the use of their belts during the rebound phase."[100]

Seat design and crash force absorption qualities play significant roles in rear-end collisions. Typically, a 0.8° to 1.6° change in the seat back residual postcrash position was observed for every 1-mph delta V increase over 20- to 25-mph collisions. This study also concluded that seat back resistance is exceeded often in rear-end collisions over 20 mph.[13] Seat back failure may protect the occupants from neck injury,[20,75] and those occupants having less weight are more vulnerable to injury.[75] A 1990 study on rear-end collisions done in France, however, concluded that the capability of the occupant's seat to absorb energy was a better restraint system than head restraints in reducing neck injuries[135] because in most cases there is too large a space between the occupant's head, and the restraint system is usually too low, thus making it ineffective. Because the head positions for people can vary up to 3.5 inches in the anteroposterior position, it has been recommended that the head restraint should be manufactured to allow a 3.9-inch forward-backward range, and thus accommodate normal variations.[43] When seats are not deformable in a crash, the head restraint system plays a more significant role, and the space between it and the head becomes more important.[135]

Do Normally Functioning Seat Belt Systems Increase Mild to Moderate Injury?

Seat belt systems are primarily designed to prevent occupant ejection for all crash types, reduce fatalities from an occupant's striking objects, lessen the risk of an occupant's striking some body part on the car interior in frontal collisions, and lessen collision velocities for the occupant by creating a ride down environment.

Current safety standards are designed to reduce injury severity and fatality risk in higher-velocity crashes. Secondary benefits include reducing the incidence of an occupant's hitting interior objects in side and rear-end collisions and being ejected in side crashes. Seat belts are designed to fit 80% of the population comfortably,[136] but occupants in the 5th and 95th percentiles (small and large) often do not fit the standard design. As mentioned earlier, trade-offs occur in the design of safety equip-

ment in automobiles. See Figure 15–18 for a summary of the effect of seat belt use on injury in hospital cases. Seat belts can create problems if the smaller body frame allows the shoulder harness to position itself close to the neck, instead of centrally located between neck and shoulder; the neck then takes additional stress in collisions.[136] Larger occupants require more belt spool-out. The junction between the shoulder harness and lap belt should never be closer than 6 inches from the body midline, because of increased risks of abdominal injury and submarining.[137]

Seat belt use has reduced overall crash fatalities in the United States in frontal crashes, because seat belts prevent occupant ejection and reduce the probability of head impact with the vehicle interior. However, head impact still occurs even with belt use, although less frequently. Depending on the study, seat belts are 29% to 50% effective in preventing moderate to critical injuries,[10,33,138,139] and 32% to 45% effective in preventing fatalities.[84,139,140] Seat belts have been found to save lives at lower-speed collisions, but not at all higher speeds.[141]

A Finnish study shows that for fatalities and survivors of crashes, seat belts were the primary cause of all injuries from the car interior.[141] A recent study in England of 120 side and frontal crash fatalities concluded that 12% of the deaths were due to seat belt usage.[142]

Those occupants who are restrained in frontal collisions need as much space as possible in front of them in which to slow down, and certain crush characteristics will have benefiting effects. For unbelted occupants, few benefiting effects are observed in crushing characteristics, such as progressive crush, and it is better for the space between the occupant and the vehicle's interior to be small.[36]

Although seat belts are effective in reducing fatality risks overall, the use of restraint systems changes the patterns of injury. Figure 15–19 illustrates these changes. There are several reasons why seat belts can increase incidence and severity of injury in some cases. Three-point belts are designed with asymmetric geometry, with one shoulder being re-

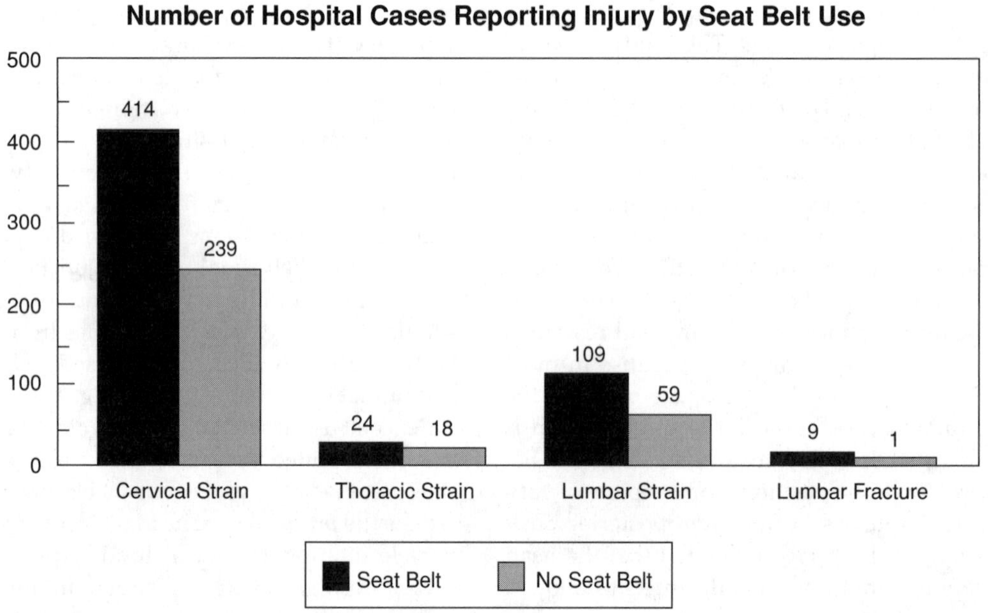

Number of Hospital Cases Reporting Injury by Seat Belt Use

Figure 15–18 Prospective study of the effect of seat belt use on injury in 1364 hospital cases. *Source:* Adapted from Olney, D.B., and Marsden, A.K., The Effect of Head Restraints in Seat Belts on the Incidence of Neck Injury in Car Accidents, *Injury*, Vol. 17, pp. 365–367, with permission of Butterworth Scientific Ltd., © 1986.

strained while the other is not, which results in additional head and shoulder rotational forces on the neck. Computer simulation shows as much as 60° of head twist in all frontal and side collisions.[40]

Loose belts can be a very serious problem in injury production for the occupant. Loose belts can be caused by the occupant's wearing bulky, loose clothing or using retractor systems that do not keep the belt snug, or in cases where the belt system is old or damaged and the system does not retract properly. Excessive slackness of restraints contributes to injury severity by magnifying the force and providing less ride down.[143] Loose belts also increase the occupant's forward excursion; velocity; and head, chest, and hip acceleration.[144]

Seat Belts and Head and Neck Injury

There have been several studies that correlated head injuries with belt usage. One such study showed that of those who used restraints, 18.4% had head and face injury, compared with 40% for those who did not use restraints.[145] The consensus of opinion is that head injuries may still occur even with seat belt use.[146] Seat belt use has consistently been found to significantly reduce the risk of head injury in lower- to moderate-velocity collisions. However, in higher-velocity crashes where the occupant is positioned close to the steering wheel, windshield, or other interior surfaces, the belt system will only have minor mitigating effects on head and face impacts incidence. Malliaris et al.[21] found that in 10- to 20-mph crashes belts significantly reduced head injury probabilities. They also concluded that in the 30- to 40-mph crashes belts only slightly reduced head injury probabilities. Head impact risk is dependent on the height of the occupant, how the occupant positions the seat for driving comfort, and vehicle size and design characteristics, which allow for

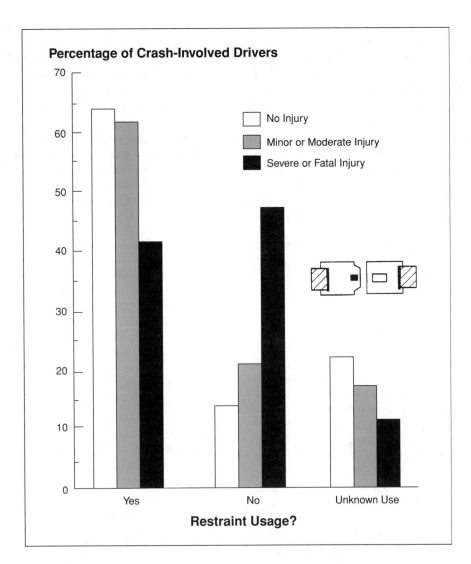

Figure 15–19 Percentage of crash-involved drivers with no injury, minor to moderate injury, and severe or fatal injury. *Source:* General Estimates System, National Highway Traffic Safety Administration, 1990.

varying occupant head and torso motion. It should be emphasized that fully restrained occupants have 1 to 2 ft of forward head motion during even modest frontal crashes.[1]

Other factors that may influence seat belt–related risks for the occupant include belt length, how the belt spools out during a crash, and occupant age and gender. In tests with dummies, 1.4 inches of extra spool-out causes the dummy head excursion to increase from about 18 inches to 21 inches at 30-mph tests.[137] Increased belt length can increase head injury risk by about 12%.[137] For every inch of added belt length, the head may have 0.25 inch of additional movement.[137] An additional 11.8 inches of seat belt webbing causes head velocity to increase about 21% and head acceleration to increase from $22g$ to $56g$.[147] Also, the three-point restraint's effectiveness may be associated with occupant age and speed of crash. One study indicates that these restraints are effective at a rate of 48% in drivers aged 18, and decline in effectiveness to 34% in drivers aged 60.[61] In crashes of over 30 mph, seat belts give less protection, according to a report by Huston and King.[40]

Most epidemiologic and automotive studies have found that seat belts increase the incidence and severity of minor (AIS-1) and moderate (AIS-2) neck injuries in automotive collisions.[33,101,126,148–150] A recent hospital study found around a 26% increase in the frequency of neck sprains, with the rear-end collision accounting for the majority of the increase. The unbelted occupants had 13.7% and the belted had 33.1% of the spinal injuries, including the neck and low back.[151] A Transport Office of Road Safety report of belt usage concludes that the use of the three-point belt increases minor whiplash injuries by 31% and moderate neck injuries by 29%, with head restraints reducing injuries.[152] It appears that there is a trade-off: in order to save lives, belt usage may cause some injury. In a recent study by Maag et al. of 3927 occupants in two-car crashes, neck injuries occurred in 21% of the belted and 14% of the unbelted occupants.[150] Several other studies have also concluded that in side and rear collisions, belted occupants suffered significantly more neck injuries.[126,150] A 1984 insurance report of 339,675 car crashes in Sweden concluded that 22.1% of belted drivers had AIS-1 neck injuries and 6.7% of the unbelted did. In another study, 4.6% of unbelted drivers in rear-end crashes had neck injuries, whereas 11.7% of belted drivers did.[33] Rutherford et al. also showed that the introduction of seat belt legislation has significantly increased the incidence of neck injuries.[153] Neck injuries occurred in 65.4% of restrained occupants versus 43.4% for unrestrained occupants in this study. The increased incidence in unrestrained occupants was believed to be due to more rotational head movement occurring as a result of the torso's being restrained.[11] An earlier report by

States et al. concluded that while belts may prevent forward pelvis motion, in the case of low headrests, they may cause the neck to hyperextend more, thus increasing neck injury frequency.[75] A surgical study on 38 MVCI patients with fractures to the C-2 pedicles found that 92% of these cases had injury from the shoulder belt's acting as a hangman's noose.[154] Neck-bruising "seat belt sign" following collision warrants close evaluation because of the risk of spinal fracture, cervical disc protrusion, and cervical cord bruising.

Seat Belts and Chest Injury

Seat belt use changes the pattern of torso injury and increases some chest injuries.[155] In a 30-mph frontal crash, the diagonal part of the shoulder belt may load 2000 lbs of force to the occupant's torso.[30] Belt anchoring during the crash causes the upper torso to move laterally and rotate.[156] Seat belt wearers have increased frequency of rupturing their distal descending aorta when there is thoracic vertebral fracture.[141] Belted front-seat passengers appear to experience lower head injury incidence than the restrained driver, but show higher numbers of chest and abdominal injuries.[70] Emergency tensioning retractors decrease the chest loading.[157] Chest-bruising "seat belt sign" following collision warrants close evaluation because of the risk of thoracic spinal fracture, rib fracture, and cardiac contusions.

Seat Belts and Abdominal, Lumbar Spine, and Pelvic Injury

The lap belt portion of the three-point seat belt system may cause injury to the occupant by acting as a fulcrum point for the rapid deceleration forces in a frontal or side collision. When this energy is focused in the pelvic area, or, if the belt slips over the front of the pelvis, the abdominal cavity contents are compressed—in some cases nearly 35% to 38%. This rapid abdominal belt compression results in the belt's approximating the anterior vertebral bodies of the occupant's spine. As a result, ligament tears, disc injuries, or spinal fracture may occur near the fulcrum point of the belt. A recent hospital study of 1364 MVCI patients found that belted occupants had approximately a 25% increase in the incidence of neck and lumbar sprain injuries.[151] A French study concluded that the lap belt was the primary cause for about 68% of the moderate- or greater-severity abdominal and torsolumbar spine injuries.[158] A 1991 German report concludes that lap belts cause about 60% of all abdominal and pelvic injuries.[159] Asbun et al.[99] report that seat belts change the pattern of injuries, with fracture/dislocations being seen because of the hyperflexion jackknifing of the occupant over the belt. The presence of the seat belt sign, which is ecchymosis along the strap site, requires hospital admission and close analysis to see whether bowel and mesentery are injured.[99] Another study found that 44% of the patients who had lumbar fracture and had been belted had associated abdominal viscous rupture injuries. In approximately 30% of the cases, the diagnosis of spinal fracture was not made for an average of 13 days.[160] In low-speed frontal crashes in which serious lumbar injuries have been reported to occur in rear-seat occupants, these cases are almost always related to excessive belt slack, poor belt position, or submarining.[143]

Submarining is usually due to rearward pelvis rotation, which allows the lap belt to slip up and over the front of the anterior superior ilium. However, it can also be due to lap belt angle, friction over clothing, and lifting by the shoulder belt.[161] Submarining may occur in collisions in which the lap belt is loose or the belt is located near the edge of the top/front pelvis, or when the occupant slides down the seat, under the belt. A mechanical seat belt pre-tensioner, which pulls up 3.9 to 5.9 inches of belt during an 8g to 15g collision, prevents injuries caused by loose belts but can create a more violent whiplash injury from more upper torso restriction.[162] A recent study using dummies in 30-mph frontal collisions

showed that in cases of submarining, the abdomen was crushed an average of 3.3 inches, with greater than a 48% incidence of severe abdominal injury.[84] If there is a 4-inch slack in the shoulder belt, it will have two times more belt loading onto the occupant.[5] If the lap belt is slack, pelvic loading is amplified 2½ times at 25 mph.[5] Submarining is infrequent if the knees hit a panel or if femurs have limited forward movement.[142] Sixty-eight percent of submarining cases, with AIS-3 (serious) or greater abdominal injuries and/or AIS-2 (moderate) or greater dorsolumbar spinal fractures, were caused by lap belt interaction.[158] Submarining can be minimized if the body is stiffened or braced, or if high seat friction is present.[158] If seat belt submarining occurs, the rearward upper torso rotation will increase 15° to 20°, causing the peak resultant head acceleration for the occupant to be increased by 22% because of the increased distance allowed for the occupant's head to move, according to the study by Viano and Arepally using dummies in 30-mph crashes.[84]

Seat Belts and Side Collisions

Although the seat belt is primarily designed for frontal collisions, the three-point seat belts do offer some protection in side collisions. Neck injuries are worse if the shoulder is anchored (vehicle being on opposite side of shoulder harness) in side collisions. In side crashes, belt use has been estimated to reduce head injury by 23.4%, face injury by 7.8%, and abdominal injury by 5.2%.[149] If the shoulder harness is on the same side as the striking vehicle, the belt holds down the shoulder, resulting in increased neck loading.[156,159] In side collisions in which the car gets hit on the opposite side of the occupant, having a seat belt is advantageous,[149] although the upper torso moves laterally and rotates.[156] About 35% of far-sided occupants who suffered minor to moderate injuries in a recent study reported having slipped out of the shoulder harness. It also has been found that in about 72% of those with mild to moderate abdominal injuries in side crashes the injuries were related to the seat belt itself.[109]

Seat Belts and Children

Seat belt systems and child restraints have been mandatory in all states since early 1990, and safety-seat usage is estimated at 81%.[139] Proper child safety seats decrease injury by an average of 61% in frontal collisions.[163] Among 229 children with MVCI, 14% of those who had been using adult lap belt–only restraints had cervical strains, and 21% of those using three-point restraints had them.[164] Children aged 4 to 9 do not configure to either child safety seats or adult restraint systems. Children are more likely to experience seat belt submarining because of their small, flat buttocks and short, underdeveloped pelvises.[165]

Seat Belt Use during Pregnancy

Fetal death as a result of seat belt use is rare, and the benefits of using safety belts outweigh the small inherent risks.[166] The primary cause of fetal death is not from belts but from maternal death. The best protection for the mother is to use the three-point harness, which will reduce the likelihood of ejection; head injury; and hitting her chest and abdomen against the steering wheel, her legs, or the seat, thus squeezing the uterus.[155] Seat belt use and proper belt placement must be emphasized by the doctor to the future mother.

Injury from Steering Wheels

The average space between the 50th percentile (representing 50% of the driving population) driver's chest and steering wheel is 14 inches.[167] Otte recently showed that around 90% of all drivers have less than 19 inches of distance between chest and steering wheel.[168] Injuries incurred by occupants' interacting with vehicle steering wheel assemblies account for 26.87% of the total economic costs to

drivers from car interior surface contacts, according to one 1982 study.[21] Steering assembly contacts caused 98.1% of the harm for shoulder injury to the driver and 0.6% for the front passenger in a study of 1979–1983 NASS data.[54] A 1991 report concludes that the steering wheel causes approximately 21% of all abdominal and pelvic injuries.[159] In the past two decades, much research has been put into designing steering wheels that will cause less injury. Energy-absorbing steering wheels, which have been introduced in recent years in the auto industry, decrease driver fatalities by 12% and reduce death and hospitalization by 38%.[163] No correlation was found in a 1982 study between frontal collision injury severity and steering rim or spoke deformation, or in the amount of energy-absorbing column compression.[169] Most of the injury takes place before deformation occurs, thus explaining the lack of correlation. A recent article concludes that the amount of steering wheel deformation is not a good indicator of chest injury.[170]

Injury from Windshield and Windows

The front, side, and rear windows in passenger cars are manufactured to minimize head and facial injuries. Current window glass in the United States has a plastic coating sandwiched between two layers of glass. This allows the glass to fragment into smaller, less injurious pieces and for the windshield to expand with the shape and force of the impacting head. There is a push to have the American glass standards follow in the steps of some of the European communities by adding a plastic coating to the inside of the glass to lessen the facial abrasions that frequently occur on direct contact with glass. Windshield impact severity was also found to decrease as the angle from the vertical increased.[171] If the collision forces are of enough magnitude to cause the occupant to hit the glass, a concussion must be suspected until ruled out. The rear window in a pickup truck is designed to act as a head restraint in rear-end collisions.

Injury from Vehicle Frame Structures

Head impacts to the A and B vehicle frame (metal structures between front windshield and side windows) are common in frontal, oblique, and side collisions, as well as rollovers. Although the rigidity of these structures is desirable with respect to roof structural strength, the same rigidity is less desirable if the structures are hit by an occupant. The head is the most common body part to hit, with less frequent impacts occurring to shoulders, arms, and other areas if the occupant is ejected. These structural members are narrower, more rigid, less padded, and uneven than windows and the padded dash. There appears to be a trade-off: strength is needed in these frame structures to avoid occupant crush, but the rigid material is more dangerous to the occupant if hit.

Injury from Knee Bolster

Knee bolster or instrument panel impacts occur commonly in frontal collisions for front-seat occupants. If a restrained occupant is in a frontal crash and no submarining occurs, knee impacts on the bolster are uncommon, unless crash velocities are high. Pike[172] recently concluded that the location of the impact on the knee can be very important. If the impact loads only the anterosuperior tibial area, rather than the knee joint and femur directly, the crash force tends to displace the tibia posteriorly with respect to the knee, thereby straining the posterior cruciate ligament—and in extreme loading rupturing it. The posterior cruciate ligament has only about ½-inch displacement tolerance, and injury to it should be suspected in the higher frontal crashes in which the occupant has struck the knee on the bolster or dash. The occupant in the right front seat has proportionally more severe lower-extremity injuries.[173] Knee bolster contacts may amplify the head velocity 6% while reducing hip and chest velocities by 6%.[5] This is one area of concern for automobile safety designers: when modifications are made in one part of the car, problems of safety may arise in others.

Injury from Armrest

Passenger car armrests, designed for occupant comfort and protection, can cause additional injury in some cases, primarily in older vehicles. This dilemma, like many in design, arises from ranges in occupant size, positioning, age, various collision vectors, and car crush extent. Design characteristics, stiffness properties, and crush patterns that help one type of population may work against another. One study on side collisions concluded that armrests could be contributors in 85% of abdominal injuries.[34] If the armrest is smooth and does not have indentations or sharp corners, the injury extent is minimized. One problem with armrests for most drivers is that they may have their arms up on the steering wheel during the crash. In side crashes the armrest will move at almost the same velocity as the striking vehicle. There is little space between the front bumper and the driver's abdomen, and little car structure to absorb crush.

REFERENCES

1. Hyde AS. *Crash Injuries: How and Why They Happen.* Florida: Hyde Associates; 1992.
2. National Safety Council. *Accident Facts.* Chicago: NSC; 1994.
3. Mackay GM. An historical perspective on impact biomechanics and some basic kinematics. In: Aldman B, Chapon A, eds. *The Biomechanics of Impact Trauma.* Amsterdam: Elsevier Science Publishers; 1984:67–80.
4. Tedford JD, Milne L. Vehicle deformation patterns in New Zealand road accidents. *Accid Anal Prev.* 1981;13(4):279–289.
5. Backaitis SH, DeLarm L, Robbins DH. Occupant kinematics in motor vehicle crashes. In: *Crash Pro-*

tection. International Congress and Exposition; paper 820247. Detroit, Mich: Society of Automotive Engineers; 1982; SP-513:107–155.

6. Carême LMM. Occupant kinematics and injury causation in side impacts: field accident experience. In: *Side Impact Occupant Protection Technologies;* paper 910316. Detroit, Mich: Society of Automotive Engineers; 1991; SP-851:1–15.

7. Rouhana SW, Foster ME. Lateral impact, an analysis of the statistics in the NCSS. In: Proceedings of the 29th Stapp Car Crash Conference; paper 851727. Washington, DC: Society of Automotive Engineers; 1985; P-167:79–98.

8. Finch PM, Gebbels DR. Side impacts. In: *Towards Safer Passenger Cars.* I Mech E Conference Publications, C185/80. London: Mechanical Engineering Publications Limited; 1980:79–82.

9. Otte D. Comparison and realism of crash simulation tests and real accident situations for the biomechanical movements in car collisions. In: Proceedings of the 34th Stapp Car Crash Conference; paper 902329. Orlando, Fla: Society of Automotive Engineers; 1990; P-236:329–347.

10. Kahane CJ. *Evaluation of Head Restraints: Federal Motor Vehicle Safety Standard 202.* Washington, DC: National Highway Traffic Safety Administration. Dept of Transportation, HS 806 108, 1982.

11. Langwieder K, Backaitis SH, Fan W, et al. Comparative studies of neck injuries of car occupants in frontal collisions in the United States and in the Federal Republic of Germany. In: Proceedings of the 25th Stapp Car Crash Conference; paper 811030. San Francisco, Society of Automotive Engineers; 1981:71–130.

12. Baker SP, O'Neill B, Karpf RS. *The Injury Fact Book.* Lexington, Mass: DC Heath and Co; 1985.

13. Strother CE, James MB. Evaluation of seat back strength and seat belt effectiveness in rear end impacts. In: Proceedings of the 31st Stapp Car Crash Conference; paper 872214. New Orleans, La: Society of Automotive Engineers; 1987:225–244.

14. Digges KH, Malliaris AC, Ommaya AK, et al. Characterization of rollover casualties. In: Proceedings of the International IRCOBI Conference of the Biomechanics of Impacts, Berlin, September 11–13, 1991:309–319.

15. Jones IS, Penny MB. Engineering parameters related to rollover frequency. In: *Accident Reconstruction: Human, Vehicle, and Environmental Factors;* paper 900104. Detroit, Mich: Society of Automotive Engineers; 1990; SP-814:73–94.

16. Mak KK, Mason RL. Selected characteristics of pole impacts. In: Proceedings of the 25th Annual Conference of the Association for the Advance-

ment of Automotive Medicine; San Francisco; 1981:43–53.

17. Otte D, Südkamp N, Appel H. Residual injuries to restrained occupants in front and rear-seat positions. In: Eleventh Technical Conference on Experimental Safety Vehicles. Washington, DC: National Highway Traffic Safety Administration; 1987:211–219. US Dept of Transportation.

18. Ryan GA, Moore VM, Dolinis J. Crash severity and neck strain in car occupants. In: International Conference on the Biomechanics of Impacts, Lyon, France; 1994.

19. Carlson WL. Crash injury loss: the effect of speed, weight, and crash configuration. *Accid Anal Prev.* 1977;9:55–68.

20. Foret-Bruno JY, Dauvilliers F, Tarriere C. Influence of the seat and head rest stiffness on the risk of cervical injuries. In: *Rear Impact,* 13th ESV Conference, Paris, France, 1991.

21. Malliaris AC, Hitchcock R, Hedlund J. A search for priorities in crash protection. In: *Crash Protection.* International Congress and Exposition; paper 820242. Detroit, Mich: Society of Automotive Engineers; 1982; SP-513:1–33.

22. Burgett A, Brubaker W. The role of the side of the motor vehicle in crash protection. In: *Crash Protection.* International Congress and Exposition; paper 820245. Detroit, Mich: Society of Automotive Engineers; 1982; SP-513:65–86.

23. Gimotty PA, Chirachavala T. Models for the prediction of severe injury. In: Proceedings of the 26th Annual Conference of the Association for the Advancement of Automotive Medicine; Ontario, Canada; 1982:63–76.

24. Verma MK, Repa BS. Pedestrian impact simulation: a preliminary study. In: Proceedings of the 27th Stapp Car Crash Conference, with International Research Committee on Biokinetics of Impacts (IRCOBI); paper 831601. San Diego, Calif: Society of Automotive Engineers; 1983:15–30.

25. White III AA, Panjabi MM. *Clinical Biomechanics of the Spine.* 2nd ed. Philadelphia: JB Lippincott Co; 1990.

26. Cooper WE, Salzberg P. Washington fatal collision research team: safety restraint usage in fatal motor vehicle crashes. In: Proceedings of the 35th Annual Conference of the Association for the Advancement of Automotive Medicine; Toronto, Canada; 1991:87–102.

27. Joksch HC. Review of the major risk factors. *J Stud Alcohol.* June 1984 (suppl 10).

28. Ernst G, Brühning E, Glaeser K-P, et al. Safety in small and large passenger cars: the compatibility problem in head-on collisions. In: Proceedings of

the International IRCOBI Conference of the Bio-mechanics of Impacts, Berlin, September 11–13, 1991:1–12.

29. Krafft M, Kullgren A, Lie A, et al. Car model safety rating based on real life accidents. In: Proceedings of the International IRCOBI Conference of the Biomechanics of Impacts, Berlin, September 11–13, 1991:25–39.

30. Grime G. *Handbook of Road Safety Research*. London: Butterworth; 1987.

31. Håland Y, Lövsund P, Nygren Å. Estimation of fatalities and disabilities in car to car side impacts—an evaluation of different risk factors. In Proceedings of the 34th Annual Conference of the Association for the Advancement of Automotive Medicine; Scottsdale, Ariz; 1990:275–287.

32. Thomas C, Faverjon G, Henry C, et al. The problem of compatibility in car-to-car collisions. In: Proceedings of the 34th Annual Conference of the Association for the Advancement of Automotive Medicine; Scottsdale, Ariz; 1990:253–267.

33. Nygren Å. Injuries to car occupants—some aspects of the interior safety of cars: a study of a five-year material from an insurance company. *Acta Laryngol Suppl*. 1984;395:1–164.

34. Tarriere C. *Injury Biomechanics*. Government/Industry Meeting and Exposition. Washington, DC: Society of Automotive Engineers; 1987; SP-731:211–221.

35. MacLaughlin TF, Saul RA, Daniel S Jr. Causes and measurement of vehicle aggressiveness in frontal collisions. In: Proceedings of the 24th Stapp Car Crash Conference; paper 801316. Troy, Mich: Society of Automotive Engineers; October 15–17, 1980:637–700.

36. Grime G. Car design and occupant safety. In: Aldman B, Chapon A, eds. *The Biomechanics of Impact Trauma*. Amsterdam: Elsevier Science Publishers; 1984:389–412.

37. Huelke DF, Sherman HW. Seat belt effectiveness: case examples from real-world crash investigations. *J Trauma*. 1987;27:750–753.

38. Ervin RD. Injury risks posed by incompatibilities between trucks and other highway users. *Bull N Y Acad Med*. 1988;64:816.

39. Harriton MB. *The Whiplash Handbook*. Springfield, Ill: Charles C Thomas, Publisher; 1989.

40. Huston RL, King TP. An analytical assessment of three-point restraints in several accident configurations. In: *Automatic Occupant Protection Systems*; paper 880398. Detroit, Mich: Society of Automotive Engineers; 1988; SP-736:55–60.

41. Cerrelli EC. Relative risk of fatal injury in vehicle to vehicle impacts involving cars of different

sizes. In: Proceedings of the 29th Annual Conference of the Association for the Advancement of Automotive Medicine; Washington, DC; 1985: 199–212.

42. Thomas C, Faverjon G, Henry C, et al. Discussion of "The problem of compatibility in car-to-car collisions," by Evans L. In: Proceedings of the 34th Annual Conference of the Association for the Advancement of Automotive Medicine; Scottsdale, Ariz; 1990:269–273.

43. Jeffery KR. Head and neck profile data for headrest design in fixed geometry seating. *Eur J Chirop*. 1984;32:197–204.

44. Anonymous. *Crash 3: Users Guide and Technical Manual*. Washington, DC: Dept of Transportation; 1981; HS 805732.

45. Robertson LS. *Injuries: Causes, Control Strategies, and Public Policy*. Lexington, Mass: DC Heath and Co; 1983.

46. Flory PJ, Otte D. Truck accidents: patterns of kinematics and injuries. In: International Association for Accident and Traffic Medicine (IAATM). Denmark, 1980:201–204.

47. Ranney TA. Accident characteristics and injury causation in accidents involving light trucks, vans, and utility vehicles. In: Proceedings of the 25th Annual Conference of the Association for the Advancement of Automotive Medicine; San Francisco, 1981;57–68.

48. Fan WRS, Jettner E. Light vehicle occupant protection: top and rear structures and interiors. In: *Crash Protection*. International Congress and Exposition; paper 820244. Detroit, Mich: Society of Automotive Engineers; 1982; SP-513:53–63.

49. Council FM, Hall WL. Large truck safety: an analysis of North Carolina accident data. In: Proceedings of the 33rd Annual Conference of the Association for the Advancement of Automotive Medicine; Baltimore; 1989:91–110.

50. Campbell KL. Fatal accident involvement rates by driver age for large trucks. In: Proceedings of the 33rd Annual Conference of the Association for the Advancement of Automotive Medicine; Baltimore; 1989:111–122.

51. Philipson LL, Rashti P, Fleischer GA. Statistical analysis of highway commercial vehicle accidents. *Accid Anal Prev*. 1981;13(4):289–306.

52. Kallberg VP. *Road Accidents of Trailer Combinations in Finland, A Case Study*. Research Report 511. Espoo, November 1987, Technical Research Centre of Finland.

53. Hertz RP. The prevalence of hours of service violations among tractor-trailer drivers. In: Proceedings of the 33rd Annual Conference of the Asso-

ciation for the Advancement of Automotive Engineers; Baltimore; 1989:123–136.

54. Malliaris AC, Hitchcok R, Hansen M. Harm causation and ranking. In: *Car Crashes*. International Congress and Exposition; paper 850090. Detroit, Mich: Society of Automotive Engineers; February 25–March 1, 1985.

55. Thomas C, Henry C, Harteman F, et al. Injury pattern and parameters to assess severity for occupants involved in car-to-car lateral impacts. In: Proceedings of the Eleventh International Technical Conference on Experimental Safety Vehicles; 1987:49–62.

56. Huelke DF, O'Day J, Mendelsohn RA. Cervical injuries suffered in automobile crashes. *J Neurosurg.* 1981;54:316–322.

57. National Safety Council. *Buckle Up.* The Safety Center, a chapter of the NSC. Sacramento, Calif: NSC; 1991:3(7).

58. States JD. Problem delineation: automobile restraint systems. *Bull N Y Acad Med.* 1988;64:684–702.

59. Lestina DC, Williams AF, Lund AK, et al. Motor vehicle crash injury patterns and the Virginia seat belt law. *JAMA.* 1991;265:1409–1439.

60. Yang KH, Wang H, Wang H-C, et al. Development of a two-dimensional driver side airbag deployment algorithm. In: Proceedings of the 34th Stapp Car Crash Conference; paper 902323. Orlando, Fla: Society of Automotive Engineers; 1990; P-236:259–266.

61. Evans L. Airbag effectiveness in preventing fatalities predicted according to type of crash, driver age, and blood alcohol concentration. In: Proceedings of the 33rd Annual Conference of the Association for the Advancement of Automotive Medicine; Baltimore; 1989:307–322.

62. Zador PL, Ciccone MA. Automobile driver fatalities in frontal impacts: air bags compared with manual belts. *Am J Public Health.* 1993;83:661–666.

63. Horsch J, Lau I, Andrzejak D, et al. Assessment of air bag deployment loads. In: Proceedings of the 34th Stapp Car Crash Conference; paper 902324. Orlando, Fla: Society of Automotive Engineers; 1990; P-236:267–288.

64. Patrick LM, Nyquist GW. Airbag effects on the out-of-position child. In: Viano DC, ed. *Passenger Car Inflatable Restraint Systems: A Compendium of Published Safety Research.* Warrendale, Pa: Society of Automotive Engineers; 1987; PT-87:271–279.

65. Vaillancourt DR, Pulling NH. Car dive and collision cost. *Accid Anal Prev.* 1983;15(3):207–214.

66. Gloyns PF, Rattenbury SJ. Cars in conflict with larger vehicles: the problem of under-run, automotive frontal impacts. International Congress and Exposition. Detroit, Mich: Society of Automotive Engineers; February 27–March 3, 1989; SP-782:1–12.

67. Brach RM. Analysis of planar vehicle collisions using equations of impulse and momentum. *Accid Anal Prev.* 1983;15(2):105–130.

68. Reed WS, Keskin AT. Vehicular deceleration and its relationship to friction. In: *Motor Vehicle Accident Reconstruction.* International Congress and Exposition; paper 890736. Detroit, Mich: Society of Automotive Engineers; 1989; SP-777: 115–120.

69. Warner CY, Smith GC, James MB, et al. Friction applications in accident reconstruction. In: Backaitis SH, ed. *Accident Reconstruction Technologies: Pedestrians and Motorcycles in Automotive Collisions*; paper 830612. Warrendale, Pa: Society of Automotive Engineers; 1990; PT-35:404–416.

70. Backaitis SH. Injury patterns and injury sources of unrestrained and three point belt restrained car occupants in injury producing frontal collisions. In: Proceedings of the 29th Annual Conference of the Association for the Advancement of Automotive Medicine; Washington, DC; 1985:365–385.

71. Hight PV, Wheeler JB, Reust TJ, et al. The effects of right side water drag on vehicle dynamics and accident causation. In: *Accident Reconstruction: Human, Vehicle, and Environmental Factors*; paper 900105. Detroit, Mich: Society of Automotive Engineers; 1990; SP-814:95–106.

72. Jakobsson L, Norin H, Jernström C, et al. Analysis of different head and neck responses in rear-end car collisions using a new humanlike mathematical model. International Conference on the Biomechanics of Impacts, Lyon, France, 1994.

73. Romilly DP, Thomson RW, Navin FPD, et al. Low speed rear impacts and elastic properties of automobiles. In: Proceedings of the 12th International Technical Conference of Experimental Safety Vehicles. Washington, DC: National Highway Traffic Safety Administration; 1989;2:1199–1204. US Dept of Transportation.

74. Matsushita K, Morita S. Relationship between vehicle front-end stiffness and dummy injury during collisions. In: Eleventh International Technical Conference on Experimental Safety Vehicles. Washington, DC: National Highway Traffic Safety Administration; 1987:529–537. US Dept of Transportation.

75. States JD, Korn MW, Masengill JB. The enigma of whiplash injury. *N Y State J Med.* December 15, 1970:2971–2977.

76. Cheng PH, Guenther DA. Effects of change in angular velocity of a vehicle on the change in velocity experienced by an occupant during a crash environment and the localized delta V concept. In: *Motor Vehicle Accident Reconstruction.* International Congress and Exposition; paper 890636. Detroit, Mich: Society of Automotive Engineers; 1989; SP-777:39–54.

77. Dvorak J, Valach L, Schmid ST. Cervical spine injuries in Switzerland. *J Manual Med.* 1989;4:7–16.

78. Jones IS, Champion HR. Trauma triage: vehicle damage as an estimate of injury severity. *J Trauma.* 1989;29:646–653.

79. Zaremba LA. Injuries to unrestrained occupants in small car-small car and large car-large car head-on collisions. *Accid Anal Prev.* 1980;12:11–29.

80. Hofferberth JE. Restraint system design and crash response. *Bull N Y Acad Med.* 1988;65:704–711.

81. Davis S, Pierce S. Van crashworthiness and aggressivity study; paper 810090. Detroit, Mich: Society of Automotive Engineers; 1981.

82. Deng YC. The importance of the test method in determining the effects of door padding in side impact. In: Proceedings of the 33rd Stapp Car Crash Conference; paper 892429. Washington, DC: Society of Automotive Engineers; 1989; P-227:79–86.

83. Breed DS, Castelli V. Trends in sensing frontal impacts. In: *Automotive Frontal Impacts.* International Congress and Exposition. Detroit, Mich: Society of Automotive Engineers; February 27–March 3, 1989; SP-782:37–49.

84. Viano DC, Arepally S. Assessing the safety performance of occupant restraint systems. In: Proceedings of the 34th Stapp Car Crash Conference; paper 902328. Orlando, Fla: Society of Automotive Engineers; 1990; P-236:301–327.

85. Mackay GM. Kinematics of vehicle crashes. *Adv Trauma.* 1987;2:21–42.

86. Siegel JH, Mason-Gonzalez S, Cushing BM, et al. A prospective study of injury patterns, outcomes, and costs of high speed frontal versus lateral motor vehicle crashes. In: Proceedings of the 34th Annual Conference of the Association for the Advancement of Automotive Medicine; Scottsdale, Ariz; 1990:289–313.

87. Daffner RH, Deeb ZL, Lupetin AR, et al. Patterns of high-speed impact injuries in motor vehicle occupants. *J Trauma.* 1988;28:498–501.

88. Weigel JA. The science of trauma. *Pa Med.* July 1988:43–44.

89. Neilson ID. The dynamics of car impact and occupant protection. In: *Toward Safer Passenger Cars.* I Mech E Conference Publications, C169/80. London: Mechanical Engineering Publications Ltd; 1980:1–6.

90. Hobbs CA. Essential requirements for an effective full scale frontal impact test. In: *Vehicle Crashworthiness and Occupant Protection in Frontal Collisions.* Detroit, Mich: Society of Automotive Engineers; February 1990; SP-807:1–19.

91. Gorski ZM, Nowak ES. Practical problems related to side impact field data accuracy and its importance to side impact protection assessments. In: *Side Impact Occupant Protection Technologies;* paper 910317. Detroit, Mich: Society of Automotive Engineers; 1991; SP-851:17–21.

92. Pauls LS. An improved side impact model for use on micro computers. In: *Side Impact Occupant Protection Technologies;* paper 910602. Detroit, Mich: Society of Automotive Engineers; 1991; SP-851:91–105.

93. Daniel RP. Biomechanical design considerations for side impact. In: *Side Impact: Injury Causation and Occupant Protection.* International Congress and Exposition. Detroit, Mich: Society of Automotive Engineers; February 27–March 3, 1989; SP-679:71–84.

94. Hultman RW, Laske TG, Chou CC, et al. NHTSA passenger car side impact dynamic test procedure-test-to-test variability estimates. In: *Side Impact Occupant Protection Technologies;* paper 910603. Detroit, Mich: Society of Automotive Engineers; 1991; SP-851:107–133.

95. Viano DC. Evaluation of the benefit of energy-absorbing material in side impact protection, I. In: Proceedings of the 31st Stapp Car Crash Conference; paper 872212. New Orleans, La: Society of Automotive Engineers; 1987; P-202:185–204.

96. Rouhana SW, Kroell CK. The effect of door topography on abdominal injury in lateral impact. In: Proceedings of the 33rd Stapp Car Crash Conference; paper 892433. Washington, DC: Society of Automotive Engineers; 1989; P-227:143–152.

97. Foret-Bruno JY, Hartemann F, Thomas C, et al. Occupant velocity change in side impact method of calculation: application to a sample of real-world crashes. In: Proceedings of the 24th Stapp Car Crash Conference; paper 801308. Troy, Mich: Society of Automotive Engineers; October 15–17, 1980:327–374.

98. Horsch JD. Occupant dynamics as a function of impact angle and belt restraint. In: Proceedings of the 24th Stapp Car Crash Conference; paper 801310. Troy, Mich: Society of Automotive Engineers; October 15–17, 1980:417–438.

99. Asbun HJ, Irani H, Roe EJ, et al. Intra-abdominal seatbelt injury. *J Trauma*. 1990;30:189–192.

100. Sharp JE, Stapp JP. Automobile seats and their role as an adjunct to restraint systems. International Congress and Exposition; paper 920129. Detroit, Mich: Society of Automotive Engineers; 1992.

101. Hobbs CA, Mills PJ. Injury probability for car occupants. In: *Frontal and Side Impacts*. Road Safety Division, Safety and Transportation Dept, Transport and Road Research Laboratory, Report No. 1124, Crowthorne, Berkshire, UK; 1984.

102. Kallieris D, Schmidt G, Mattern R. Vertebral column injuries in 90 degrees collisions: a study with post-mortem human subjects. In: Proceedings of the International IRCOBI Conference on the Biomechanics of Impacts, Birmingham, UK; 1987: 189–202.

103. Kallieris D, Schmidt G. Neck response and injury assessment using cadavers and the US-SID for far-side lateral impacts of rear seat occupants with inboard-anchored shoulder belts. In: Proceedings of the 34th Stapp Car Crash Conference; paper 902313. Orlando, Fla: Society of Automotive Engineers; 1990; P-236:93–100.

104. Thomas P, Bradford M. Side impact severity: the use of discriminant analysis to classify injury. In: Proceedings of International IRCOBI Conference on the Biomechanics of Impacts, Bergisch, Germany; 1988:131–148.

105. Bendjellal F, Tarriere C, Gillet D, et al. Head and neck responses under high G-level lateral deceleration. In: Proceedings of the 31st Stapp Car Crash Conference; paper 872196. New Orleans, La: Society of Automotive Engineers; 1987; P-202:29–48.

106. Faeber E. Interaction of car passengers in frontal, side, and rear collisions. In: Proceedings of the 26th Stapp Car Crash Conference; paper 821167. Ann Arbor, Mich: Society of Automotive Engineers; 1982:335–352.

107. Carême LMM. Thoraco-abdominal impact tolerance levels in side impact accidents: collection of field data and mathematical models. In: *Side Impact: Injury Causation and Occupant Protection*. International Congress and Exposition. Detroit, Mich: Society of Automotive Engineers; February 27–March 3, 1989; SP-679:61–70.

108. Rouhana SW. Abdominal injury prediction in lateral impact: an analysis of the biofidelity of the Euro-SID abdomen. In: Proceedings of the 31st Stapp Car Crash Conference; paper 872203. New Orleans, La: Society of Automotive Engineers; 1987; P-202:95–104.

109. Mackay GM, Parkin S, Hill J, et al. Restrained occupants on the non-struck side in lateral collisions. In: Proceedings of the 35th Annual Conference of the Association for the Advancement of Automotive Medicine; Toronto, Canada; 1991; 119–132.

110. Schuller E, Beier G, Steiger T. Injury patterns of restrained car occupants in near-side impacts. In: *Side Impact: Injury Causation and Occupant Protection*. International Congress and Exposition. Detroit, Mich: Society of Automotive Engineers; February 27–March 3, 1989; SP-769:1–5.

111. Rimel RW, Alves W, Jane JA. A prospective study of severity of CNS trauma and vehicular accidents. In: Proceedings of the 26th Annual Conference of the Association for the Advancement of Automotive Medicine; Ontario, Canada; 1982: 1–14.

112. Cooperrider NK, Thomas TM, Hammoud SA. Testing and analysis of vehicle rollover behavior. In: *Accident Reconstruction: Human, Vehicle, and Environmental Factors*; paper 900366. Detroit, Mich: Society of Automotive Engineers; 1990; SP-814:125–134.

113. Orlowski KF, Bundorf RT, Moffatt EA. Rollover crash tests: the influence of roof strength on injury mechanics. In: Proceedings of the 29th Stapp Car Crash Conference; paper 851734. Washington, DC: Society of Automotive Engineers; 1985; P-167:181–204.

114. Habberstad JL, Wagner RC, Thomas TM. Rollover and interior kinematics test procedures revisited. In: Proceedings of the 30th Stapp Car Crash Conference; paper 861875. San Diego, Calif: Society of Automotive Engineers; 1986:1–12.

115. Obergefell LA, Kaleps I, Johnson AK. Prediction of an occupant's motion during rollover crashes. In: Proceedings of the 30th Stapp Car Crash Conference; paper 861876. San Diego, Calif: Society of Automotive Engineers; 1986; P-189:13–26.

116. Thomson RW, Romilly DP, Navin FPD, et al. Dynamic requirements of automobile seatbacks; paper 930349. Warrendale, Pa: Society of Automotive Engineers; 1993.

117. McConnell WE, Howard RP, Guzman HM, et al. Analysis of human test subject kinematic responses to low velocity rear end impacts; paper 930889. Detroit, Mich: Society of Automotive Engineers; 1993:21–30.

118. Geigl BC, Steffan H, Leinzenger P, et al. The movement of head and cervical spine during rearend impact. International Conference of the Biomechanics of Impacts, Lyon, France, 1994.

119. Matsushita T, Sato TB, Hirabayashi K, et al. X-ray study of the human neck motion due to head inertia loading; paper 942208. In: Proceedings of the 38th Stapp Car Crash Conference. Detroit, Mich: Society of Automotive Engineers; 1994.

120. Svensson MY, Lövsund P, Håland Y, et al. Rear-end collisions: a study of the influence of backrest properties on head-neck motion using a new dummy neck; paper 930343. Warrendale, Pa: Society of Automotive Engineers; 1993:129–142.

121. Scott MW, McConnell WE, Guzman HM, et al. Comparison of human and ATD head kinematics during low-speed rearend impacts; paper 930094. Warrendale, Pa: Society of Automotive Engineers; 1993:1–8.

122. Fox JC, Williams JF. Mathematical model for investigating combined seatback-head restraint performance during rear-end impact. In: *Medical and Biological Engineering.* May 1976:263–273.

123. McKenzie JA, Williams JF. The dynamic behavior of the head and cervical spine during "whiplash." *J Biomech.* 1971;4:477–490.

124. Blaisdell DM, Levitt AE, Varat MS. Automotive seat design concepts for occupant protection; paper 930340. Detroit, Mich: Society of Automotive Engineers; 1993.

125. Warner CY, Stother CE, James MB, et al. Occupant protection in rear-end collisions, II: the role of seat back deformation in injury reduction; paper 912914. Warrendale, Pa: Society of Automotive Engineers; 1991.

126. Olsson I, Bunketorp O, Carlsson G, et al. An in depth study of neck injuries in rear end collisions. International IRCOBI Conference on the Biomechanics of Impacts; Bron, France; 1990:269–280.

127. Ono K, Kanno M. Influences of the physical parameters on the risk to neck injuries in low impact speed rear-end collisions. In: International Conference on the Biomechanics of Impacts, Eindhoven, Netherlands; 1993.

128. Emori RI, Horiguchi J. Whiplash in low speed vehicle collisions. In: *Vehicle Crashworthiness and Occupant Protection in Frontal Collisions.* Detroit, Mich: Society of Automotive Engineers; February 1990; SP-807:103–108.

129. Lövsund P, Nygren Å, Salen B, et al. Neck injuries in rear end collisions among front and rear seat occupants. In: Proceedings of International IRCOBI Conference on the Biomechanics of Impacts, Bergisch, Germany, 1988: 319–326.

130. Ommaya AK. The neck: classification, physiopathology and clinical outcome of injuries to the neck in motor vehicle accidents. In: Aldman B, Chapon A, eds. *The Biomechanics of Impact Trauma.* ICIS. Amsterdam: Elsevier Science Publishers; 1984:127–138.

131. Ameis A. Cervical whiplash: considerations in the rehabilitation of cervical myofascial injury. *Can Fam Physician.* 1986;32:1871–1876.

132. McLean AJ, Simpson DA, Cain CMS, et al. Head and neck injuries in passenger cars: a review of the literature. NH & MRC Road Accident Research Unit, University of Adelaide, Report No CR 59; Federal Office of Road Safety; Adelaide, Australia; September 1987.

133. Sances A Jr, Myklebust JB, Maiman DJ, et al. The biomechanics of spinal injuries. *CRC Crit Rev Biomed Eng.* 1984;11:1–76.

134. Carroll C, McAfee PG, Riley LH Jr. Objective findings for diagnosis of whiplash: comprehensive care can bring long-term relief. *J Musculoskeletal Med.* March 1986:57–76.

135. Foret-Bruno JY, Tarriere C, Le Coz JY, et al. Risk of cervical lesions in real-world and simulated collisions. In: Proceedings of the 34th Annual Conference of the Association for the Advancement of Automotive Medicine; Scottsdale, Ariz; 1990:373–389.

136. Ziegler PN. The relationship between shoulder belt fit and occupant protection. In: Proceedings of the 26th Annual Conference of the Association for the Advancement of Automotive Medicine; Ontario, Canada; 1982:267–278.

137. Pritz HB, Ulman MS. National Highway Traffic Safety Administration. FMVSS 208 belt fit evaluation: possible modification to accommodate larger people. In: *Automotive Frontal Impacts.* International Congress and Exposition. Detroit, Mich: Society of Automotive Engineers; February 27–March 3, 1989; SP-782:121–131.

138. American Medical Association Council on Scientific Affairs. Automobile-related injuries: components, trends, prevention. *JAMA.* 1983;249:3216–3222.

139. National Highway Traffic Safety Administration. Occupant protection trends in 19 cities (November 1989). Office of Driver and Pedestrian Research. In: *Use of Automatic Safety Belt Systems in 19 Cities (February 1990).* Washington, DC: NHTSA; 1990. Data used in National Safety Council *Accident Facts,* 1990 edition.

140. Evans L. Motorized two-point safety belt effectiveness in preventing fatalities. In: Proceedings of the 34th Annual Conference of the Association for the Advancement of Automotive Medicine; Scottsdale, Ariz; 1990:187–201.

141. Arajärvi E. *Maxillofacial, Chest and Abdominal Injuries Sustained in Severe Traffic Accidents.* Division of

Orthopaedic Surgery and Traumatology, Surgical Hospital, University Central Hospital, Helsinki, Finland, 1989, Liikenneturva.

142. Mackay GM. Abdominal injuries to restrained front seat occupants in frontal collisions. In Proceedings of the 26th Annual Conference of the Association for the Advancement of Automotive Medicine; Ontario, Canada; 1982:146–148.

143. Green RN, German A, Gorski ZM, et al. Misuse of three-point occupant restraints in real-world collisions. In: Proceedings of International IRCOBI Conference on the Biomechanics of Impacts, Birmingham, UK; 1987:102–112.

144. Verace J. Occupant kinematics in motor vehicle crashes, discussion for paper 820247. In: *Crash Protection*. International Congress and Exposition. Detroit, Mich: Society of Automotive Engineers; 1982; SP-513:198–199.

145. McLean AJ. Head first? The causes, consequences, and relative importance of head injuries in urban crashes. In: Proceedings of the 25th Annual Conference of the Association for the Advancement of Automotive Medicine; San Francisco; 1981:15–27.

146. Federal Office of Road Safety. Vehicle Occupant Protection in Australia, Report No. OR 10, March 1988.

147. Viano DC, Culver CC, Prisk BC. Influence of initial length of lap-shoulder belt on occupant dynamics: a comparison of sled testing and MVMA-2D modeling. In: Proceedings of the 24th Stapp Car Crash Conference; paper 801309. Troy, Mich: Society of Automotive Engineers; 1980:375–416.

148. Bourbeau R, Desjardins D, Maag U, et al. Neck injuries among belted and unbelted occupants of the front seat of cars. *J Trauma*. 1993;35:794–799.

149. Jones IS. Injury severity versus crash severity for front seat car occupants involved in front and side impacts. In: Proceedings of the 26th Annual Conference of the Association for the Advancement of Automotive Medicine; Ontario, Canada; 1982: 17–36.

150. Maag U, Desjardins D, Bourbeau R, et al. Seat belts and neck injuries. In: International IRCOBI Conference on the Biomechanics of Impacts, Bron, France, 1990:1–13.

151. Orsay EM, Dunne M, Turnbull TL. Prospective study of the effect of safety belts in motor vehicle crashes. *Ann Emerg Med*. 1990;19:258–61.

152. Cameron MN. *Effect of Seat Belts and Head Restraints on Neck Injury*. Dept of Transport Australia, Office of Road Safety, CR 19, 1981.

153. Rutherford WH, Greenfield T, Hayes HRM, et al. The medical effects of seat belt legislation in the United Kingdom. Department of Health and So-

cial Security Research Report No. 13. London: Her Majesty's Stationery Office; 1985;78:151.

154. Lesoin F, Thomas CE, Lozes G, et al. Has the safety-belt replaced the hangman's noose? *Lancet*. June 8, 1985:1341.

155. Wiechel JF, Sens MJ. Critical review of the use of seat belts by pregnant women. In: *Automotive Frontal Impacts*. International Congress and Exposition. Detroit, Mich: Society of Automotive Engineers; February 27–March 3, 1989; SP-782:61–69.

156. Horsch JD, Schneider DC, Kroell CK, et al. Response of belt restrained subjects in simulated lateral impact. In: Proceedings of the 23rd Stapp Car Crash Conference; paper 791005. San Diego, Calif: Society of Automotive Engineers; 1979:71–103.

157. Grösch L, Katz E, Marwitz H, et al. New measurement methods to assess the improved injury protection of airbag systems. In: Proceedings of the 30th Annual Conference of the Association for the Advancement of Automotive Medicine; Montreal, Canada; 1986:235–246.

158. Leung YC, Tarriére C, Lestrelin D, et al. Submarining injuries of 3 point belted occupants in frontal collisions: description, mechanisms, and protection. In: Proceedings of the 26th Stapp Car Crash Conference; paper 821158. Ann Arbor, Mich: Society of Automotive Engineers; 1982:173–206.

159. Kramer F. Abdominal and pelvic injuries of vehicle occupants wearing safety belts incurred in frontal collisions: mechanisms and protection. In: Proceedings of the International IRCOBI Conference of the Biomechanics of Impacts, Berlin, September 11–13, 1991:297–308.

160. Green DA, Green NE, Spengler DM, et al. Flexion-distraction injuries to the lumbar spine associated with abdominal injuries. *J Spinal Disord*. 1991;4(3):312–318.

161. Horsch JD, Hering WE. A kinematic analysis of lap-belt submarining for test dummies. In: Proceedings of the 33rd Stapp Car Crash Conference; paper 892441. Washington, DC: Society of Automotive Engineers; 1989:281.

162. Zuppichini F. Effectiveness of a mechanical pretensioner on the performance of seat belts. In: Proceedings of International IRCOBI Conference on the Biomechanics of Impacts, Stockholm; 1989:93–98.

163. Kahane CJ, Clar CC, Khadilkar A. Evaluation of child safety seats based on sled tests. In: Proceedings of the 31st Stapp Car Crash Conference; paper 872210. New Orleans, La: Society of Automotive Engineers; 1987; P-202:171–184.

164. Agran PF, Winn D. Traumatic injuries among children using lap belts and lap/shoulder belts in motor vehicle collisions. In: Proceedings of the 31st Annual Conference of the Association for the Advancement of Automotive Medicine; New Orleans, La; 1987:283–296.

165. Huelke DF. The rear seat occupant in car crashes. *AAAM Q J.* 1987;9(4):21–24.

166. Walz FH. Lower abdomen and pelvis: anatomy and types of injury. In: Aldman B, Chapon A, eds. *The Biomechanics of Impact Trauma. ICTS.* Amsterdam: Elsevier Science Publishers; 1984: 279–288.

167. Cohen DS, Jettner E, Smith WE. Light vehicle frontal impact protection. In: *Crash Protection.* International Congress and Exposition; paper 820243. Detroit, Mich: Society of Automotive Engineers; 1982; SP-513:35–51.

168. Otte D. Change in injury situation for belted front-seat car passengers in the course of development in vehicle construction. In: Proceedings of the 32nd Stapp Car Crash Conference; paper 881718. Atlanta, Ga: Society of Automotive Engineers; 1985; P-215:125–138.

169. Huelke DF. Steering assembly performance and driver injury severity in frontal crashes. In: *Occupant Crash Interaction with the Steering System.* International Congress and Exposition; paper 820474. Detroit, Mich: Society of Automotive Engineers; 1982; SP-507:1–30.

170. Christensen LL, Ross SE, O'Malley KF. The effectiveness of the mechanisms of injury in the triage of patients to trauma centers. In: Proceedings of the 34th Annual Conference of the Association for the Advancement of Automotive Medicine; Scottsdale, Ariz; 1990:457–461.

171. Browne AL. Windshield impact response: an empirical study of the standard three-ply construction. In: Proceedings of the 33rd Stapp Car Crash Conference; paper 892434. Washington, DC: Society of Automotive Engineers; 1989; P-227:153–176.

172. Pike JA. *Automotive Safety: Anatomy, Injury, Testing, and Regulation.* Warrendale, Pa: Society of Automotive Engineers; 1990.

173. Huelke DF, O'Day J, States JD. Lower extremity injuries in automobile crashes. *Accid Anal Prev.* 1982;14(2):95–106.

Chapter 16

Injury Tolerance and Injury Factors

Lawrence S. Nordhoff, Jr.

TOLERANCE DEFINED

Historically, efforts have been made to establish human injury tolerances and their relationship to injury level, risk of injury, and injury severity.[1] A specified tolerance level is how much loading of a type of tissue or part will produce a predicted specific type and severity level of injury.[2] However, there is no exact correlation between the amount of mechanical loading and human injury severity.[3] Viano and Arepally suggest using tolerance levels that involve the response at which about 25% of the tested population will experience serious injury.[4] Certainly, human tolerance is age dependent and varies with differing individual factors. Tolerance risk levels typically are shown on a sigmoidal curve. The diversity is seen, for example, in the human spine and its muscular and ligamentous attachments, being a nonhomogeneous biomechanical structure, with some structures (such as the spine) that are rigid and others (such as discs) that are deformable. Therefore, overall mechanical responses to forces are not linear[5] and may vary, depending on the type of tissue loaded.

Various tests performed on animals, dummies, and cadavers or, more recently, in computer crash programs give ranges for human tolerances for such injuries. However, the reader should remember that the figures in tolerance tests discussed throughout this chapter are only estimates. Many of the cadavers used in tolerance tests are older people. Also, cadavers do not have the living fluid and tissue dynamics that might influence tolerances in ways the tests cannot determine. In addition, an occupant's individual physical condition will influence his or her tolerance.

FORCES OF ACCELERATION OR DECELERATION (*g* FORCES)

Injury may happen simply from inertial loading, as a result of rapid acceleration or deceleration, which is spoken of in terms of *gravity*, or *g* forces. For example, when you drive around a corner as fast as you can in a car, the feeling of pull against your body is a gravity force of about 1*g*.

A velocity change of 30 mph in 130 milliseconds, which is a typical duration of collision into a rigid barrier, results in a deceleration of

330 ft/s², or 10*g*, since 1*g* = 33 ft/s². Examples of *g* forces are panic braking and rollercoaster riding, which produce approximately 0.8*g* to 4*g*. Astronauts experience 4*g* to 11*g*, or 1600 lbs. A moderately slow crash of 30*g* deceleration involving a 150-lb occupant may produce 4500 lbs of force.[6] A recent US Department of Transportation guide shows that forces for unrestrained occupants in collisions may range from 80*g* to 100*g*, or about 15,000 lbs.[7] When one is trying to relate *g* forces to an occupant, it is important to remember that each body part will have different *g* forces due to mass size differences, time of motion, and variables such as seat belt system interaction. Trimble writes about studies on live human volunteers who experienced different forces to various regions of the body, ranging from 9*g* at the neck to 23*g* at the forehead in rear-end collisions of about 10 mph.[8]

In practical terms, it is difficult for the physician, claims adjuster, attorney, or lay person outside a crash laboratory to equate *g* forces with injury. Tests of *g* forces are more useful to the safety engineer. Unless the person has been on a simulated crash sled there is little real-world experience to which the person can equate these forces. Explaining that the acceleration forces in a 30-mph collision is equivalent to falling out of a third-story building onto concrete pavement is more understandable.

HEAD AND SPINE TOLERANCE

In mild head, neck, and back injury, there are only limited practical ways for the clinician to determine tolerance levels. Knowing the crash speed levels that have been correlated with injury, how much abdominal compression is necessary for lumbar spine injury, and what the normal ranges of motion are, and whether they were exceeded, may help the physician. Spine range-of-motion normalized standards have been developed and need no further expansion in this text. Simply put, if the neck, thoracic, or lumbar spine joints move beyond their anatomic limits, injury of some degree will occur.

Head Injury Tolerance

The human head can probably tolerate a 10-mph impact into a well-padded, rigid object without sustaining severe injury.[9] Malliaris et al. found that at a 10-mph change in velocity (delta V), a mild Abbreviated Injury Scale 1 (AIS-1) head injury would occur, with every additional 5 mph of speed causing an increase of one higher AIS head injury severity level.[10] Hobbs and Mills[11] showed that in collisions having a delta V of 10 mph, 57% of the belted occupants and 16% of the unbelted occupants had AIS-1 head injury. At a delta V of 20 mph, 85% of the unbelted occupants and 48% of the belted occupants had AIS-1 head injury.[11] One study shows that 80% of AIS-4 (severe) to AIS-6 (fatal) head injuries occur at a delta V of less than 25 mph.[9] Fan and Jettner found that 19% of severe to fatal head injuries occur at a delta V of less than 20 mph, and 50% occur at a delta V of less than 30 mph.[9] In another study, the average delta V for an AIS-1 (mild) brain, skull, or spinal cord injury averaged 15.4 mph, and for AIS-2 (moderate) injury it averaged 18.4 mph.[12] In a study on light vehicles in frontal collisions for unrestrained occupants, serious head/face injury was associated with a mean delta V of approximately 27 mph.[13] A recent study by Otte[14] showed that at a delta V of up to 18.6 mph, about 29% of occupants had head injury in side impacts and 16% had head injury in frontal impacts.

Spine Injury Tolerance

There are several basic principles that the physician must consider when determining the tolerance or criteria for when certain car crash injuries may occur. Practically speaking, consider the following:

- Evaluate the degree of spine motion. Did motion or the potential for motion result in the occupant's exceeding normal anatomic limits (i.e., 60° of cervical extension or 20° of lumbar flexion)? Was the head restraint low enough and the occupant tall enough to allow the head to move beyond limits?

- Evaluate the rate of motion, as each tissue has its own unique loading characteristics. Does rate exceed ability of myofascial, tendon, ligament, and disc ability to stretch and/or move fluids? Consider the occupant's age, gender, pre-existing conditions/traumas, physical condition, and genetic or acquired characteristics of joints and soft tissue—there is no typical human or typical crash.

- Evaluate and correlate crash studies that explore and quantify risk of injury to change in crash velocity. This is a very practical method to utilize.

- Look at crash studies that compare risk of injury to vector of collision.

Neck Injury Tolerance

As a general rule, increased crash velocities correlate with higher incidences and more severe injuries; however, this rule relates only to probability or risk. Neck injury tolerance has been shown to be correlated with vector of crash, gender, and age of the occupant, with the rear-end collision producing significantly more neck injuries at lower crash speeds than both frontal and side crashes. A 1993 report concludes that 4- to 5-mph low-speed rear-end collisions appear to be the threshold for cervical strain injury.[15] One study, by Langwieder et al.,[16] evaluating crash data from both the United Kingdom and United States, indicates that a collision having a delta V of 20 mph is the threshold for a critical to fatal neck injury. A study by States et al.[17] concluded that significant neck injury can occur in rear-end collisions of 10 mph. Foret-Bruno et al.[18] found that rear impacts having a delta V of less than 15.5 mph

have about 16.7% probability of AIS-1 neck injury. Foret-Bruno et al. conclude that in side collisions having a delta V of greater than 30 mph there is risk for cervical fracture.[18]

Thorax and Thoracolumbar Spine Injury Tolerance

Thoracolumbar injury tolerance can be determined by the amount (distance) of compression required from either side door structures or a belt system that causes injury or by collision velocities. McConnell et al.[15] report that 4- to 5-mph low-speed rear-end collisions appear to be the threshold for minor thoracic and lumbar muscle strains and/or vertebral joint microcontusional injuries. One report found that if the occupant's delta V reached about 24 mph in frontal crashes, there was approximately a 50% risk of the occupant's having an AIS-2 (moderate) thorax injury.[19] In a study of light-vehicle frontal collisions for unrestrained occupants, serious chest injury was seen if the delta V was about 27 mph.[13]

Lumbar spine injuries generally are included in the abdominal tolerance section because of proximity and injury association. In frontal and lateral crashes, the average abdominal penetration limit was approximately 5 inches before actual spine contact. In humans, 60% frontal compression and 45% lateral compression in the abdomen equal spine contact.[20] Lumbar flexion dynamic loading of 175 nm (1 millisecond) may result in ligament failure.[21]

Mackay[22] concludes that rib fracture is the threshold for significant chest injury in frontal crashes in loading by either the steering wheel or a seat belt. This rule does not apply to side impacts, in which thoracic injury can occur without rib fracture.[22] An anterior chest compression depth of 35% has been shown to have a 25% probability of causing a severe thorax injury.[23] In side collisions, 31% to 38% compression will result in a 25% chance of having severe thorax injury.[24,25]

HUMAN FACTORS INFLUENCING INJURY

The physical and physiologic characteristics of the occupant will influence his or her tolerance to injury. As doctors well know, human characteristics can vary dramatically. Numerous factors can make some individuals more prone to injury and affect the reparative outcome. This section is important for the doctor to understand and, when appropriate, educate the patient about these various factors.

Human factors become useful for the doctor in four cases: (1) explaining to the patient why the injury was as bad or not as bad as it was, (2) justification for further testing or special treatment procedures, (3) explaining to the patient why the pain/disability is unusually severe and protracted, and (4) for legal purposes for the insurance carrier and/or attorney involved.

Age and Its Effect on Injury

Older drivers are more prone to injury, since they have decreased reserve capacity, decreased bone strength, decreased organ sinew, less adaptable brain tissue, and decreased blood vessel flexibility.[26,27] Older people also have decreased muscle mass,[28] decreased intracellular fluid volume,[28] decreased brain weight,[28] and decreased brain size, primarily because of extracellular fluid loss,[29] as well as decreased nerve conduction velocity.[29] The connective tissues have increased density and decreased water as one ages.[29] There is strong evidence that there is also a decreased capacity for repair.[30] Older people also have less effective homeostatic mechanisms, which may increase their vulnerability to the environment.[31] Lesser traumas are not as easily repaired,[30] and the negative balance between synthesis and degradation may change the metabolic balance of youth. Other changes may include decreased strength and speed of muscle contraction, decreased numbers of functional motor units,[30] decreased tissue elasticity, calcification of tendons and ligaments, increased fibrous tissue, and generalized weakening of osseous and ligamentous structures.[30,32]

It appears from one animal study that age has a bearing on where ligaments will tear. In young animals, ligaments mature earlier than the ligament-bone junction; therefore, an injury will tear the junction first. After maturity the midligaments will weaken first, resulting in tearing at the midligament area.[33]

Child occupants up to the age of 10 have been shown to have about one sixth the risk of sustaining neck injury as that for adult occupants.[16] A Lövsund et al.[34] study of rear-end crashes found that children were less prone to sustaining neck injuries but had similar trends as adults in other regions of the body. When comparing adults to children (aged 0 to 14), this study found that 18.6% of front-seated children and 12.3% rear-seated children reported neck injury. This compared to adults, who reported neck injury in 35% of front-seated adults and 21.3% in back-seated adults.

Elderly occupants have substantially poorer prognoses, particularly for mild to moderate injuries.[35] Sjogren[36] found that once the driver is over age 60, women have no increased injury frequency, whereas men have increased injury frequency as they continue to age. Age is more significant than velocity in motor vehicle crash injury (MVCI) outcome.[37] Other studies show that injury severity is related to age of the occupant and the magnitude of the delta V.[38] There is a positive linear relationship between occupant age and injury severity.[39] Viano et al.,[40] in a laboratory study, concluded that after age 40 tolerance to impact decreases. Older patients have slower rates of nerve regeneration, according to Deehan and Wilson.[41]

Potentiating Effects of Alcohol

Few problems plague our society and drain our economy in costs, deaths, and disability as does the combination of alcohol and driving. It has been estimated that by eliminating this combination we would see a decrease in MVCI fatalities of 32% and in serious injury of 12%.[42] The myth that drunks die less often, tolerate injury better, and survive crashes that no one else could have survived is belied by medical and automotive literature that shows increased deaths and injuries with worsened healed residual outcome among intoxicated occupants in motor vehicle accidents.[42-47]

The most significant recent study, by Waller et al.,[45] evaluating 1 million MVCI cases where other factors that could influence injury outcome were eliminated, concluded that the potentiating effects of alcohol were seen primarily in the low-speed and low-damage collision. This study also showed that alcohol increased the vulnerability of the occupant to injury in any given crash, and that the intoxicated driver has four times the risk of fatality.[45] A Finland hospital study of 14,995 trauma patients concluded that alcohol had potentiating effects on MVCI and falls down stairs, but had no significant effect on other types of injuries.[48]

It appears from the literature that the potentiating effects of alcohol on injury are of relatively short duration. An MVCI victim who is intoxicated will have significant increased risk of death at the injury site or death on arrival.[49] Substantially higher numbers of those having an elevated blood alcohol content (BAC) died during the first 30 minutes to 1 hour after injury, compared with those not having elevated levels.[50,51] This may explain why some studies that look at the potentiating effects of alcohol several hours after injury show little difference between intoxicated and nonintoxicated patients.

Intoxicated drivers have shorter survival periods[52] and are more likely to be seriously hurt or killed regardless of speed, age, crash type, belt use, or gender. Highly intoxicated occupants may have less recuperative ability[53] and have longer hospitalizations.[54]

Brain and Spinal Cord Injury and Alcohol

Motor vehicle accidents cause most central nervous system (CNS) head and spinal cord injuries. Alcohol intoxication has been found to potentiate CNS trauma[44,46,55] and worsen functional recovery[56] in animal studies in which cerebral injury was induced. After intoxication, 12 cats of 14 were totally paraplegic, whereas none in the control group were.[57] In another study, among 43 mice only 5% of the group survived, compared with 67% of the nonintoxicated group. Intoxicated mice had 5% survivors, whereas a nonintoxicated group had 67% survival in 8 days.[58] Anderson and Viano[42] found postcontusion recovery of spinal cord injuries due to excessive bleeding within the cord associated with intoxication. Injuries that would normally result in moderate spasticity caused permanent paralysis in those with an elevated BAC.[42] Even low levels of alcohol may affect recovery of conduction after mechanical injury to nerve axons.[42]

Blunt Chest/Heart Injury and Alcohol

Drivers frequently hit their chests on the steering wheel, suffering blunt chest trauma. The right ventricular chamber is most likely to be affected by blunt chest injury.[59] Sudden fatality from even a minor cardiac injury, such as a small bruise on the right ventricle, is not rare.[60] Acute intoxication significantly increases immediate or delayed death after chest impacts. In animal tests, BAC levels of 65 mg/dL prior to injury resulted in a 66% mortality rate within 1 hour, compared with the nonintoxicated group having only transient arrhythmias.[42] Nicholas and DeMuth reported a 90% mortality rate for cardiac impacts on animals if they were intoxicated.[61] Viano[62] found that mortality from chest impacts was 17% at 0.06 BAC, 50% at 0.12 BAC, and 71% at 0.18 BAC.

Why Does Alcohol Potentiate Injury?

Flamm et al.[57] suggested that poor head injury outcome in intoxicated patients possibly was due to modifications in membrane-bound enzymes, altered clotting mechanisms, and changes in cell membranes through abnormal free radical reactions. The study by Anderson and Viano[42] on head injuries hypothesized that "alcohol reduces membrane stability directly, thus increasing local hemorrhage, impairing restoration of electrolyte gradients necessary for recovery of axonal conduction and rendering membranes more accessible to proteolytic or peroxidative degradation."[42] Alcohol potentiation of spinal cord injury was thought to be due to increased hemorrhage and decreased ability of the axon to recover.[56] One study on 124 cats with spinal cord trauma concluded that alcohol acts synergistically with mechanical energy to amplify the injury response by increasing the extent of edema.[63] Higher fatalities may be due to decreased platelet aggregation[64] and prolonged bleeding times.[65,66] It is possible that the increased hemorrhage may cause MVCI patients to incur more rapid and extensive shock. Nicholas and DeMuth concluded that in cardiac trauma under intoxication there was significant uncoupling of the oxidative phosphorylation of cardiac mitochondria, resulting in alterations in the heart energy metabolism.[61] Viano thought that the increased rate of cardiac complications was due to decreased pumping effectiveness of the heart due to electrical-mechanical decoupling or dissociation.[62] Other authors believe that alcohol will cause actin and myosin dissociation,[67] or depression of the calcium uptake and binding by the cardiac sarcoplasmic reticulum.[68] All lead to decreased cardiac function, and alcohol intoxication is capable of producing life-threatening arrhythmias and cardiovascular collapse.[67] Pre-existing cardiac pathology results in less favorable outcome.[67] A laboratory study on awake, bleeding, intoxicated dogs concluded that groups that were intoxicated required significantly less blood loss to induce shock and lower blood pressures.[69]

Clark et al.[70] suggest that trauma is a symptom of alcoholism and therefore advise that all intoxicated persons who enter the emergency department should be evaluated for alcoholism. All patients brought to emergency departments after an automobile collision should have BAC tested. Screening for alcoholism will give more information on injury severity, as intoxication may mask or overrepresent injury extent, as well as prompt appropriate alcoholism counseling. If the driver is intoxicated at the time of impact, and the injury extent or functional outcome is worsened as a result, the person should be advised that a portion of his or her problems may be due to contributory negligence.

Occupant Size and Height

The stiffness of the human frame coincides with a person's size or mass. Generally speaking, the larger the occupant's mass, the less the chance of injury in a collision. It takes more force to accelerate a larger occupant. It is evident in the crash literature that size may dictate occupant dynamics in a crash. For example, smaller, unrestrained drivers in frontal crashes usually will have their heads propelled through the windshield first, whereas a large driver's head usually will hit the steering wheel first, then move to the windshield. Smaller occupants usually will have their seats closer to the windshield or steering wheel than larger counterparts, resulting in a higher incidence of chest impacts onto the steering wheel and dash.[71] The smaller-sized occupant will have higher head injury levels as the result of having less body mass, incurring less belt stretch and higher head acceleration.[72,73] Additionally, if the shoulder harness for the small occupant is positioned close to the neck, the injury level will be greater.[73] Rebound into the seat is more severe for tightly belted occupants and larger-sized occupants.[71] Taller occupants also may have higher risk of incurring neck injury (Figure 16–1).

Occupant Gender and Injury

There is general agreement in the literature that, compared with men, women incur more

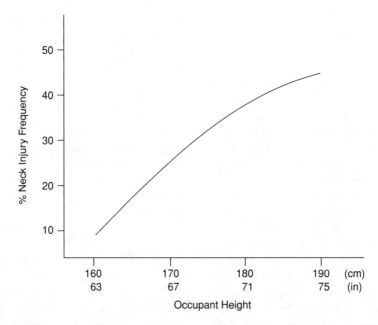

Figure 16–1 Taller occupants may incur higher frequency of neck injury than their shorter counterparts in rear-end collisions. *Source:* Reprinted from Carlsson, G., et al., Neck Injuries in Rear-End Collisions, International Research Committee on Biomechanics of Impacts/Association for the Advancement of Automotive Medicine, Conference on the Biomechanics of Impacts, Gotenborg, with permission of the IRCOBI, © 1985.

injuries, require more treatment for the same injuries, and are significantly more likely to have long-term pain and/or disability. Several automotive and clinical studies show that women have significantly higher risk for neck injury in all crash types than their male counterpart.[18,34,74–78] A 1994 large nationwide insurance claims report finds that in bodily injury states 46% of claims were made by men and 54% were made by women. In no-fault states 41% of claims were made by men and 59% were made by women.[79] In 1992 a large consumer survey of 133,570 households in the United States was performed, finding that 60% of those involved in an auto accident were female.[80] A recent study of 1197 crashes, after which every occupant was monitored, found that 18.3% of women and 12.5% of men had neck injury.[77] Another recent automotive study of 15,000 occupants in MVCI found that in rear collisions, 42% of women had cervical injuries, compared

with 21% of men. In frontal collisions 17% of women had neck injuries and 7.5% of men, and in side collisions 13% of women had neck injuries and 6.5% of men.[75] One study shows that the risk of having 8 days of disability after car accidents is 1.4/1,000 per year for men and 6.7 for women. This represents more than four times the incidence for men.[78] One study concluded that women recover more slowly from MVCI than do men.[81] Figure 16–2 compares the incidence of neck injuries in men and women.

Women may be more vulnerable to injury because they have weaker neck muscles, longer necks, smaller head size, and less body weight.[17,82] One small study comparing men and women found that women averaged 1.58 inches less neck circumference than men and had 0.59 inch smaller circumference heads[17]; thus they had less muscle mass in the neck,[75] meaning that more head acceleration would occur, primarily in extension.[83]

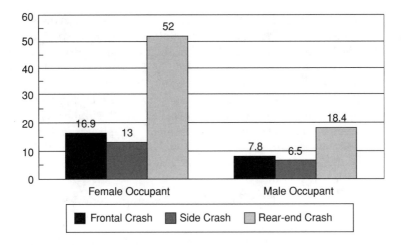

Figure 16–2 Frequency and comparison of neck injuries AIS ≥ 1 by gender and vector of collision in a study of 9789 injured occupants. *Source:* Data from Foret-Bruno, J.Y., Tarriere, C., Le Coz, J.Y., et al., Risk of Cervical Lesions in Real-World and Simulated Collisions, in 34th Proceedings, Scottsdale, Arizona, Association for the Advancement of Automotive Medicine, 1990.

Physical Condition of Injured

The physical condition of the patient prior to the MVCI plays a significant role in the extent of injury and recovery outcome. Patients who are very athletic and have good muscle tone, flexibility, and endurance will recover faster and will have fewer residual problems after the repair process. Nevertheless, even athletes have had difficulty or inability returning to preinjury athletic skills after car collisions. The person who exhibits good overall physical condition, however, will have higher tolerance to injury. Thus higher speeds or impact vectors with more serious consequences are required to cause serious injury. This means that in a car with multiple occupants, if one of the occupants is in much better physical condition, the treatment schedule and length of treatment time should reflect that fact.

BENEFITS OF BRACING BEFORE COLLISION

In most frontal and side collisions the occupant is aware of the striking vehicle. The driver frequently will grasp the steering wheel and push the feet down against the brake. In crashes in which the occupant is unaware of the impending impact, usually rear-end impacts, the occupant is relaxed. In the surprised, relaxed occupant, neck reflex responses to collisions take about 57 to 170 milliseconds, depending on the study, which is far too slow to produce any significant reducing load or acceleration benefits.[2,84,85] Most injuries to occupants occur at approximately 30 milliseconds. It is important to note that occupant bracing will lessen head motion extent,[86] thus reducing neck injury stretch and tearing.[87,88] Bracing will reduce peak head acceleration in lower-speed crashes, but as the collision velocity increases, the beneficial effects become insignificant. In a crash study using live human subjects, persons who braced themselves prior to collision showed joint locking until 75 milliseconds, at which point the joints unlocked.[89] This study concluded that bracing significantly attentuates peak head angular acceleration.[89] One study showed that if the occupant braced, an 80-millisecond delay in brain activity could occur, resulting in more energy being transmitted through the lower extremities.[84] A computer biomechanical model study, which included the muscular elements of the cervical spine during collisions, found that tensed neck muscles will reduce bending and give increased stability to the cervical spine during low accelerations, with the trade-off of increases in the axial compressive stresses of the passive structures, such as the disc and zygapophyseal joints, and also increasing axial tensile stresses in the neck neuromusculature.[83] If the occupant is braced, it is rare for temporomandibular joint injuries to occur because of inertial loading. Upper-extremity injury often will be worse for the occupant who braces, which is the trade-off for lessening the extent of spinal injuries.

OCCUPANT ORIENTATION AND SEATING POSITION

The orientation of the occupant's head and torso to the car interior and the striking vehicle's vector may play significant roles in the injury outcome. For example, if a person in the 12-o'clock position is rear-ended, muscular and bony elements on both sides of the spine share equal stresses, whereas if the head or torso is turned, one side takes most of the forces.

In general, in all crashes, rear-seat occupants incur less injury.[90] The rear-seated occupant does not have a windshield, dash, or steering wheel to contend with. In addition, the rear seats have different design characteristics. Carlsson et al.[90] found that in rear-end crashes, the frequency of neck injuries was 35% for drivers, 25% for front-seat passengers, and 22% for rear-seat occupants.

PRE-EXISTING COMPLICATING CONDITIONS

Patients who have clinically significant pre-existing complicating medical conditions may have more severe injuries, slower recoveries, and poorer prognoses. For example, endo-crine conditions such as diabetes mellitus and hypothryoidism cause peripheral nerves to be more prone to injury[91] and to heal more slowly. The patient, as well as the doctor, may become frustrated at the slow rate of healing unless the presence of complicating factors is revealed. The insurance carrier should be informed, as well. Pre-existing spinal, nutritional, physical, and emotional problems can all cause problems.

Pre-Existing Cervical Spinal Joint Spondyloarthrosis

Spinal joints with pre-existing degenerative joint changes that are subjected to rapid, high-force traumas, such as a vehicle hyperextension-hyperflexion injury, not only will have more severe injuries but also will have more residual problems. Several authors conclude that a pre-existing arthritic cervical spine will cause an MVCI to result in more serious injury than the same amount of force would create in the absence of arthritis.[39,92–94] Degenerative diseases of the spine may predispose the individual to injury.[95] Mild neck injuries in occupants having cervical spondylosis may give rise to radicular symptoms.[96]

In cases where the intervertebral foramina have narrowed due to osteophytes, minor neck injury may cause nerve root edema, and with the irregular surface to glide over, trivial activities such as driving or riding in a car can worsen the condition.[96] Cervical spondylosis may result in a relaxation of the attaching annular and capsular ligaments, allowing more movement to occur in flexion.[96] Minor trauma can lead to serious spinal cord injury if the occupant has pre-existing degenerative spinal disease.[97] One study on ankylosing spondylitis concluded that most spine injuries occurred as a result of minor trauma or MVCI, primarily affecting the C-5 and T-1 areas.[98] Osteoarthrosis is primarily due to aging and mechanical insult.[30] Jeffreys and McSweeney report that in cases of cervical spondylosis, there may be fibrous or bony ankylosis between vertebral bodies, resulting in more strain on the anterior longitudinal ligament and posterior longitudinal ligament before normal ranges of motion are reached, causing a lowered tolerance level.[93]

A study by Sances and Yoganandan[99] compared degenerated cervical joints and disc strength, concluding that normal intervertebral joints resisted higher failure loads and absorbed more external energy than degenerated joints.

Cervical spondylosis is a degenerative process that many authors believe begins in the intervertebral disc. As the disc ages it becomes dehydrated and its normal space narrows. Cracking and fissuring of the disc occur, allowing the soft disc to bulge or extrude.[100] Moskovich[101] reports that the vulnerability of the cervical discs to rupture increases as degeneration, annular fissuring, and nucleus pulposus desiccation progress, resulting in a situation in which a trivial trauma may cause disc rupture. Older cartilage has lesser capacity to repair its matrix.[30] Degenerative discs have less proteoglycan concentration. In cartilage, normal amounts of proteoglycans retard the rate of sudden tensile stretch, and in the degenerated disc the collagen fibrils may be more easily damaged.[102] Also, a nucleus with decreased proteoglycans would allow the inner annulus collagen lamellae to sag into the nuclear space when the disc is subjected to modest rotational loading,[102] leading to damage equivalent with those having no nucleus.

Pre-Existing Fibromyalgia, Fibrositis, and Myofascial Fibrosis

One of the more common pre-existing problems seen in younger patients is varying degrees of subclinical or clinical myofascial anatomic alterations acquired either from prior trauma, microtrauma, or endocrine abnormalities. Fibrosis is an alteration of the normal structural and functional capacity of a group of muscles that normally are not pain sensitive. These areas usually involve the postural muscles, such as the trapezius, rhomboid, levator scapulae, scalene, and paraspinal muscles. Microtrauma from sustained posture or previous macrotraumas have occurred in the past. Sustained postural muscle contraction leads to cellular ischemia, metabolic buildup, and eventually an inflammatory reaction that leads to adhesion formation. Either way, the person develops pre-existing excessive scar tissue formation in these regions. These tissues may be asymptomatic prior to the car crash, but a minor trauma can initiate severe pain and/or disability. In the acute injury, pre-existing myofascial adhesions are easily diagnosed. However, if the patient is examined 3 to 4 months after MVCI the etiology is less clear.

Pre-Existing Cervical Stenosis

Trimble thinks that about 10% of the population have tight cervical spinal cord canals, which may make these people vulnerable to injuries.[8] Cervical stenosis, due to either degenerative changes or genetic history, may cause anterior or posterior cord compression, venous congestion, ischemia, intervertebral fascial narrowing, or nerve root sleeve fibrosis,[93] creating an environment in which roots may develop intraneural fibrosis and wallerian degeneration. Minor trauma may set off clinical pain due to the overstretching of the fibrotic nerve root sleeves and ligaments.

Pre-Existing Genetic Conditions

Genetic conditions are seen with enough frequency in an average practice that they should be discussed. Cervical dysphagias, such as in the Klipple-Feil syndrome, platybasia (malformed occipital and/or sphenoid bones), and the Arnold-Chiari malformation warrant close screening by the doctor. The consensus of opinion is that in these genetic conditions many types of tissues are anomalous. Not only are bony tissues abnormal in size, shape, and function, but also ligaments and muscles may vary immensely in their architecture, size, and attachment sites. This results in a generalized weakness and altered biomechanics, resulting in a loss of the elasticity and strength that would be present in a normal spine. Spinal stenosis in the cervical or lumbar spine may complicate injuries. The normal spacing of the vertebral structures provides a safety margin and allows for the body to withstand most normal activities or injuries. In stenosis, minor to moderate disc bulges, which would not normally be symptomatic, result in neurologic deficits and pain syndromes that respond slowly to treatment. Neurovascular and muscular variations in the thoracic outlet and cervical spine lead to atypical symptom presentations, and require modifications of treatment if success is to be achieved. Pizzutillo et al.[103] report that in patients with Klippel-Feil syndrome biomechanical hypomobility in the upper neck and hypermobility in the lower cervical spine were seen on stress radiographic analysis.

Pre-Existing Postsurgical Conditions

Previous surgeries, such as spinal fusions or laminectomies in the neck and back, can complicate and magnify injury extent, recovery time, and prognosis. A postsurgical case study concluded that bilateral resection of more than 50% of the cervical facet joints after facetectomy significantly compromised the shear strength of the cervical spine.[104] Biomechanical studies of human cadavers show that unilateral facetectomy resulted in a 32% decrease in strength and bilateral facetectomy a 50% decrease in strength of the spine to withstand increasing loads.[105] In conditions such as

fusion for scoliosis, or fusions for herniated discs, stenosis, and cord involvement, the result is that fewer joints absorb traumatic forces, meaning more damage. One recent study concluded that there is a compensatory increase in motion in segments adjacent to surgically fused segments,[106] leading to compensatory instability.

Pre-Existing Autoimmune Diseases

Autoimmune diseases such as rheumatoid arthritis can seriously complicate even the minor MVCI. This is especially true in patients with previous serious juvenile afflictions with subsequent spinal ligamentous instability. Fortunately, these conditions are not very common, but they still need to be screened for and treated carefully. It is important to educate the patient about these conditions as well.

CONCLUSION

Car crash injury victims present the clinician with a unique challenge. Even with the best knowledge currently available there is much we do not understand about dealing with human variables. The reader may consider the variability in crash characteristics between different car models in the world and ask why a Volvo occupant has significantly less injury than a Hyundi occupant, but maybe we can understand human variables even though we have no control over manufacturing design and aging. We insure millions of people in the United States for injuries, accepting each individual as he or she is and sharing the risk, yet still we must consider each person unique.

REFERENCES

1. Eppinger RH, Shaibani S. Examination of the theoretical bases of current injury indices and considerations for the future. In: Proceedings of International Research Committee on Biomechanics of Impacts; Stockholm, 1989:183–194.

2. Goldsmith W, Ommaya AK. Head and neck injury criteria and tolerance levels. In: Aldman B, Chapon A, eds. *The Biomechanics of Impact Trauma.* Amsterdam: Elsevier Science Publishers; 1984: 149–190.

3. Hoefs R. *Injury Biomechanics*. Government/Industry Meeting and Exposition. Washington, DC: Society of Automotive Engineers; 1987; SP-731: 13–14.

4. Viano DC, Arepally S. Assessing the safety performance of occupant restraint systems. In: Proceedings of the 34th Stapp Car Crash Conference; paper 902328. Orlando, Fla: Society of Automotive Engineers; 1990; P-236:301–327.

5. Yoganandan N, Myklebust JB, Ray G, et al. Mathematical and finite element analysis of spine injuries. *CRC Critical Rev Biomed Eng.* 1987;15(1): 29–93.

6. McSwain NE Jr, Martinez JA, Timberlake GA. *Cervical Spine Trauma: Evaluation and Acute Management.* New York: Thieme Medical Publishers; 1989.

7. Holden JA, Cristoffel T. *A Course on Motor Vehicle Trauma: Instructor's Guide: Final Users Manual.* Washington, DC: US Dept of Transportation; OST/P-34/86-050; September 1986.

8. Trimble MR. *Post-Traumatic Neurosis: From Railway Spine to Whiplash.* Chichester, UK: John Wiley & Sons; 1981.

9. Fan WRS, Jettner E. Light vehicle occupant protection: top and rear structures and interiors. In: *Crash Protection.* International Congress and Exposition; paper 820244. Detroit, Mich: Society of Automotive Engineers; 1982; SP-513:53–63.

10. Malliaris AC, Hitchcock R, Hedlund J. A search for priorities in crash protection. In: *Crash Protection.* International Congress and Exposition; paper 820242. Detroit, Mich: Society of Automotive Engineers; 1982;SP-513:1–130.

11. Hobbs CA, Mills PJ. Injury probability for car occupants in frontal and side impacts. Transport and Road Research Laboratory Report No 1124, Crowthorne, Berkshire, UK, Road Safety Division, Safety and Transportation Department; 1984.

12. Scott WE. *Epidemiology of Head and Neck Trauma in Victims of Motor Vehicle Accidents: Head and Neck Injury Criteria, a Consensus Workshop.* Washington, DC: US Government Printing Office; July 1983: 1–6.

13. Cohen DS, Jettner E, Smith WE. Light vehicle frontal impact protection. In: *Crash Protection.* International Congress and Exposition; paper 820243. Detroit, Mich: Society of Automotive Engineers; 1982; SP-513:35–51.

14. Otte D. Comparison and realism of crash simulation tests and real accident situations for the biomechanical movements in car collisions. In: Proceedings of the 34th Stapp Car Crash Conference; paper 902329. Orlando, Fla: Society of Automotive Engineers; 1990; P-236:329–347.

15. McConnell WE, Howard RP, Guzman HM, et al. Analysis of human test subject kinematic responses to low velocity rear end impacts; paper 930889. Warrendale, Pa: Society of Automotive Engineers; 1993.

16. Langwieder K, Backaitis SH, Fan W, et al. Comparative studies of neck injuries of car occupants in frontal collisions in the United States and in the Federal Republic of Germany. In: Proceedings of the 25th Stapp Car Crash Conference; paper 811030. San Francisco: Society of Automotive Engineers; 1981:71–130.

17. States JD, Korn MW, Masengill JB. The enigma of whiplash injury. *N Y State J Med.* December 15, 1970:2971–2977.

18. Foret-Bruno JY, Tarriere C, Le Coz JY, et al. Risk of cervical lesions in real-world and simulated collisions. In: Proceedings of the 34th Annual Conference of the Association for the Advancement of Automotive Medicine; Scottsdale, Ariz; 1990:373– 389.

19. Foret-Bruno JY, Hartemann F, Thomas C, et al. Occupant velocity change in side impact method of calculation: application to a sample of real-world crashes. In: Proceedings of the 24th Stapp Car Crash Conference; paper 801308. Troy, Mich: Society of Automotive Engineers; October 15–17, 1980:327–374.

20. Stalnaker RL, Ulman MS. Abdominal trauma: review, response, and criteria. In: Proceedings of the 29th Stapp Car Crash Conference; paper 851720. Washington, DC: Society of Automotive Engineers; 1985; P-167:1–16.

21. Osvalder A-L, Neuman P, Aldman B, et al. Methods for studying effects on the spine under different loads. In: Proceedings of the International Research Committee on Biomechanics of Impacts. Birmingham, UK; 1987:239–249.

22. Mackay M. Biomechanics and the regulation of vehicle crash performance. In: Proceedings of the 33rd Annual Conference of the Association for the Advancement of Automotive Engineers; Baltimore, 1989:323–326.

23. Viano DC, Lau IV. A viscous tolerance criterion for soft tissue injury assessment. *J Biomech.* 1988;21:387–399.

24. Cavanaugh JM, Walilko TJ, Malhotra M, et al. Biomechanical response and injury tolerance of the thorax in twelve sled side impacts. In: Proceedings of the 34th Stapp Car Crash Conference; paper 902307. Orlando, Fla: Society of Automotive Engineers; 1990;23–38.

25. Weiss DS, Kirsner R, Eaglstein WH. Electrical stimulation and wound healing. *Arch Dermatol.* 1990;126:222–225.

26. Lishman WA. Physiogenesis and psychogenesis in the "post-concussional syndrome." *Br J Psychiatry*. 1988;153:460–469.

27. Pike JA. The elderly and vehicle-related injury; paper 881753. In: *Effects on Aging of Driver Performance*. Warrendale, Pa: Society of Automotive Engineers; 1988.

28. Kenny RA. Physiology of aging. *Clin Geriatr Med*. 1985;1:37–59.

29. Berman R, Haxby JV, Pomerantz RS. Physiology of aging, I: normal changes. *Patient Care*. January 15, 1988:20–36.

30. Masoro EJ. The biology and physiology of aging. In: Nelson CL, Dwyer AP, eds. *The Aging Musculoskeletal System: Physiological and Pathological Problems*. Lexington, Mass: DC Heath and Co; 1984.

31. Abrass IB. The biology and physiology of aging. *West J Med*. 1990;153:641–645.

32. Cotta H, Puhl W, Koester G. Aging process of the musculoskeletal system. In: Karacoloff L, et al., eds. *Orthopedics: Clinical Handbooks in Physical Therapy Management*. Gaithersburg, Md: Aspen Publishers, Inc; 1987: chap 7.

33. Woo SL-Y, Orlando CA, Gomez MA, et al. Tensile properties of the medial collateral ligament as a function of age. *J Orthop Res*. 1986;4:13–41.

34. Lövsund P, Nygren Å, Salen B, et al. Neck injuries in rear end collisions among front and rear seat occupants. In: Proceedings of International Research Committee on Biomechanics of Impacts, Bergisch, Germany; 1988:319–326.

35. Baker SP, O'Neill B, Karpf RS. *The Injury Fact Book*. Lexington, Mass: DC Heath and Co; 1985.

36. Sjogren H. Injuries in the elderly sustained in the traffic environment. In: Proceedings of the 34th Annual Conference of the Association for the Advancement of Automotive Medicine; Scottsdale, Ariz; 1990:41–55.

37. Petrucelli E, States JD, Hames LN. The Abbreviated Injury Scale: evolution, usage, and future adaptability. In: Proceedings of the International Association for Accident and Traffic Medicine, Denmark, 1980:163.

38. Verma MK, Repa BS. Pedestrian impact simulation: a preliminary study. In: Proceedings of the 27th Stapp Car Crash Conference and International Research Committee on Biokinetics of Impacts; paper 831601. San Diego, Calif: Society of Automotive Engineers; 1983:15–30.

39. Gorman W. Whiplash: a neuropsychiatric injury. *Ariz Med*. 1974;31:414–416.

40. Viano DC, Culver CC, Evans L, et al. Involvement of older drivers in multivehicle side-impact crashes. *Accid Anal Prev*. 1990;22:177–188.

41. Deehan MR, Wilson RL. Diagnosis and management of carpal tunnel syndrome. *J Musculoskeletal Med*. 1989;6:47–60.

42. Anderson TE, Viano DC. Effect of acute alcohol intoxication on injury tolerance and outcome. In: Noordzij PC, Roszbach R, de Gier JJ, et al., eds. *Alcohol, Drugs, and Traffic Safety*. Proceedings of the 10th International Conference on Alcohol, Drugs, and Traffic Safety. Amsterdam: Excerpta Medica; 1987; T-86:251–254.

43. Evans L, Frick MC. Alcohol's influence on fatality risk, given that a crash has occurred. In: Proceedings of the 35th Annual Conference of the Association for the Advancement of Automotive Medicine; Toronto, Canada; 1991:179–195.

44. Luna GK, Maier RV, Sowder L, et al. The influence of ethanol intoxication on outcome of injured motorcyclists. *J Trauma*. 1984;24:695–700.

45. Waller PF, Stewart JR, Hansen AR, et al. The potentiating effects of alcohol on driver injury. *JAMA*. 1986;256:1461–1466.

46. Waller PF, Stewart JR, Hansen AR, et al. Alcohol as a potentiating factor in motor vehicle crash injury. In: Noordzij PC, Roszbach R, de Gier JJ, et al., eds. *Alcohol, Drugs, and Traffic Safety*. Proceedings of the 10th International Conference on Alcohol, Drugs, and Traffic Safety. Amsterdam: Excerpta Medica; 1987;T-186:255.

47. Warren RA, Simpson HM, Buhlman MA, et al. Relationship of driver blood alcohol to injury severity. In: Proceedings of the 25th Annual Conference of the Association for the Advancement of Automotive Medicine; San Francisco; 1981:133–141.

48. Honkanen R, Smith GS. Impact of acute alcohol intoxication on the severity of injury: a cause-specific analysis of non-fatal trauma. *Injury*. 1990; 21:353–357.

49. Dischinger PC, Soderstrom CA, Shankar BS, et al. The relationship between use of alcohol and place of death in vehicular fatalities. In: Proceedings of the 32nd Annual Conference of the Association for the Advancement of Automotive Medicine; Seattle, Wash; 1988:299–312.

50. Fell JC, Hertz ES. The effects of blood alcohol concentration on time of death for fatal crash victims. In: Proceedings of the 34th Annual Conference of the Association for the Advancement of Automotive Medicine; Scottsdale, Ariz; 1990:69–81.

51. Stewart JR. Estimating the effects over time of alcohol on injury severity. In: Proceedings of the 32nd Annual Conference of the Association for the Advancement of Automotive Medicine; Seattle, Wash; 1988:319–326.

52. Stewart JR. Estimating the effects over time of alcohol on injury severity. *Accid Anal Prev.* 1989;21:575–579.

53. House EG, Waller PF, Stewart JR. Blood alcohol level and injury in traffic crashes. In: Proceedings of the 26th Annual Conference of the Association for the Advancement of Automotive Medicine; Ontario, Canada; 1982:349–359.

54. Jehle D, Cottington E. Effect of alcohol consumption on outcome of pedestrian victims. *Ann Emerg Med.* 1988;17:953–956.

55. Albin MS, Bunegin L. An experimental study of craniocerebral trauma during ethanol intoxication. *Crit Care Med.* 1986;14:841–846.

56. Anderson TE. Effects of acute alcohol intoxication on spinal cord vascular injury. *Cent Nerv Syst Trauma.* 1986;3:183–192.

57. Flamm ES, Demopoulos HB, Seligman ML, et al. Ethanol potentiation of central nervous system trauma. *J Neurosurg.* 1977;46:328–335.

58. Franco CD, Spillert CR, Spillert KR, et al. Alcohol increases mortality in murine head injury. *Nat Med Assoc.* 1988;80:63–65.

59. Sutherland GR, Calvin JE, Driedger AA. Anatomic and cardiopulmonary responses to trauma with associated blunt chest injury. *J Trauma.* 1978;21:1.

60. Lasky N. Traumatic non-penetrating heart disease: a review. *Med Times.* 1963;91:917.

61. Nicholas GG, DeMuth WE Jr. Blunt cardiac trauma: the effect of alcohol on survival and metabolic function. *J Trauma.* 1980;20:58–60.

62. Viano DC. *Scope of Current Biomechanics Research: Introduction into Injury Biomechanics.* SP-731. Warrendale, Pa: Society of Automotive Engineers; November 1987.

63. Brodner RA, VanGilder JC, Collins WF Jr. Experimental spinal cord trauma: potentiation by alcohol. *J Trauma.* 1981;21:124–129.

64. Horak JK, Brandon TA, Ribeiro LG, et al. Effects of ethanol and hemolysis on in vivo and in vitro platelet aggregation. *J Cardiovasc Pharmacol.* 1982;4:1037–1041.

65. Elmer O, Goransson G, Zoucas E. Impairment of primary hemostasis and platelet function after alcohol ingestion in man. *Haemostasis.* 1984;14:223–228.

66. Waller PF, Hansen AR, Stutts JC, et al. Alcohol: a potentiating factor in motor vehicle crash injury. In: *Alcohol, Accidents, and Injuries.* paper 860184. Warrendale, Pa: Society of Automotive Engineers; 1986; P-173:53–61.

67. Desiderio MA. Effects of acute, oral ethanol on cardiovascular performance before and after experimental blunt cardiac trauma. *J Trauma.* 1987;27:267–277.

68. Swartz MH, Repke DI, Katz AM, et al. Cardiac microsomes: effects of ethanol on calcium binding and uptake. *Biochem Pharmacol.* 1974;23:2369.

69. Zink BJ, Syverud SA, Dronen SC, et al. The effect of ethanol on survival time in hemorrhagic shock in an unanesthetized swine model. *Ann Emerg Med.* 1988;17:15–19.

70. Clark DE, McCarthy E, Robinson E. Trauma as a symptom of alcoholism. *Ann Emerg Med.* 1985; 14:127.

71. Backaitis SH, DeLarm L, Robbins DH. Occupant kinematics in motor vehicle crashes. In: *Crash Protection.* International Congress and Exposition; paper 820247. Detroit, Mich: Society of Automotive Engineers; 1982; SP-513:107–155.

72. Mackay GM. Abdominal injuries to restrained front seat occupants in frontal collisions. In: Proceedings of 26th Annual Conference of the Association for the Advancement of Automotive Medicine; Ontario, Canada; 1982:146–148.

73. Ziegler PN. The relationship between shoulder belt fit and occupant protection. In: Proceedings of the 26th Annual Conference of the Association for the Advancement of Automotive Medicine; Ontario, Canada; 1982:267–278.

74. Faverjon G, Henry C, Thomas C, et al. Head and neck injuries for belted front occupants involved in real frontal crashes: patterns and risks. In: Proceedings of the International Research Committee on Biomechanics of Impacts, Bergisch, Germany; 1988:301–318.

75. Foret-Bruno JY, Dauvilliers F, Tarriere C. Influence of the seat and head rest stiffness on the risk of cervical injuries in rear impact. In: Proceedings of the 13th ESV Conference, Paris, France; 1991.

76. Larder DR, Twiss MK, Mackay GM. Neck injury to car occupants using seat belts. In: Proceedings of the 29th Annual Conference of the Association for the Advancement of Automotive Medicine; Washington, DC;1985:153–165.

77. Otremski I, Marsh JL, Wilde BR, et al. Soft tissue cervical spinal injuries in motor vehicle accidents. *Injury.* 1989;20:349–351.

78. Schutt CH, Dohan FC. Neck injury to women in auto accidents: a metropolitan plague. *JAMA.* 1968;206:2689–2692.

79. Insurance Research Council. *Auto Injuries: Claiming Behavior and Its Impact on Insurance Costs.* Oak Brook, Ill: IRC; 1994.

80. Insurance Research Council. *Paying for Auto Injuries: A Consumer Panel Survey of Auto Accident Victims.* Oak Brook, Ill: IRC; 1994.

81. Greenfield J, Ilfeld FW. Acute cervical strain: evaluation and short term prognostic factors. *Clin Orthop.* 1977;122:196–200.

82. Kahane CJ. Evaluation of head restraints: Federal motor vehicle safety standard 202. Washington, DC: National Highway Traffic Safety Administration. US Dept of Transportation HS 806 108, 1982.

83. Pontius UR, Liu YK. *Neuromuscular Cervical Spine Model for Whiplash;* paper 760769. Warrendale, Pa: Society of Automotive Engineers; 1976.

84. Begeman PC, King AI, Levine RS, et al. Biodynamic response of the musculoskeletal system to impact acceleration. In: Proceedings of the 24th Stapp Car Crash Conference; paper 801312. Troy, Mich: Society of Automotive Engineers; October 15–17, 1980:481–509.

85. Melvin JW, Weber K. Review of the biomechanical impact response and injury in the automotive environment. Ann Arbor, Mich: University of Michigan Transportation Research Institute; 1985.

86. Reid SE, Raviv G, Reid SE Jr. Neck muscle resistance to head impact. *Aviat Space Environ Med.* 1981;52:78–84.

87. Cailliet R. *Neck and Arm Pain.* 3rd ed. Philadelphia: FA Davis Co; 1991.

88. Fox JC, Williams JF. Mathematical model for investigating combined seatback-head restraint performance during rear-end impact. *Med Biol Eng Comput.* May 1976;263–273.

89. Seemann MR, Lustick LS, Frisch GD. Mechanism for control of head and neck dynamic response. In: Proceedings of the 28th Stapp Car Crash Conference; paper 841669. Chicago: Society of Automotive Engineers; 1984; P-152:207–222.

90. Carlsson G, Nilsson S, Nilsson-Ehle A, et al. Neck injuries in rear end car collisions. In: Proceedings of International Research Committee on Biomechanics of Impacts/Association for the Advancement of Automotive Medicine Conference on the Biomechanics of Impacts, Göteborg, Sweden, 1985.

91. Bluestone R. A practical approach to hand pain: the common causes and their distinctive patterns. *J Musculosekeletal Med.* 1984;1:66–73.

92. Green J. *Common Head, Neck, and Back Injuries.* Malabar, India: Robert E Krieger; 1988.

93. Jeffreys E, McSweeney T. *Disorders of the Cervical Spine.* London: Butterworth, 1980.

94. Nicholson MW. Whiplash: fact, fantasy, or fakery. *Hawaii Med J.* 1974;33:168–170.

95. Sances A Jr, Maiman DJ, Myklebust JB, et al. Biodynamics of vehicular injuries. In: Peters GA, Peters BJ, eds. *Automotive Engineering and Litigation.* New York: Garland Law Publishing; 1984:1:449–550.

96. Batzdorf U. Differential diagnosis of arm and thoracic radicular pain and sensory disturbance. *Spine State Art Rev.* 1988;2:565–583.

97. Watson N. Road traffic accidents, spinal injuries, and seat belts. *Paraplegia.* 1983;21:63–64.

98. Detwiler KN, Loftus CM, Godersky JC, et al. Management of cervical spine injuries in patients with ankylosing spondylitis. *J Neurosurg.* 1990;72:210–215.

99. Sances A Jr, Yoganandan N. *The Societal Impact of Biomechanics.* Special Symposium on Maturing Technologies and Emerging Horizons in Biomedical Engineering; New Orleans, 1988:115–122.

100. Schmidek HH. Cervical spondylosis. *Am Fam Physician.* 1986;33:89–99.

101. Moskovich R. Neck pain in the elderly: common causes and management. *Geriatrics.* 1988;43:65–70.

102. Oegema TR, Bradford DS. The inter-relationship of facet joint osteoarthritis and degenerative disc disease. *Br J Rheumatol.* 1991;30(suppl 1):16–20.

103. Pizzutillo PD, Woods M, Nicholson L, et al. Risk factors in Klippel-Feil syndrome. *Spine.* 1994; 19(18):2110–2116.

104. Raynor RB, Pugh J, Shapiro I. Cervical facetectomy and its effect on spine strength. *J Neurosurg.* 1985;63:278–282.

105. Cusick JF. Yoganandan N, Myklebust JB, et al. Biomechanics of cervical spine facetectomy. In: Proceedings of 15th Annual Meeting of the Cervical Spine Research Society; Washington, DC; December 2–5, 1987.

106. Shirasaki N, Fuji T, Hirayama N, et al. Structural characteristics predisposing cervical instability after anterior spinal fusion. *Neurol Orthop.* 1991; 10:97–109.

Chapter 17

Cost Effectiveness and Efficacy in Management of Car Crash Injuries, Headaches, and Low Back Pain

Lawrence S. Nordhoff, Jr. and Malik Slosberg

INTRODUCTION

Managed health care with cost containment forces are continuing to push forward at a rapidly accelerating pace in the United States in an attempt to control the enormous costs associated with health care. Motor vehicle collision injuries (MVCIs) present a unique challenge to the managed care system because of the following:

- the enormous cost associated with this type of injury
- the occurrence of nearly 2 million disabling MVCIs annually[1]
- the lack of sound documentation for therapeutic indicators and effectiveness of treatment
- the inconsistencies in clinical diagnosis criteria

In an attempt to broaden the perspective of the reader on larger public health care issues, the authors will discuss car crash injuries, headaches, and low back pain management. We will first summarize the 1995 Quebec Task Force report on whiplash injuries. Then we will look at MVCI, low back pain, and headache health care issues facing America. We

will discuss how doctors perceive themselves when treating these injuries, how the consumer views the doctor, and will give recommendations in how to improve the current management model. Lastly, the authors will discuss economic issues relating to MVCI, headaches, and low back pain. The reason for discussing these three common functional disorders in this chapter is to confront the historical controversies associated with the spinal manipulation. The authors will attempt to give a brief overview of the literature, realizing that there are inherent differences in these conditions. However, there is one uniting and similar reality: the vast majority of MVCIs, headaches, and low back pain are biomechanical functional disorders. The MVCI patient is uniquely different in that the victim typically has multiple injuries and has more rapid acceleration forces, and therefore has a more complex repair process and larger probability of permanent disability.

QUEBEC TASK FORCE ON WHIPLASH-ASSOCIATED DISORDERS

This text would not be complete without summarizing the 1995 $1.5 million (Canadian dollars) report findings of the Quebec Task Force on whiplash-associated disorders (WAD).[2] A total of 4,766 individuals who submitted claims from motor vehicle crashes were included in this study. The Quebec Automobile Insurance Society (SAAQ) developed a comprehensive task force to analyze whiplash epidemiology and its related disability and treatment costs. They were to develop realistic strategies for providing the highest scientific treatment standards focused on preventing chronicity and lessening the economic burden. Other issues of concern focused on diagnostic, therapeutic, and rehabilitation inconsistencies. The task force research team collected bibliographic information on 10,382 titles and abstracts for the preliminary screening. Independent task force reviewers concluded that only 62 MVCI studies were both "relevant and scientifically meritorious." The task force conclusions were:

- Few valid scientific publications were found on MVCIs.
- Whiplash management excess was not as common as low back pain.
- 31% of crash events were documented as rear-end crashes.
- A 6- to 8-km/h impact, which subjects the cervical spine up to 4.5g, is recommended as the threshold for cervical strain injury.
- 91% of whiplash injury victims were wearing seat belts, and seat belt use may increase risk for neck injury.
- 43% of whiplash victims sustained multiple injuries.
- 53.8% of whiplash injuries were reported from collisions where the speed limit was below 60 km/h.
- Whiplash claims were notably higher in women.
- 21% of whiplash subjects had delays in symptoms.
- Those occupants with a higher probability of reporting prolonged disability in-

cluded women, people who sustained multiple injuries, older individuals, people who have a higher number of dependents, and those who were involved in a rear-end crash.

- Rear-end collisions resulted in higher rates of relapses or recurrences of symptoms.
- Injury repair takes up to 6 weeks with remodelling up to 1 year.
- A-P, A-P open mouth, and lateral X-rays are considered baseline views.
- Prolonged cervical immobilization will worsen recovery.
- Prolonged bed rest is contraindicated.
- Persistent complaints and residual disability after 45 days are important warnings of chronicity.
- There is no proven value for physiotherapy.
- Early interventions that promote mobilization, manipulation, and exercises in combination with limited use of medications are recommended.

MVCI ECONOMIC COSTS AND DISABILITY

In a comprehensive total economic cost analysis, motor vehicle collisions cost the United States about $333 billion in 1988[3] (Figure 17–1). Several studies confirm that about half of these MVCI patients will suffer some level of disability,[4-6] and about 50% of all of the total economic costs from auto accidents, including minor to fatal injury costs, involve a minor car crash injury.[6] About 6% to 12% of all MVCI patients develop chronic, ≥10% ratable, disability of some type, most involving the neck and back (see Chapter 10).

Retrospective studies consistently report that the most dominant injuries to occupants in motor vehicle crashes involve soft tissue damage, with 53% of consumers and 62% of insurance claimants reporting neck sprain/ strains and 45% of consumers and 56% of in-

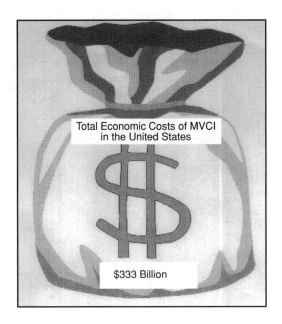

Total Economic Costs of MVCI
in the United States

$333 Billion

Figure 17–1 Total annual economic costs associated with MVCI in the United States. *Source: Data from Miller, T.R., Costs and Functional Consequences of U.S. Roadway Crashes, Accident Analysis & Prevention, Vol. 25, No. 5, pp. 593–607, Elsevier Science Ltd., 1994.*

surance claimants reporting back sprain/strains as a result of car crashes.[4,5] Consumers also report that, in terms of the seriousness of injuries suffered, 55% felt that the sprain/strains were the most grave.[3] This study also evaluated fractures, lacerations, head injuries, and other types of injuries. In addition, we know that a vast majority of all types of crash injuries seen in clinical practice by physicians outside the hospital environment present with no pathologic findings.

TYPES OF PROFESSIONALS SEEN

Balla[7] reports that 94% of MVCI patients see more than one type of health care provider during the course of treatment. A nationwide consumer study shows that about two thirds of all crash victims go to a hospital emergency department, about half see a medical doctor outside the emergency department, 26% see

chiropractors, 27% see physical therapists, and 19% see other health care professionals.[3] A large nationwide study of insurance claims reviewed[4] the types of health care professionals (Figure 17–2) giving health care, with the typical patient seeing two providers. Since 1987, MD/DO practitioners outside the hospital environment have had the same share of the market. Both chiropractors and physical therapists have enlarged their share of the market by about 6% to 7%.

MVCI CASES: PATHOLOGIES OR FUNCTIONAL DISORDERS?

Car crash injuries, headaches, and low back pain syndromes present similar difficulties in differential diagnosis and management. In these types of conditions the identification of distinct pathologies responsible for the clinical presentation usually is lacking or is out of proportion to objective signs; yet significant, even disabling, levels of pain and disability are frequent. Most authors have concluded that the pathology underlying acute or chronic whiplash pain syndromes currently is unknown or poorly defined.[8,9] We find similar lack of diagnostic pathology in the literature on low back pain, as well.[10] Here, too, there is considerable difficulty identifying a pathology in most chronic low back pain sufferers.

When the classic reductionistic medical model approach to disease is used for diagnosing and curing the MVCI, the chronic car crash injury patient often will fail to meet the criteria for a "disease state."[9] When the patient fails to meet the pathology criteria many physicians may feel frustrated or inept, leading the clinician to consider that the pain may be psychologic[9] or due to litigation or compensation neurosis. The nonorganic opinion has been substantiated by several authors, including a recent physician survey on whiplash syndromes in which 31% of family practitioners, 29.4% of neurologists, 39.8% of neurosurgeons, and 46.8% of orthopedists felt that the origin of prolonged whiplash symptoms

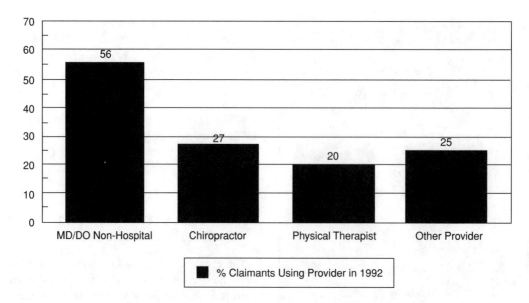

Figure 17–2 Percentage of claimants in the United States utilizing types of health care providers in 1992 in bodily injury states. *Source:* Data from *Auto Injuries: Claiming Behavior and Its Impact on Insurance Costs* , Insurance Research Council, 1994.

was psychogenic.[11] This study revealed several other findings, including the following: (1) 13% to 18% of these physicians felt that emotional factors were most responsible for the symptoms; (2) most physicians do not believe that effective treatment is available for whiplash syndromes and postconcussion syndrome; and (3) the physicians believed that litigation was responsible for many of the complaints.

EVALUATION OF HEALTH CARE PROVIDERS IN MANAGED CARE SYSTEMS

Although managed care is in its infancy, many studies either have been done or are slated to begin soon looking at ways to cut treatment costs. Each type of health care provider and type of therapy used will be evaluated in terms of their effectiveness in treating these functional disorders. Those who provide postinjury treatment will be evaluated by the following criteria:

- Clinical outcome trials (effectiveness by type of treatment and provider type)
- Patient (consumer) satisfaction with type of health care provider and type of treatment
- Total economic costs (direct and indirect) associated with the health care provider's management plan
- Risk of provider's patients' developing temporary or permanent disability
- Extent and costs associated with provider's patients' disability
- Treatment complications (risk of reinjury, new injury, further disability, and adverse medication reactions)

NUMBER OF OFFICE VISITS BY TYPE OF PROFESSIONAL SEEN

Consumers report that the average number of office visits for specific car crash strain/sprain conditions at the 75th percentile was 35 for chiropractors, 30 for physical therapists, 10 for other health care providers, and 8 for medical doctors/osteopaths outside the emergency department.[4] The Insurance Research Council's study of insurance claims found that the average claimant saw a medical doctor outside a hospital for 8 visits, a chiropractor for 25 visits, and a physical therapist for 19 visits in bodily injury states. Claimants in no-fault states averaged more visits than those in bodily injury states.[5] The authors point out that these averages represent several crash vectors, both genders, and various injury severities and should be used only as a guide.

AUTO INJURIES AND LOW BACK PAIN COSTS ASSOCIATED WITH PROVIDER SEEN

Several studies have found that chiropractic is cost effective in managing low back pain.[12–15] Stano[15] did a retrospective statistical analysis of 2 years of insurance claims nationwide that provided data on 395,641 patients with one or more of 493 neuromuscular codes of the *International Classification of Diseases*, 9th revision, *Clinical Modification* (ICD-9-CM), comparing patients seeing medical doctors and chiropractors. This study found that when only outpatient services were considered, MD patient costs were slightly lower than DC patient costs; however, when inpatient services were accounted for, MD patient costs were higher over the 2 years.[15]

Two 1994 auto accident reports, one a large consumer study and the other a study of insurance claims, have tabulated economic costs by type of provider. The nationwide consumer report[4] looked at auto accident victims and the total economic costs associated with the provider. The second, an insurance claims study of 61 of the larger insurance carriers in the United States, looked only at provider treatment bills, excluding diagnostic studies, rehabilitation, spiraling costs, disability costs, and other economic factors.[4] These two studies are summarized in Figure 17–3, which clearly shows that MVCI patients seeing a chiropractor have significantly lower associated total economic costs.

SPIRALING COSTS ASSOCIATED WITH PROVIDERS

When evaluating costs by type of health care professional, the reader needs to consider associated indirect costs. Indirect costs include the additional expenditures not associated with direct costs of care. These costs include expenses for referrals for diagnostic testing, medications, physical therapy, etc. The study by Manga et al.[13] found that for every dollar paid to the primary treating chiropractor, 25 cents in additional costs were generated. For every dollar paid to the primary treating medical doctor, an additional 4 to 5 dollars in additional costs were generated.[13] To shed some insight into some of the factors that affect spiraling costs in the medical system, a recent survey of physicians involved in the management of whiplash and concussion syndromes found that 9% to 17% of family practitioners, neurologists, neurosurgeons, and orthopedists performed tests such as computed tomography, magnetic resonance imaging, electroencephalography, and neuropsychologic evaluations to reassure patients; 12% to 16% had these tests done for litigation purposes.

PATIENTS' CONFIDENCE IN DOCTORS

Studies that compare chiropractors with medical doctors in terms of patient satisfaction for management of low back pain consistently indicate significantly greater satisfaction with chiropractic care. Cherkin and MacCornack[16] found in their study that 25% of patients seeing medical doctors and 60% of patients seeing chiropractors felt that their provider was comfortable and confident in dealing with their problems. Because of the similarities in the structure of the various regions of the spine and similarities in studies evaluating the time required for tissue repair,

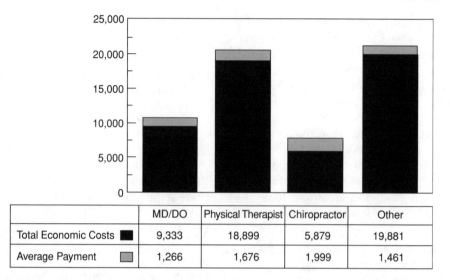

	MD/DO	Physical Therapist	Chiropractor	Other
Total Economic Costs ■	9,333	18,899	5,879	19,881
Average Payment ▨	1,266	1,676	1,999	1,461

Figure 17–3 Costs of providing reimbursement to health care providers for treatment and total economic costs associated with specific providers. Claimants may have seen more than one provider. *Source:* Data from *Paying for Auto Injuries: A Consumer Panel Survey of Auto Accident Victims,* and from *Auto Injuries: Claiming Behavior and Its Impact on Insurance Costs,* Insurance Research Council, 1994.

inferences may be made regarding functional disorders such as those resulting from car crash injuries.

DOCTORS' SELF-CONFIDENCE LEVELS

A comparative study of family physicians and chiropractors was conducted with several types of cases. One case stipulates that a 52-year-old man was seen after a minor car accident; he had low back pain and sciatica with a depressed ankle reflex and a positive straight-leg-raising test. The responses to the question of whether the doctors would be able to hasten significantly the patient's recovery were MDs, 74%; DCs, 97%. When asked whether they would be comfortable in dealing with this type of case, 43% of MDs and 86% of DCs responded positively; 59% of MDs and 23% of DCs reported feeling frustrated by patients who wanted them to "fix" them.[17] Confidence may account for why many patients see a chiropractor for more office visits.

PATIENTS' SATISFACTION WITH PROVIDERS

Several studies have been published regarding consumer satisfaction by provider type for care received for functional disorders such as whiplash injuries or low back pain. The 1-month retrospective study by Balla and Iansek[18] of 190 whiplash injury patients reported the following results in terms of treatment satisfaction:

- 100% chiropractor
- 100% acupuncturist
- 91% tranquilizer
- 81% cervical collar
- 77% advice and analgesia
- 63% physiotherapy
- 63% ultrasound
- 50% short wave
- 28% traction

A recent survey of more than 70,000 consumers reports about their experiences with their medical doctors.[19] The findings illustrate the need for all physicians to work more effectively with patients. This survey found that the most dissatisfied patients were those having chronic ailments such as back pain, headaches, broken bones, and torn ligaments. Problems consumers had with their medical doctors included:

- 29% did not explain how the patient could improve health with lifestyle changes.
- 26% did not explain possible side effects of medications.
- 20% did not encourage questions about condition or treatment.

Low back pain studies also look at consumer satisfaction. The study by Cherkin and MacCornack[16] found that 66% of patients whose low back pain was managed by chiropractors were very satisfied, compared with only 22% of patients whose pain was managed by medical doctors.

MOST COMMON SOURCES OF CHRONIC MVCI PAIN

A recent study concludes that cervical zygapophyseal joint pain is the most common single cause of whiplash pain, finding prevalence between 54% and 85%.[20]

Other authors have concluded that myofascial pain (fibromyalgia) is one of the most common causes of chronic pain following whiplash injury.[9,21,22] Chester[21] found in a 7-year postinjury study that 50% of his cases developed fibromyalgia.

Chronic low back pain[23] and chronic neck pain syndromes are frequently caused by a downward spiral of inactivity, biomechanically weak neck and backs, and reduced functional capacity.

We have identified three primary causes for development of chronic neck and back pain following MVCI. For each area there appears to be one or two primary options currently available that may have long-term benefits.

Other methods, such as medications and other therapies, may help the clinician achieve better outcome.

1. Synovial fold entrapments (biomechanically alter spinal joint motion)
   (a) Spinal manipulation and mobilization techniques
2. Poor physical conditioning syndromes, mechanical neck and back syndromes, or unstable back regions
   (a) Gentle isometric muscle contractions and stretching starting 1 to 2 days after injury,[9] in pain-free regions, intensity and frequency of isotonic exercises progressively increasing
   (b) Ergonomic and postural changes[9]
3. Myofascial pain (trigger points)
   (a) Deep myotherapy and trigger-point work.[24] Wolfe evaluated satisfaction with treatment outcome among patients with fibrositis; 47% to 65% found rest or relaxation to be effective; 46% found chiropractic to be effective; and medication, physical therapy, and other treatment measures were found to be less effective.[25]

Ultimately, managed health care for MVCI will focus on who provides manipulation, myotherapy, and exercise/stretching in an effective and cost-efficient manner for these patients. The following questions will be addressed:

- Which providers treat these conditions?
- How many providers does it take to treat these conditions?
- Which providers are best suited to fit the whiplash model?
- Should providers be permitted to manage these conditions if they do not provide comprehensive care?

CONFIDENCE OF HEALTH PROFESSIONALS ABOUT TREATMENT

Low back pain studies shed some light on practitioners' confidence about treatment. In a survey evaluating attitudes of family physicians and chiropractors, Cherkin and MacCornack found that MDs felt considerably more frustrated in managing patients with low back pain, felt inadequately trained, and felt that they could do less to prevent acute back pain from developing into chronic back pain.[16] In comparing chiropractors with medical doctors, a recent survey found that only a small minority of family physicians, neurologists, orthopedists, and neurosurgeons believed that whiplash syndromes are well defined and that there are effective treatments available.[11]

BED REST AFTER NECK AND BACK INJURY

There is little clinical or scientific evidence supporting the efficacy of bed rest for uncomplicated neck or back injuries,[26,27] and some authors believe that bed rest may be deleterious, actually delaying the patient's recovery.[27,28] "Resting the neck for too long may itself have detrimental effects and may actually prolong subsequent disability."[8] Waddell and others believe there is strong evidence that prolonged bed rest may be the most harmful treatment ever devised and a potent cause of iatrogenic disability.[24,25,27] There is a growing trend toward early mobilization of patients with these injuries to promote earlier recovery and reduce subsequent disability.[8] In fact, the newly released Agency for Health Care Policy and Research guidelines on the management of acute low back problems in adults suggests that bed rest be minimized and that even in patients suffering from sciatica it should be limited to 2 to 4 days.[29]

RISK OF DEVELOPING CHRONIC SYMPTOMS OR DISABILITY WITH PROFESSION SEEN

Comparative studies of low back pain are the best way to evaluate the risk of chronic symptom development. One report concludes that 48% of patients seeing MDs and 17% of those seeing DCs were restricted for more than 1 week.[15] Ebrall reports that when workers' compensation cases of low back injury are managed chiropractically there is 6 times less likelihood that patients will progress to chronicity (only 1.9% of patients), compared with those receiving medical care (11.6%).[30] Another report found that 57% of MDs and 98% of DCs felt that they could do much to prevent patients with acute low back pain from developing chronic pain.[17] Cherkin and MacCornack[16] report that the average low back chiropractic patient averaged 10.8 days of disability, compared with 39.7 days of disability for patients seeing medical doctors. The study by Jarvis et al.[31] of management costs associated with back injury claims with identical diagnostic codes by MDs and DCs showed that the number of work days lost by patients under medical care was nearly 10 times higher than that for patients receiving chiropractic care. Wolk studied 10,652 patients receiving workers' compensation for low back injuries treated by MDs and DCs and found that the chiropractic patient had about 50% less temporary total disability duration, less than half of the number of hospitalizations, and significantly less costs than the medically treated patient.[32]

Hurwitz[33] did a comparative outcome study of 187 patients seeing medical doctors and 103 patients seeing chiropractors for the same 15 musculoskeletal diagnostic codes over a period of 3 months. The study found that at the end of 3 months the patients seeing chiropractors had twice the rate of reported successful recovery than those seeing medical doctors.

SAFETY AND EFFECTIVENESS OF SPINAL MANIPULATION

Several authors and large reports have concluded from either experience, actual analysis of the literature, or in controlled studies that spinal manipulation is a safe and/or effective therapy for many musculoskeletal conditions such as whiplash injuries, neck pain, headaches, and low back pain.[2,13,19,34–37] The US Agency for Health Care Policy and Research, Public Health Service, Department of Health and Human Services released its December 1994 study of various practitioners and therapies used in the treatment of low back pain. Spinal manipulation and oral medications were the only favorable recommendations.[29] Chila et al.[38] feel that manipulation may be indicated for various musculoskeletal asymmetries, abnormal range-of-motion, and soft tissue texture changes. Meade et al.[39] in a study of chiropractic manipulation and hospital outpatient treatment for low back pain, including bracing and standard physical therapy modalities, found that chiropractic therapy was more effective than conventional therapy having long-term benefits. Koes et al.[40] found that manipulative therapy for neck and back complaints was more effective than physiotherapy after 12 months. The recent Quebec Task Force report on whiplash-associated disorders concluded that manipulation and mobilization were recommended.[2] A recent study comparing manipulative therapy to amitriptyline for treatment of chronic tension-type headaches also concludes that spinal manipulation patients have significantly better long-term results than those using medications.[37]

TREATMENT TYPES THAT INCREASE RISK OF REINJURY OR DEVELOPMENT OF MORE CHRONIC SYMPTOMS

Chapter 11 discusses several treatment types that may lead to prolonged symptoms or poorer prognosis. Use of cervical collars for more than 2 weeks has been implicated. About 50% to 70% of medical doctors recommend cervical collars for whiplash injuries, and 13% to 30% recommend collar use for 4 weeks or more.[11]

Use of ice can speed repair, but surveys show that MDs advise use of heat more frequently than do DCs.[11] About 70% to 80% of all MDs surveyed recommend the use of heat. About 96% to 99% of MDs recommend nonsteroidal anti-inflammatory drugs to their patients, as well as other medications. The use of these medications hastens a sense of well-being and by doing so increases the time frame of reinjury vulnerability. Leadbetter[41] feels that these medications may increase the injured patient's susceptibility to injury by reducing pain and inflammation quickly but not accelerating actual tissue healing. As a result, athletes feel pain free and healthy substantially earlier than when the tissues are actually healed enough to be able to tolerate the types of stresses and strains associated with rigorous athletic activity.[41]

TYPES OF PATIENT CARE NEEDED FROM THE HEALTH CARE PROVIDER

In acute injury, the care provided to the injured patient must begin early, with an emphasis on early patient education, early use of cryotherapy, controlled activity and exercise, and focus on active participation of the patient from the beginning. This will ensure a more active role for patients, encouraging in them a sense of control over their own health and a sense of shared responsibility for their outcome. This will promote less long-term patient dependence and reduce the risk of patients' developing a passive coping style as well as reducing the costs of overutilization.[34] Active care, in order to be justified in managed care, should hasten functional recovery. This means that the doctor should focus on types of care that improve and maintain normal neuromusculoskeletal function during the repair process so that healing can be enhanced and less residual disability will occur.

In chronic injury, the emphasis needs to be multifaceted. This treatment should include patient education, restoration of soft tissue and joint function, and exercise, including flexibility and strengthening exercises that promote general fitness and aerobic capacity. In addition, ergonomic and postural factors should be addressed.

The doctor who utilizes a single or limited approach to MVCI management will be at a disadvantage. The system will eventually favor the type of management that is the most cost effective, that is, the type of provider and care that provide all the necessary steps to maximize recovery most cost effectively.

Waddell[27] believes that the standard medical advice for the patient to rest, stay off work, and avoid physical activity has promoted fear of pain, poor coping, and disability.

THE ROLE OF CHIROPRACTIC

The Center for Studies in Health Policy has concluded that the chiropractor is considered to be a primary care provider, can be considered a generalist, and can be considered a gatekeeper when a patient enters the health care service system. This includes diagnostic differentiation, assessment, treatment, and referral.[42] Chiropractors have clearly been shown to provide safe and effective treatment for several functional disorders such as low back pain and MVCI, obtain good patient satisfaction, and are very cost effective, primarily in the area of reducing economic costs associated with disability. The chiropractic profession must continue to strive for better outcome measures such as functional capacity tests, promote more comparative studies, and remember that these MVCI patients deserve the best care.

CONCLUSION

Several large 10- to 15-million dollar studies need to be performed in the United States that evaluate treatment, legal, administrative, and diagnostic resource consumption. We need to establish and standardize injury diagnosis severity at a nationwide provider level. We need to evaluate the legal costs of representing claimants versus financial benefits to the victim. Attorneys and physicians that state that they specialize in personal injury cases must take courses that certify them. Physicians must be educated on the benefits of prevention management and how to avoid chronicity. Diagnostic standards need to be developed for radiology, electrodiagnosis, and other diagnostic tests. Controlled treatment outcome studies of conventional and nonconventional therapeutics are needed that evaluate long-term results (using scientific measures), what forms of treatment are associated with reduced disability, chronicity, and resource consumption. The trend toward a more multidisciplinary approach to chronic management needs further scrutiny. The chiropractor, family practitioner, general practitioner, or other specialist who has taken specialized courses in MVCI must be allowed to be a primary gatekeeper in treating the minor to moderate injury.

Consumers and public policy makers must demand safer car designs to lessen injury. Abuses within the medical and legal system need to be identified and confronted with public policy changes. Excess expenditures associated with unnecessary tests, expensive and perhaps unnecessary interventionist procedures such as surgery, and clinical interventions without adequate documentation of beneficial outcomes all must be evaluated critically.

REFERENCES

1. National Safety Council. *Accident Facts*. Chicago: NSC; 1994.

2. Spitzer WO, Skovron ML, Salmi LR, et al. Scientific monograph of the Quebec task force on whiplash-associated disorders: redefining "whiplash" and its management. *Spine*. 1995;20S(8S):1S–73S.

3. Miller TR. Costs and functional consequences of U.S. roadway crashes. *Accid Anal Prev*. 1994; 25:593–607.

4. Insurance Research Council. *Paying for Auto Injuries: A Consumer Panel Survey of Auto Accident Victims*. Oak Brook, Ill: IRC; 1994.

5. Insurance Research Council. *Auto Injuries: Claiming Behavior and Its Impact on Insurance Costs*. Oak Brook, Ill: IRC; 1994.

6. Luchter S. *Traffic Related Disabilities and Impairments and Their Economic Consequences*. Warrendale, Pa: Society of Automotive Engineers. paper 860505; 1986.

7. Balla JI. The late whiplash syndrome. *Aust N Z J Surg*. 1980;50:610–614.

8. Barnsley L, Lord S, Bogduk N. The pathophysiology of whiplash. *Spine State Art Rev*. 1993;7:329–353.

9. Teasell RW, McCain GA. Clinical spectrum and management of whiplash injuries. In: Tollison CD, Satterthwaite JR, eds. *Painful Cervical Trauma: Diagnosis and Rehabilitative Treatment of Neuromusculoskeletal Injuries*. Baltimore: Williams & Wilkins; 1992.

10. Delitto A. Are measures of function and disability important in low back care? *Phys Ther*. 1994; 74:452–462.

11. Evans RW, Evans RI, Sharp MJ. The physician survey on the post-concussion and whiplash syndromes. *Headache*. 1994;34:268–274.

12. Dean DH, Schmidt RM. A comparison of the costs of chiropractic versus alternative medical practitioners. Arlington, Va: FCER and Virginia Chiropractic Association, 1992.

13. Manga P, Angus DE, Papadopoulos C, et al. *A Study to Examine the Effectiveness and Cost-Effectiveness of Chiropractic Management of Low Back Pain*. Ontario, Canada: Ministry of Health, Government of Ontario, 1993.

14. Schifrin LG. Mandated health insurance coverage for chiropractic treatment: an economic assessment, with implications for the Commonwealth of Virginia. Arlington, Va: FCER and Virginia Chiropractic Association, 1992.

15. Stano M. A comparison of health care costs for chiropractic and medical patients. *J Manipulative Physiol Ther*. 1993;16:291–299.

16. Cherkin DC, MacCornack FA. Patient evaluations of low back pain care from family physicians and chiropractors. *West J Med*. 1989; 149:351–355.

17. Cherkin DC, et al. Managing low back pain: a comparison of the beliefs and behaviors of family physicians and chiropractors. *West J Med*. 1989; 149:475–480.

18. Balla JI, Iansek R. Headaches arising from disorders of the cervical spine. In: Hopkins A, ed. *Headache: Problems in Diagnosis and Management*. London: WB Saunders; 1988.

19. How is your doctor treating you? *Consumer Reports*. February 1995:81–83.

20. Lord S, Barnsley L, Bogduk N. Cervical zygapophyseal joint pain in whiplash. *Spine State Art Rev*. 1993;7:355–372.

21. Chester JB. Whiplash, postural control, and the inner ear. *Spine*. 1991;16:716–720.

22. Fricton JR. Myofascial pain and whiplash. *Spine State Art Rev*. 1993;7:403–422.

23. Mikheev M. 1993 World Chiropractic Congress. In: Chapman-Smith D, ed. *The Chiropractic Report*. July 1–6, 1993.

24. Hong C-Z, Chen Y-C, Pon CH, et al. Immediate effects of various physical medicine modalities on pain threshold of an active myofascial trigger point. *J Musculoskeletal Pain*. 1993;1:37–53.

25. Wolfe F. The clinical syndrome of fibrositis. *Am J Med*. 1986;81(S3A):7–14.

26. Fitz-Ritson D. The chiropractic management and rehabilitation of cervical trauma. *J Manipulative Physiol Ther*. 1990;13:17–25.

27. Waddell G. 1993 World Chiropractic Congress. In: Chapman-Smith D, ed. *The Chiropractic Report*, July 1–6, 1993.

28. Ameis A. Cervical whiplash: considerations in the rehabilitation of cervical myofascial injury. *Can Fam Physician*. 1986;32:1871–1876.

29. Bigios S, Bowyer O, Braen G, et al. Acute low back problems in adults. Clinical Practice Guidelines No. 14, AJCPR publication no 95-0642. Rockville, Md: Agency for Health Care Policy and Research, Public Health Service, US Dept of Health and Human Services, December 1994.

30. Ebrall PS. Mechanical low back pain: a comparison of medical and chiropractic management within

the Victorian workcare scheme. *Chirop J Aust.* 1992;22(2):47–53.

31. Jarvis KB, Phillips RB, et al. Cost per case comparison of back injury claims of chiropractic versus medical management for conditions with identical diagnostic codes. *J Occup Med.* 1991;33:847–852.

32. Wolk S. Chiropractic versus medical care: a cost analysis of disability and treatment for back-related workers' compensation cases. Arlington, Va: FCER; 1988.

33. Hurwitz EC. The relative impact of chiropractic versus medical management of low back pain on health status in a multispecialty group practice. *J Manipulative Physiol Ther.* 1994;17:74–82.

34. Haldeman S, Chapman-Smith D, Petersen DM Jr. *Guidelines for Chiropractic Quality Assurance and Practice Parameters: Proceedings of the Mercy Center Consensus Conference.* Gaithersburg, Md: Aspen Publishers, Inc; 1993.

35. Shekelle PG, Adams A, et al. *The Appropriateness of Spinal Manipulation for Low-Back Pain.* Santa Monica, Calif: RAND Corporation; 1992.

36. Shekelle PG. Spine update spinal manipulation. *Spine.* 1994;19:858–861.

37. Boline PD, Kassak K, Bronfort G, et al. Spinal manipulation vs. amitriptyline for the treatment of chronic tension-type headaches: a randomized clinical trial. *J Manipulative Physiol Ther.* 1995; 18:148–154.

38. Chila AG, Jeffries RR, Levin SM. Is manipulation for your practice? *Patient Care.* May 15, 1990.

39. Meade TW, Dyer S, et al. Low back pain of mechanical origin: randomized comparison of chiropractic and hospital outpatient treatment. *Br Med J.* 1990;300:1431–1437.

40. Koes BC, Bouter LM, et al. Randomized clinical trial of manipulative therapy and physiotherapy for persistent back and neck complaints: results of one year follow up. *Br Med J.* 1992;304:601–605.

41. Leadbetter WB. Cell-matrix response in tendon injury. *Clin Sports Med.* 1992;11:533–578.

42. Gonyea MA. The role of the doctor of chiropractic in the health care system in comparison with doctors of allopathic medicine and doctors of osteopathic medicine. Washington, DC: Center for Studies in Health Policy, FCER 1993.

Appendix A

Glossary of Terms

Acceleration: Temporal rate of change of velocity is acceleration, expressed in feet per second per second. As explained in Newton's law, an external force changes the velocity of a body and produces three types of acceleration:

1. **Rotational/angular acceleration:** Unless otherwise specified, an acceleration indicates the rate of velocity change in a translational motion. If the motion is rotational and the velocity changes, the rate of change is rotational, or angular, acceleration, expressed in degrees per second per second or radian per second per second. Involves a change in both speed and direction simultaneously. Combines translational and rotational acceleration. Seen where vehicle spins or rolls; movement around center of gravity (*cg*).

2. **Linear acceleration:** An acceleration in which only a change in velocity is involved in a straight line.

3. **Translational acceleration:** Movement of a body part in relation to a fixed point in a straight line.

Association for the Advancement of Automotive Medicine (AAAM): AAAM Headquarters at 2340 Des Plaines Avenue, Suite 106, Des Plaines, IL 60018. Phone (708) 390-8927. Annual fall conferences are held.

Axial: Characteristic to or along an axis, such as axial flow, axial velocity, etc. (contrary to rotational).

Deceleration: If the external force is applied to slow down the motion of a body, the temporal change of its velocity becomes negative. The negative acceleration is called deceleration, the unit being feet per second per second. Measured in gravitational units (*g*) in seconds.

Deformation: Refers to permanent or temporary structural changes; produced by external forces of loads that act on nonrigid or elastic bodies. Longitudinal deformations are lengthening or shortening of the body, and angular deformations are changes of angle between faces within the body. Plastic deformation results in permanent structural alterations, whereas elastic deformation results in no outward permanent structural changes after loading has occurred.

Delta V, velocity change: Delta V can apply to the change of velocity of a vehicle or occupant in collision. If two vehicles with a same mass, both traveling at 50 mph, collide head-on and stop, both vehicles have a delta V of 50 mph. If a vehicle hits a rigid barrier at 20 mph and rebounds at 10 mph, the delta V is 30 mph.

Dynamic crush: Maximum exterior deformation suffered by a vehicle during a collision with another object. Because of an elastic rebound of vehicle structure, the maximum deformation is often 10% to 20% greater than deformation as observed after the collision.

Elastic behavior: Elasticity is the ability of a material to restore to its original configuration when external forces are removed. Because of elastic character, some rebound observed of vehicle deformation after collision. (*See* Restitution, coefficient of.)

Energy: A moving vehicle possesses kinetic energy that must be completely dissipated to stop the vehicle. Energy is the product of force and distance and expressed in lb(ft/sec)^2 or ft–lbf. To dissipate the energy, force must be applied either by braking or hitting into a solid wall if the vehicle is to stop in a very short distance. The kinetic energy is one half of the product mass and velocity squared; hence, if the prebraking speed is doubled, the braking distance is quadrupled.

Force: Force deforms a body and/or causes acceleration of the body. In case of accelerating the body, the force is equal to the mass of the body multiplied by the acceleration. (See Newton's second law.) Since the acceleration of a vehicle in an accident is sometimes very large, the impact force on the vehicle also becomes surprisingly large. For example, if a vehicle of 3000 lb hits a concrete wall squarely at 60 mph, the maximum deceleration of the vehicle may become as high as 25g and the maximum force on the

vehicle approximately 40 tons. It has a vector quantity having both magnitude and direction. One pound of force will accelerate 1 lb of mass by 32.2 ft/s^2. The force is directly proportional to the mass and to the acceleration. Force is inversely proportional to the time and distance traveled during linear acceleration or deceleration.

Frictional force: Frictional force is the resistive force as observed when two solid surfaces slide or tend to slide toward each other.

Friction, coefficient of: Friction increases with normal force, which presses two sliding surfaces together; the coefficient of friction is defined as the frictional force divided by the normal force. The coefficients are sensitive to the surface finish, sliding speed, temperature, existence of liquid film, etc. The coefficient of tire friction, for example, is as high as 1.0 in a good operating condition, but decreases with vehicle speed. On an icy surface, it drops as low as 0.1.

***g* acceleration:** All bodies on the earth are under the influence of gravitational acceleration of the earth, which is commonly denoted by the letter g. Under the influence of gravity alone, and if all other effects such as air resistance are disregarded, all falling bodies increase velocity with the rate of g. The standard value of g is 32.1740 ft/s/s (or 9.80665 m/s/s in metric system) as measured at sea level and latitude 45°. Sometimes acceleration is expressed in terms of g; i.e., maximum deceleration of the struck vehicle in the accident is 40g. This is similar to Mach number to express the speed of aircraft, which is a multiple of the speed of sound.

Inertia: Inertia is the property of a body to hold its state of rest or motion unless acted on by an external force. (See Newton's first law of motion.) A fundamental property of mass. The inertial resistance during an acceleration from a car crash manifests itself as weight. The inertial effects of the human body during acceleration or deceleration cause the physiologic body changes.

International Research Committee on the Biomechanics of Impacts (IRCOBI): European equivalent to annual United States Stapp Car Crash Conferences (Society of Automotive Engineers) held in the fall. 109 Avenue Salvador Allende, 69500 Bron, France.

Kinetic energy: Amount of energy a moving mass has because of its velocity. One foot-pound of force is the amount of energy (work) used to raise 1 lb of mass 1 ft. A vehicle weighing 3290 lbs traveling 30 mph has a kinetic energy of 167,000 ft lb force. Doubling the speed increases the kinetic energy four times greater, which has four times the potential for causing damage.[1]

Magnification of acceleration: When a striking elastic object contacts another elastic surface, such as two cue balls or two bumpers in low-speed crashes, having no permanent deformation, energy is not only transferred (due to its momentum) from the striking surface into the struck elastic object, but the struck object can be propelled with greater speeds than the striking object. This can be seen in rear-end crashes where the seat back and occupant may achieve rebound velocities up to 150% more than the striking vehicle.[2]

Mass: Mass and weight are used often ambiguously and incorrectly to mean the same thing. Weight becomes zero in a weightless environment such as on a satellite, and on the moon it becomes one-sixth of that on earth. Mass of the body is the weight divided by the gravitational acceleration; hence the mass does not depend on the environment, but is a unique property of the body. The unit of the mass is expressed in pounds, while the unit of weight is expressed in pounds of force.

Momentum: Momentum is the product of mass and velocity. In a linear collision of two bodies, such as head-on vehicle collision, the vehicle with larger momentum pushes back the other. In other words, even a light vehicle can push back a heavy vehicle if the light vehicle has a high velocity to offset the weight disadvantage. The unit is pounds per foot per second. (Momentum should not be confused with the moment of a force, which is the product of the force and its lever arm.)

Motor vehicle collision injury (MVCI): Any single or multiple injury or its subsequent symptoms, biomechanical, or biochemical alterations, or diagnostic entities subsequent to a car crash.

National Accident Sampling System (NASS): Under the umbrella of the NHTSA. Police-reporting samples of several million crashes annually.

National Highway Traffic Safety Administration (NHTSA): An agency created by Congress, under the Department of Transportation. This organization has the responsibility for developing, promulgating, maintaining, and enforcing new motor vehicle safety standards. It was founded in 1966 to reduce collisions, injuries, and deaths related to crashes. Its director is a political appointment.

Newton's Laws of Motion

First law: A body remains at rest or in uniform motion in the same straight line unless an external force is applied on the body. As an example, if a vehicle collides into a solid wall, the passengers continue the precollision motion and fly forward unless fastened by a restraint device such as a seat belt and acted on by an external force.

Second law: An external force acting on a body causes an acceleration of the body in the direction of the force. The acceleration is proportional to the force and inversely proportional to the mass of the body. As an example, a mild braking takes a long distance to stop a vehicle; that is, the deceleration (negative acceleration) is small. In order to obtain a large deceleration to stop a vehicle in a few feet, you can run into a solid wall to apply a large external force on the vehicle.

Third law: When two bodies are in contact, one of the bodies applies a force to the other, called action. There is always a reaction, that is, an opposing force offered by the second body to the first at all times as long as the two bodies are in contact. Example: since action and reaction are same in magnitude and opposite in direction, both vehicles in an accident suffer almost the same damage if they have similar structural configuration. For every action there is an equal and opposite reaction. This means that for every accelerative force there is an equal and opposite inertial force. The accelerative force is caused by the force of another object acting on the body, i.e., car seat; whereas the inertial force is the resistance of the body acting against the accelerative force.

5th Percentile population: Represents the percentage of distribution of 5% or less of total population characteristics and physical sizes. If standing height is taken as characteristic, the fifth percentile includes very small people.

50th Percentile population: Represents 50% of the population and is the average common practice; weight about 150 lbs.

80th Percentile population: Represents 80% of the normal population; 5 ft, 10 in tall occupant.

95th Percentile population: Represents 5% of the larger-sized population; a 95th percentile dummy may weigh 250 lb or more.

Plastic behavior: Plasticity is the property of material that maintains a permanent deformation after external forces are removed. Vehicle damages are mostly due to plastic behavior or material, except small elastic rebound. (*See* Elastic behavior.)

Reaction time: The time of human reaction after perception of a hazardous situation. Even if one expects an event such as a pistol shot at the start of a 100-m dash, the reaction time in 0.1 to 0.2 second. If the event is not expected, such as a car accident, the reaction time becomes much larger.

Rebound: Ratio of rebound velocity to impact velocity; a measure of rebound or bounce. (See Restitution, coefficient of.)

Resistance: Opposing or retarding force on a moving body. In the case of a running vehicle, resistances are tire friction, friction of moving mechanical parts, and aerodynamic force. The unit is pounds of force, same as force.

Restitution, coefficient of: When two masses come into collision on a straight line, the coefficient of restitution is defined as the ratio of relative speed of the two masses after the collision to that before the collision. The coefficient becomes 1.0 for perfectly elastic bodies, such as billiard balls, and 0 for plastic bodies such as clay or lead balls. The coefficient of the restitution in a high-speed vehicle collision is 0.1 to 0.2, indicating small rebound. The value is also applicable to vehicle-to-bicycle, -motorcyle or -pedestrian collisions. The coefficient is nondimensional.

Rural community: 5,000 or less population.

Society of Automotive Engineers (SAE): 400 Commonwealth Drive, Warrendale, PA 15096–0001; phone (412) 776–4970. Holds annual conference proceedings.

Shearing stress: If a rod is twisted, shearing stress is generated in the rod; if the stress exceeds the durable stress of the material, the rod is sheared off. The unit is pounds of force per square inch.

Speed: The rate of object motion, magnitude only.

Static crush: Amount of deformation measured in a vehicle after a crash has ended.

Stiffness: Resistive character to deflection under load.

Stopping distance: Necessary distance to stop a running vehicle. The stopping distance is the sum of coasting distance before braking force is generated on wheels, due to delay time after the driver sees the hazard, and the braking distance. The delay time includes human reaction time, change of foot on pedals, pressing brake pedal, and movement of mechanical parts in brake system, all summing to 0.8 to 1.0 second even if the driver expects a hazard ahead of time, as in the case of a tailgater.

Submarining: Term used for a lap belt slipping over pelvis onto lower abdominal structures.

Tension forces: Pulling or distracting forces.

Torque: A force that acts to produce rotation by its lever arm. Torque is the force times the lever arm and is expressed in lbf-ft. Torque and moment mean the same, but the torque is used commonly in engineering practice, such as engine torque, while the moment is used in dynamic and kinetic description, such as moment subjected by the neck in hyperextension.

Torsion: Twisting of a body, in which not only shear stress but also tensile and compressive stresses are generated in general.

Urban community: More than 5000 population.

Vector: A quantity that has both magnitude and direction, usually expressed by an arrow, such as velocity. In an anatomical application, x vector means lateral, y vector means superior-inferior, and z vector means anterior-posterior.

Velocity: Velocity is the temporal rate of change of location of a body. Speed and velocity are sometimes used in the same manner, but in engineering, the speed indicates only magnitude whereas the velocity includes the magnitude and the direction. In other words, the velocity is a vector and the speed is a scalar, both expressed in feet per second. It has a vector, which includes both magnitude and direction. The velocity of the car or body changes in direction or speed. Angular velocity is measured in radians/second; linear velocity is measured in feet per second or meters per second.

Viscous response: Velocity of deformation over time and body compression to soft tissues. It measures the instantaneous injury risk induced by compression and rate of body deformation.[3] Used to evaluate injury tolerances in areas such as thorax and abdominal areas. It is the instantaneous probability of sprain/strain rate in soft tissue undergoing dynamic deformation and correlated biomechanics with neural trauma.[4] The viscous criterion is related to higher-speed compression, a rate-dependent deformation that exceeds the energy-dissipation capability of tissues.

Weight: $W = m \times g$. The force exerted on a given mass by the pull of gravity. Weight is a force; mass is a quantity. Weight changes, depending on gravitational field, whereas mass is always constant.

REFERENCES

1. White AA III, Panjabi MM. *Clinical Biomechanics of the Spine.* 2nd ed. Philadelphia: JB Lippincott Co; 1990.

2. Romilly DP, Thompson RW, Navin FPD, et al. Low speed rear impacts and elastic properties of automobiles. In: Proceedings of the 12th International Technical Conference of Experimental Safety Vehicles. Washington, DC: NHTSA; 1989.

3. Lau IV, Viano DC. The viscous criterion-bases and applications of an injury severity index for soft tis-

sues. In: Proceedings of the 30th Stapp Car Crash Conference; paper 861882. Detroit, Mich: Society of Automotive Engineers; 1986.

4. Viano DC. Biomechanics of head injury: toward a theory linking head dynamic motion, brain tissue deformation, and neural trauma. In: Proceedings of the 32nd Stapp Car Crash Conference, paper 881708. Detroit, Mich: Society of Automotive Engineers; 1988.

Appendix B

Velocity Conversion Tables

Miles per hour (mph)	Kilometers per hour (km/h)	Meters per second (m/s)	Feet per second (ft/s)
1	1.6093	0.4470	1.467
0.6818	1.097	0.3048	1
0.6214	1	0.2778	0.9113
2.237	3.6	1	3.281
3.1	5	1.4	
6.2	10	2.8	
9.3	15	4.2	
12.4	20	5.6	
15.5	25	6.9	
18.6	30	8.3	
21.7	35	9.7	
24.9	40	11.1	
28.0	45	12.5	
31.1	50	13.9	
34.2	55	15.3	
37.3	60	16.7	
40.4	65	18.1	

Index

---

final diagnosis, 203
medicolegal report, 248–249
multidisciplinary evaluation, 200–202
    examination, 202
    team members, 201–202
procedures, 61
rationale, 1–2
surgery, 203–204
typical crash, 2–3
typical patient, 2–3
visual symptom, 16–17
working diagnosis, 202
Diathermy, 165
Diffuse axonal injury. *See* Mild head injury
Disability, 205–223. *See also* Specific type
crash factors, 210
defined, 206–207
diagnosis, problems, 220–222
headache, 213–214
human factors, 210
independent medical examination, 222–223
initial injury/symptom severity, 210–213
predicting disability outcome, 209–210
socioeconomic factors, 209
specific conditions, 213–215
vehicle factors, 210
Disability rating scale
multiple injury functional capacity
    questionnaire, 215, 217–219
    modifiers, 220
    scoring, 215–220
types, 215–220
Dizziness, 15–16
Documentation. *See also* Chart; Medicolegal
report
Double-crush syndrome, 45
Drug use, 271–272
Drug-induced headache, 20
Dynamic crush, defined, 356

E

Elastic behavior, defined, 356
Elbow injury, 43–44
Electrical cellular stimulation, 165
Electrical nerve stimulation, 164
Electromyography, neck injury, 126–128
Energy, defined, 356
External body injury, evaluation, 85

F

F wave study, neck injury, 126
Facet arthrosis
computed tomography, 118–119
magnetic resonance imaging, 118–119
Fatality, velocity, 282
Fibromyalgia, 50–56
disorders mimicking, 56
disorders perpetuating, 56
pre-existing, 337
Fibromylagia, disability, 213
Fibrositis, pre-existing, 337
Foot injury, 47, 48
Force, defined, 356
Forces of acceleration, 328–329
Forces of deceleration, 328–329
Frictional force, defined, 356
Frontal collision
collision dynamics, 291–298
    offset, 294–298
    restrained occupant, 292–294
    unrestrained occupant, 294
statistics, 279
Functional capacity loss, defined, 206–207
Functional capacity testing, medicolegal report,
248

G

G force, 328–329
defined, 356
Galvanic current, 164
Gender, 333–334
motor vehicle collision injury, 272–274
Genetic condition, pre-existing, 337–338
George's line, 97–98

H

Handicap, defined, 207
Head impact, neck injury, 31–32, 33
Head injury
algorithm, 177
headache, 17
home instruction form, 178
mechanisms, 10
mild. *See* Mild head injury
seat belt, 314–316